Cystic Fibrosis: Advanced Researches

Cystic Fibrosis: Advanced Researches

Edited by **Jeffrey Swann**

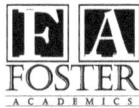

FOSTER
ACADEMICS

New Jersey

Published by Foster Academics,
61 Van Reypen Street,
Jersey City, NJ 07306, USA
www.fosteracademics.com

Cystic Fibrosis: Advanced Researches
Edited by Jeffrey Swann

International Standard Book Number: 978-1-63242-104-3 (Hardback)

Contents

Preface

The main aim of this book is to educate learners and enhance their research focus by presenting diverse topics covering this vast field. This is an advanced book which compiles significant studies by distinguished experts in the area of analysis. This book addresses successive solutions to the challenges arising in the area of application, along with it; the book provides scope for future developments.

Living a healthy life is one's ultimate goal, but the genetics behind the creation of each human is not same. As a curse of human suffering, certain people are born with congenital defects in their menu of the genome. The complexity of cystic fibrosis condition has impacts on several organ systems of the human body perplexing further with secondary infections. It is a complicated disease and scientists across the globe are still trying to comprehend it and formulate a cure because though they narrowed it down to a single target gene, the effects of this disease reach several unfamiliar corners of the human body. Decades of scientific research in the field of chronic diseases like this certainly escalated the level of life expectancy. Scientists and researchers from across the globe have contributed significant information in this all-inclusive book which encompasses three broad sections namely, cystic fibrosis- a system, genetics and biochemistry, and microbiology and immunology.

It was a great honour to edit this book, though there were challenges, as it involved a lot of communication and networking between me and the editorial team. However, the end result was this all-inclusive book covering diverse themes in the field.

Finally, it is important to acknowledge the efforts of the contributors for their excellent chapters, through which a wide variety of issues have been addressed. I would also like to thank my colleagues for their valuable feedback during the making of this book.

Editor

Part 1

Cystic Fibrosis – A Complex Syndrome

The Prognosis of Cystic Fibrosis – A Clinician's Perspective

Patrick Lebecque

Cliniques St-Luc, Université de Louvain, Brussels
Belgium

1. Introduction

Looking at the prognosis of Cystic Fibrosis (CF) from the clinician's point of view is very relevant. Median predicted survival age of CF increased from 6 months when the disease was first described (1938) to 12 years in 1970 and over 35 years in 2010 in the United States of America (Davis, 2006). Three types of factors weigh on this prognosis, which is conditioned by lung disease: factors linked to the quality of care management, to genetics and to the environment. It has been estimated from studies in twins and siblings that the relative influence of the latter two is roughly equivalent. Though pollution may have increased in certain areas, and lighter forms of CF are now being detected by neonatal screening and in clinics where nasal potential measurements are widely available, their impact is limited and can not account for the spectacular changes in life expectancy. Thus, this improvement is due essentially to a better care management. Quality of care is the main determinant of CF prognosis.

The question of prognosis is almost invariably the very first that parents of a newly diagnosed CF infant will ask their physician, whose task to answer in a sensitive and sensible fashion is by no means easy. This question is also at the heart of daily concerns of the clinician, who has to take its determinants into consideration not so much in view of their fascinating underlying mechanisms (e.g. modifier genes) but rather to the extent they can give grip to improved care.

2. How to express CF prognosis? Median predicted survival: Facts, limitations and hopes

CF is a serious disease, which reduces life expectancy. Parents have often already found on the internet the associated 'Median predicted survival', which is the estimated duration of time until 50% of a given population dies. This given number of years has the effect of a guillotine and haunts their thoughts. For CF patients in 2008, it was 37.4 years in the US (CFF Registry, 2008), 38.8 years in the UK (UK CF Registry, 2008) and 46.6 in Canada (44.8 years after excluding adult diagnoses) (Canadian CFF, 2008). However, for a number of methodological issues, it is difficult to compare results of national registries. Evaluating cohorts on the basis of the presence or absence of pancreatic insufficiency was recently suggested as a way to help to overcome some of the current limitations (Buzzetti *et al.*, 2009).

Limiting the analysis to patients homozygous for the *F508del* mutation could be even 'cleaner' (Zelin *et al.*, 2010; Lebecque *et al.*, 2010). It is important to note that over the past 60 years, median predicted survival has actually increased in a continuous fashion by almost 6 years every decade (Davis, 2006). Part of this improvement is probably linked to the increased detection of milder forms of the disease. As proposed for the comparison of registries, it would be interesting to study the data of only those patients homozygous for the *F508del* mutation. For four reasons developed below, this brutal landmark has limited value in an individual patient.

2.1 Cohort effects

Cohort survival curves consistently show that survival continues to improve with each successive birth cohort over the decades. However, this effect is not taken into account by current survival curves. As a result, advice based on the latter could be unduly pessimistic. This has led authors to model the trend observed in cohort survival curves and to extrapolate a median survival for recent cohorts. Accordingly, a median life expectancy of the order of 40 years was predicted for newborns in 1990 in the UK (Elborn *et al.*, 1991). This proved to be realistic and updated extrapolation for the birth cohort of the year 2000 predicts a median survival of 50 years (Dodge *et al.*, 2007). Recent work has further validated this approach (Jackson *et al.*, 2011).

2.2 Wide heterogeneity of the disease

Median predicted survival does not take into account the vast heterogeneity of CF. Yet the latter has long been recognized, even amongst patients homozygous for the *F508del* mutation (Kerem *et al.*, 1990; Johanssen *et al.*, 1991). When diagnosing a new patient carrying 2 CF-causing mutations, this variability renders precise individual prognosis almost always impossible.

2.3 Quality of life

The raw median predicted survival rate says nothing about quality of life. In CF, pulmonary function is often used as a surrogate for survival, with FEV_1 remaining the single most useful parameter (Kerem *et al.*, 1992). Though insensitive to early stages of the disease, spirometry is widely available, inexpensive, non-invasive and very reproducible. It can usually be performed from the age of 5 and upwards. FEV_1 has the advantage of reflecting pulmonary involvement, thereby conditioning prognosis, throughout the whole course of the disease. The rate of FEV_1 decline might be an even stronger surrogate for survival (Liou *et al.*, 2001; Schluchter *et al.*, 2002; Rosenbluth *et al.*, 2004).

Quality of life is at least as important as its length. For every human being, it is largely conditioned by how an individual handles the careful balance of renunciations, and accepts these. Its precise and fine perception inevitably escapes all questionnaires. Specific tools developed over the past 20 years cannot presume to its assessment but can help discern the impact of new treatment modalities and are increasingly being used in this context (Abbott *et al.*, 2011). This also implies that, given the choice between equally efficient treatments, the least invasive treatment and follow-up modalities are to be favoured (Wainwright *et al.*, 2011). Under close supervision and for adequately selected patients, home intravenous antibiotic treatment is a less disruptive alternative to hospital admissions. Though fatigue can be worse for home participants, home treatment has been associated to improvement in quality of life (Balaquer *et al.*, 2008). At all stages of this complex long-term disease, a holistic approach of the care management of both the patient and his family is essential (Bush *et al.*, 2006; Cohen-Cymberknoh *et al.*, 2011).

2.4 Hope for a curative treatment

Predicting survival of a disease based on the past and present data bypasses the possibility of discovering a cure. Despite all prognostic improvements linked to progress in follow-up and symptomatic treatment of CF, it remains imperative to discover a cure for respiratory disease of CF, for at least 3 reasons: i) current treatment is increasingly cumbersome, 'devouring' about 2 hours every day on average; ii) the cost of CF treatment is constantly rising, leading to fears that there may be increasing limitations as to its availability, even in richer countries; iii) some patients still experience a much more rapid FEV1 decline. The approach favoured today is that of the search for pharmacological agents capable of circumventing the consequences of genetic anomalies as determined by CFTR gene class mutations (Amaral, 2011; Rogan *et al.*, 2011). The principle is to interrupt 'the source' of the cascade of events that leads from an ionic transport anomaly in the respiratory epithelium to lung destruction. Treatment tailored to the type of mutation appears today reasonably within reach (Accurso *et al.*, 2010). Should this eventuality become a reality, the prognosis of patients still free of significant pulmonary lesions would be radically transformed.

3. Causes of death in CF

Over 95% of known causes of death in CF (including data following lung transplantations of CF patients) are linked to involvement of the respiratory system (CFF Registry, 2000). Amongst the specific and much rarer causes of death, feature complications of liver disease, dehydration and intestinal obstruction in countries where physicians have little knowledge of CF (Verma *et al.*, 2000).

4. Prognostic factors

A pragmatic way of looking at prognostic factors of CF is to distinguish those that are linked to the quality of care management and those on which care management has little (e.g. environmental factors) or no grip (genetic factors) (Wolfenden *et al.*, 2009). Figure 1 gives an overview of prognostic factors in CF.

Three aspects of the discussion are worth mentioning i) interactions between factors are numerous and their complex statistical evaluation study has probably been too shallow in many publications; ii) the evaluation of the role of certain less easily quantifiable factors, such as treatment adherence, escapes usual means of analysis; iii) our choice is to focus on factors that appear essential to a clinician. The complexity of interactions between the different factors is clearly illustrated by the example of the impact of passive smoking on respiratory function. Although the deleterious effects of passive smoking are well established, they vary according to CFTR genotype and certain alleles of modifying genes (Collaco *et al.*, 2008). Moreover, several studies demonstrated a link between passive smoking and socio-economic status (Smyth *et al.*, 1994).

One example of 'the clinician's choice' in the discussion is not to dwell on the often reported issue of a 'female disadvantage' (Rosenfeld *et al.*, 1997; Mehta *et al.*, 2010; Olesen *et al.*, 2010), which may not concern adult diagnosed CF patients (Nick *et al.*, 2010). Numerous hypotheses have been brought forward to account for it, without any practical impact to date. Furthermore, though this might have been achieved at the price of a higher burden of treatment in females (Olesen *et al.*, 2010), there is evidence that modern intensive treatment may result in similar key clinical parameters for the two genders (Verma *et al.*, 2008; Olesen *et al.*, 2010).

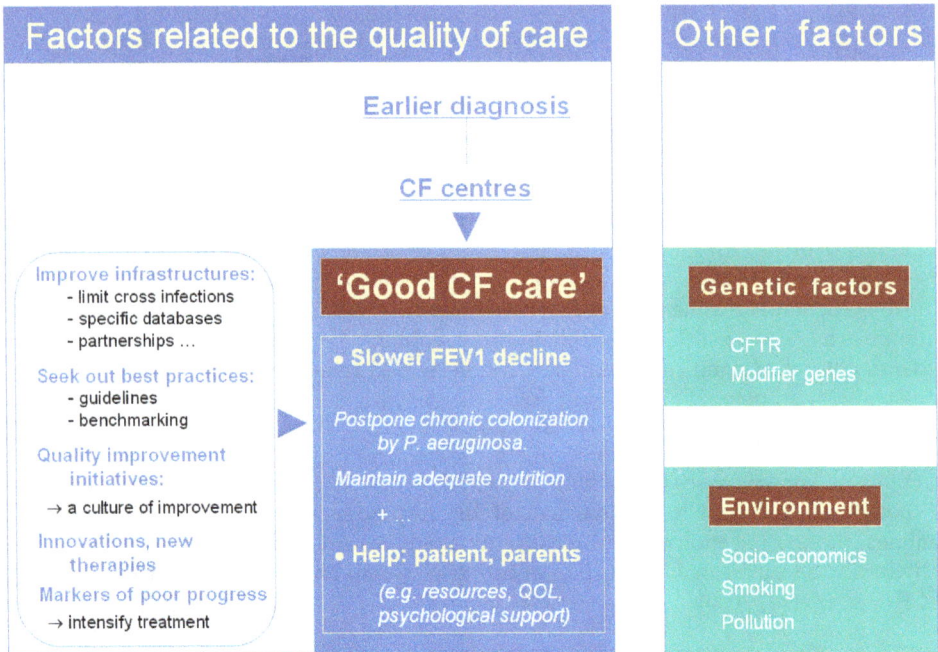

Fig. 1. Prognostic factors in CF

5. Good care management of CF

Early and mostly optimal management of CF is thus the principal reason for the improved prognosis observed over the past decades. Comprehensive follow-up and progress in symptomatic treatment proved essential. Antibiotics are the mainstay of CF therapy. In view of the complexity of this multisystemic and in many ways unique pathology, optimal management is only possible in truly specialized structures. Limiting the impact of economic status on treatment is an important issue. Most impressively, a pioneer clinician had already specifically stressed the importance of every single one of the above-named factors as early as 1974 (Crozier, 1974).

Taken in isolation and often combined to other factors (see discussion below), several complications can be linked to an accelerated rate of FEV_1 decline. Their awareness, prevention or early detection followed by optimal management carries the potential to reduce the rate of FEV_1 decline. This is well illustrated by the case for CF-related diabetes (CFRD) over the past 20 years. At one large CF centre, early detection and optimal management of CFRD resulted in a decrease on its impact on mortality and the disappearance of a sex difference in mortality (Moran *et al.*, 2009).

Two factors in particular, chronic airway colonisation by *Pseudomonas aeruginosa* (PA) and malnutrition, have such spontaneous prevalence and such prognostic impact, that their prevention constitutes one of the major objectives of CF care management.

Several medications have been associated to slowing down the rate of FEV_1 decline: dornase alpha (Konstan *et al.*, 2011), ibuprofen (Konstan *et al.*, 1995; Konstan *et al.*, 2007), azithromycin (Hansen *et al.*, 2005) and inhaled corticosteroids (De Boeck *et al.*, 2011). This does not mean that *all* patients will benefit from them. In addition, possible side-effects in the long-term have to be kept in mind (cf. e.g. ibuprofen). Also, it cannot be inferred that other drugs are necessarily ineffective: they may simply not have been subjected to appropriate studies, which occasionally may be due to commercial reasons or ethical concerns (e.g. physiotherapy).

5.1 Early diagnosis: CF newborn screening (NBS)

A number of studies using bronchoalveolar lavage (BAL) markers of infection and inflammation, lung function tests or computed tomography of the chest have documented that significant lung damage occurs very early in many, even asymptomatic, infants (Khan *et al.*, 1995; Ranganathan *et al.*, 2001; Davis *et al.*, 2007; Mott *et al.*, 2009). The results of two recent studies concerning very young infants who were investigated routinely after CF diagnosis by NBS are particularly striking (Sly *et al.*, 2009; Stafler *et al.*, 2011). Unsuspected positive cultures were found in 21-27% of them, there was evidence of airways inflammation with BAL neutrophilia in most patients and CT evidence of bronchial dilatation in 18.6%.

CF is a progressive disease for which symptomatic treatment has proven to have a real impact albeit of partial efficiency. So, starting treatment as early as possible is meaningful. CF NBS is now available throughout the USA and in many European countries. For those newborns carrying a genotype clearly associated with the disease, benefits of neonatal screening has long been proven in nutritional terms. Respiratory benefits have only recently been acknowledged (Accurso *et al.*, 2005; Rosenfeld *et al.*, 2010), as these were temporarily obscured by a publication indicating an increased risk of early chronic colonisation by PA in screened newborns (Farrell *et al.*, 2003). This increased risk was eventually linked to the lack of measures aiming to limit cross infections in that particular centre and subsequent studies failed to confirm it (Siret *et al.*, 2003; Sims *et al.*, 2005; Baussano *et al.*, 2006; Collins *et al.*, 2008). In countries with a high level of medical care, neonatal screening enables clinicians to diagnose CF in infants before the age of 2 months, with demonstrable benefits (Sims *et al.*, 2007).

5.2 The case for CF care centres

5.2.1 CF centres are necessary

CF NBS is universally coupled with immediate referral to a specialist centre. Guidelines and international consensus all emphasize this to be the key to efficiency for all CF programs

(Castellani *et al.*, 2009; Comeau *et al.*, 2007). Even outside the context of CF NBS, early referral to a specialist healthcare centre is considered as a major prognostic factor as highlighted in consensus reports on optimal management of CF (Littlewood, 2000; Kerem *et al.*, 2005; Colombo *et al.*, 2011). Though this has long been supported by a number of common sense reasons and has been mentioned as a model for the management of complex diseases (Schechter *et al.*, 2005), most published studies concerning the impact of this centralization on lung disease are either biased due to comparison with historical controls, and/or probably underpowered (Hill *et al.*, 1985; Nielsen *et al.*, 1988; Walters *et al.*, 1994; Collins *et al.*, 1999; Merelle *et al.*, 2001; Van Koolwijk *et al.*, 2002).

Two studies avoid these pitfalls. Mahadeva *et al.* compared two groups of adults who had either received continuous care from paediatric and adult CF centres (n=50) or had received neither paediatric nor adult centre care for their CF (n=36). Excluding body mass index as a covariate, FEV_1 was significantly better in the first group (Mahadeva *et al.*, 2000). More recently, a Belgian retrospective multicentre study clearly showed that earlier referral of children suffering from CF to specialist care was associated with significant pulmonary benefits (Lebecque *et al.* , 2009). Children referred 'early' (less than 2 years after diagnosis) had a better FEV_1 (86.7% pred. ± 19.4 *vs.* 77.2% ± 22.4, p=0.01) and a lower prevalence of PA (17.5% *vs.* 38.6 %, p<0.05) than carefully matched patients referred later.

5.2.2 CF centres might not be sufficient

Large differences between outcome variables obtained from the different centres have been recognized for a long time (Bauernfeind *et al.*, 1996) and are now drawing considerable attention as they may provide an opportunity to develop quality improvement initiatives. Striking illustrations of this outcome heterogeneity are provided by recent data from the 2007 US Registry (CFF Registry, 2007 – public data), allowing for comparisons between centres: i) mean FEV_1 (% predicted) for CF children aged 6-17 years ranged from 75 to 103% (national average: 92.6%, reference values: Wang & Hankinson) ii) the percentage of patients under 20 years of age with a BMI < 5th percentile ranged from 32 to 83% (national average: 52.7%) iii) MRSA infection rate ranged from 6 to 42% (national average: 21.2%). These differences persisted after taking into account socio-economic factors. Similar features can be derived from the CF German Registry where a quality management program with an overall coverage of 82% for the year of 2005 confirmed considerable differences between centres in terms of key parameters (Stern *et al.*, 2008). For instance, the percentage of children (6-18 years) with an FEV_1 above 80% of the predicted value ranged from 20 to 100% in centres treating less than 50 patients and from 35% to 100% in larger centres. Globally, the mean FEV_1 in this age group was 88% of the predicted value. A recent Belgian multicentre study confirmed the broad outcome differences between reference centres within this small country, where corresponding values for FEV_1 in children reportedly ranged from 74% to 95% predicted (Lebecque *et al.*, 2009) while the prevalence of PA (last visit of the year) ranged from 5 to 46% and the mean weight expressed as percentage of ideal body weight ranged from 88% to 100%.

5.2.3 Marked differences in clinical results between CF centres: Why?

One report of 18,411 patients followed in 194 North American centres in 1995 showed that close monitoring and heavier treatment (more frequent antibiotics in particular) clearly characterized those north-American centres with better clinical results (Johnson *et al.,* 2003). It is interesting to note that this more intensive management included two modalities which do not correspond to standard management: frequent prescription of nedocromil and more common prophylactic prescription of inhaled antibiotics, particularly in patients with still little pulmonary involvement. The use of nedocromil in CF is not well documented in the literature, neither is the potential of giving prophylactic inhaled antibiotics, which is discussed a little further in this chapter. Another North American study concerned 837 children aged 6 to 12 years (Padman *et al.,* 2007), whose CF centres were classified according to the children's FEV_1 values in 2003. The analysis also suggested that closer follow-up starting before the age of 3 years was characteristic of those centres with the best functional results. This 'more attentive and more active 'attitude' is in line with current standards of care, which are derived as much as possible from evidence-based medicine (Littlewood, 2000; Kerem *et al.,* 2005; Littlewood, 2005; Tiddens, 2009).

In 2002, the CFF launched an innovative Quality Improvement (QI) initiative, which included the vision statement that within 5 years, life expectancy of CF patients could be extended by 5-10 years through the consistent implementation of existing evidence-based clinical care (Quinton, 2007). However, evidence-based medicine has its limitations and possible stumbling blocks (Driever, 2002; Saarni *et al.,* 2004; Miles *et al.,* 2008; Shahar, 2008; Miles *et al.,* 2011), in particular when it concerns diseases as complex as CF for which numerous therapeutic modalities have simply not yet been adequately studied (Cheng *et al.,* 2000; David, 2001; Briggs *et al.,* 2006; Kraynack *et al.,* 2009). Best practice remains individualized in part, although a coherent foundation of evidence-based medicine is absolutely necessary.

One comparative study of 3 CF centres illustrates how even beside care standards, clinician intuition can lead to potentially judicious choices that deserve prospective studies. A better nutritional status was indeed linked to the prescription of dornase alpha (Pulmozyme ®) under the age of 2 years (Padman *et al.,* 2008), whereas the effects of Pulmozyme in this age group have only been reported in one limited study (Berge *et al.,* 2003) where 9 infants were given the drug for 2 weeks. The necessity to conceive and study new strategies stems from the fact that current ones are relatively powerless in preventing pulmonary lesions in early diagnosed infants (Stick *et al.,* 2009).

Information concerning the standards of CF care is widely available as are new drugs in rich countries. Differences in clinical results between various CF centres must therefore have a different origin. One can suspect subtle combinations of several factors resulting in small differences in interventionist attitudes. Beside adequate means i.e. infrastructures and human resources, optimal care requires a careful organisation (structure of the centre, coherence of attitudes, multiple fail safe systems etc.) necessitating considerable long-term thoughtful investment of all those involved.

5.2.4 Variability of outcomes in CF centres: Benchmarking as a right to patients

It is not possible for a CF clinic to function without landmarks. Specific databases prove to be very precious by giving immediate access to progress over time and by age group of essential parameters, thereby constituting a sort of 'compass' for measures that could be taken to improve care management. Although limiting the objective to FEV_1 improvement would be reductive, it clearly remains an essential parameter. The FEV_1 of patients aged 6-18 years old (Figure 2) is a particularly relevant landmark for the 3 following reasons: i) very few patients die or require transplantation prior to that age ii) a significant proportion of adults has not benefited from immediate specialized care iii) adolescence is a particularly high risk time period with regard to deterioration of respiratory function. Appropriate indicators to define nutritional outcomes are also necessary (Lai et al., 2008). If they are to be used to compare CF centres, these indicators have to be adjusted for risk factors - which does not change the overall outcome variability of CF centres (Schechter et al., 2002) - and several years should be taken into consideration, in order to appreciate their coherence and tendencies.

Mean FEV1 (% pred.) – children (6 to 17 years)   Percentage of children with a FEV1 ≥ 90% pred.

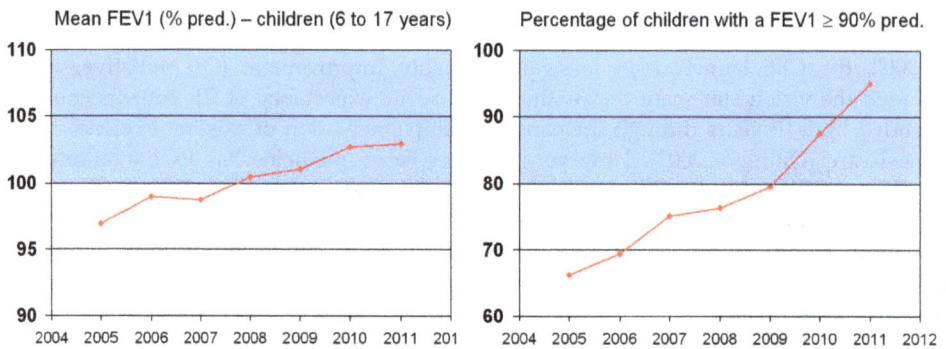

Fig. 2. Lung function in children followed-up at St Luc (last visit of the year, reference equations from Wang et al. for females through age 15 and males through age 17, and Hankinson et al. at older ages) (Wang et al., 1993; Hankinson et al., 1999).

The differences in mean FEV_1 observed in children from various CF centres can exceed 20% of predicted values. Recent data can help to perceive the implications of such differences: i) some centres now report a mean annual FEV_1 decline around 1% (Que, 2006) ii) in terms of FEV_1 (expressed in % pred.), improvements from baseline observed in two major randomized controlled trials of inhaled dornase alfa and tobramycin were less than 4% and 5% respectively (Fuchs et al., 1994; Ramsey et al., 1999) iii) in the USA, from 1990 to 2008, median FEV_1 at 12 years of age increased by 14 % predicted. Thus the prognostic significance of the differences between centres is major, also in terms of life expectancy. For this reason, public access to these data can be considered as a right to the patient and/or parents. In 2006, the outcomes data from the CF Foundation registry became public on the foundation's website, with an accompanying warning against simplistic interpretations. This choice bore witness to the priority given to the patients. Their health is at stake, and keeping them informed has to take precedence over the risk of embarrassing some physicians. In the USA, the fear that some patients may leave CF centres with average performance has not materialised: patients and their family maintain their trust once they realize that everything is done to improve results (Quinton, 2007).

5.2.5 'Good enough' care for CF does not exist: Towards a culture of improvement

Benchmarking, which is the process of identifying practices associated with the best results, may help to understand why certain centres obtain better clinical results. Not only can it be considered a right to the patients, it can also serve as an incentive to CF centres to increase their efforts to improve quality of care delivery. In the USA, most CF healthcare providers actually accepted it as a call to action (Schechter *et al.*, 2005). Public release of meaningful adjusted clinical outcomes data has been used in other fields of medicine, such as cardiac surgery, as a means to stimulate improvement efforts within the medical profession (Ferris *et al.*, 2010). Others have advocated 'softer' uses of benchmarking which do not require to be channelled via public data (Stern *et al.*, 2011). In the field of CF, benchmarking is not an easy task. It is possible when based on well-established CF registries but issues related to quality control and missing data obviously remain crucial (van der Ent, 2008). A number of methodological issues make it even harder to compare data from different countries. These include (but are not limited to) the population coverage level, the choice of reference equations, the type of subjects included in the registry (an increasing number of patients with milder forms of the disease are now being identified in some countries through wide access to CFTR gene sequencing and nasal potential difference measurements, or via CF NBS), a lack of uniform definitions of specific items (FEV_1 has been recorded as the last, the best, the mean or the average of the best value for each quarter of the year; normal FEV_1 has been defined as $\geq 80\%$ or $\geq 90\%$ of the predicted value in different registries) or of clinical conditions (hepatopathy, CF-related diabetes, pulmonary exacerbation), differences in age stratification (in the UK, adults are defined as patients ≥ 16 years old), inclusion or exclusion of lung transplanted patients ('another disease'), wide heterogeneity of CFTR mutations throughout the world, etc. There is indeed an obvious need for standardization in data collection if we are to compare different registries meaningfully. The ever present need to 'always try to do better' that animates so many clinicians and paramedics involved in caring for CF patients has led to the development of several QI initiatives. The latter have tended to improve key indices concerning either nutrition or respiratory function, but can also have other objectives such as a greater involvement of patients as partners in care, by sending them for example a copy of their own medical records (Treacy *et al.*, 2008). Guidelines and evidence-based medicine provide the directions in which changes for QI should be made. Various strategies can be put into place as part of these QI initiatives (Quinton, 2004; VandenBranden, 2004; Schechter, 2004; Quinton *et al.*, 2007; Britton *et al.*, 2008; Schechter *et al.*, 2010; Kraynack *et al.*, 2009; Quon *et al.*, 2011). They all rely on adequate infrastructures, the acknowledgement that changes are needed, relevant and quantifiable objectives identified on the basis of the centre's known clinical outcomes, the deployment of the necessary means and an objective evaluation of the various steps undertaken. Taking into consideration identified obstacles to optimal treatment (Zemanick *et al.*, 2010), trends of medication use over time (Konstan *et al.*, 2010), and the considerable differences in treatment practices (Borsje *et al.*, 2000) or in clinical approach between specialized CF centres (Kraynack *et al.*, 2011) could nurture reflection and help to identify and better discern the objectives and means to be put into place.

5.3 Tools and challenges

The range of responsibilities of a team dedicated to CF patients is vast, in keeping with the complexity of this chronic disease. Close and comprehensive follow-up enables an early start of an efficient symptomatic treatment. Guidelines and specific databases belong to those tools that are essential to the clinicians. The importance of the latter can not be overemphasized (Kerem *et al.*, 2005; Quinton *et al.*, 2007; Leal *et al.*, 2007; Tiddens, 2009).

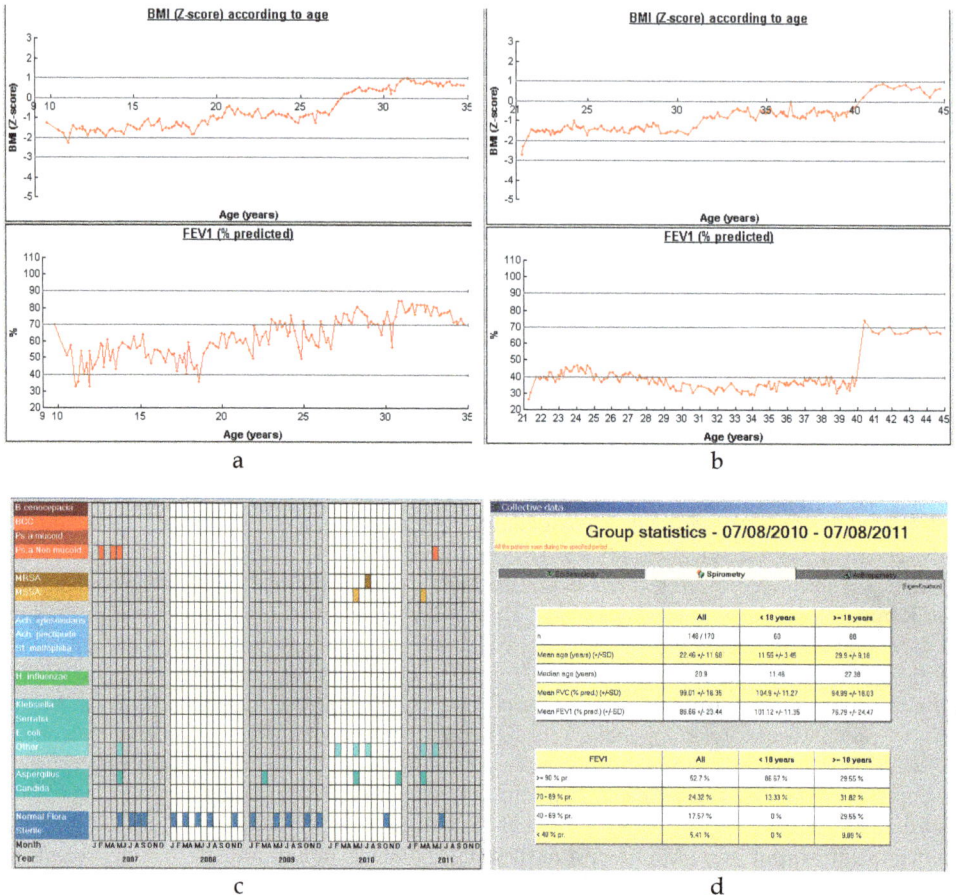

Fig. 3. Specific database provide instant access to critical information at the individual level and at the level of the clinic as a whole. *a.* Current treatment modalities occasionally lead to sustained very long-term improvement of both FEV$_1$ and BMI. *b.* They can also allow prolonged survival in stable conditions despite severe pulmonary lesions (this patient eventually benefited from a lung transplant following recurrent life-threatening haemoptysis). *c*: This screen summarize bacteriological findings of a given patient over 5 years, also allowing to determine at a glance the state of *Pseudomonas aeruginosa* infection according to a meaningful classification (Lee *et al.*, 2003). *d*: Instant access to key parameters at the scale of the whole clinic.

In the setting of the clinic, visualizing with a simple click trends of essential parameters such as FEV$_1$ or BMI can help the patient to fully understand the need for treatment modifications.

Regularly updated guidelines and in-depth reviews are essential resources. They cover most areas including standards of care (Kerem *et al.*, 2005), diagnosis (Farrell *et al.*, 2008), adult management (Yankaskas *et al.*, 2004), care of infants diagnosed by CF NBS (Accurso *et al.*, 2009; Sermet-Gaudelus *et al.*, 2010), nutrition (Sinaasappel *et al.*, 2002; CF Trust, 2002; Stallings *et al.*, 2008), antibiotic therapy (CF Trust, 2009), respiratory infections (Ramsey *et al.*, 2003), by *Pseudomonas aeruginosa* in particular (Döring *et al.*, 2000; Saiman *et al.*, 2003; Döring *et al.*, 2004; CF Trust , 2004; Hoiby *et al.*, 2005), microbiology laboratory standards (CF Trust 2010), pregnancy management (Edenborough *et al.*, 2008; Lau *et al.*, 2010) or complications such as Allergic BronchoPulmonary Aspergillosis (ABPA) (Stevens *et al.*, 2003), diabetes (Moran *et al.*, 2010), pneumothorax or haemoptysis (Flume *et al.*, 2010).

5.3.1 Challenge 1: Postpone chronic colonisation by *Pseudomonas aeruginosa*

The reasons for which PA has a predilection for the lungs of CF patients are still unclear (Gibson *et al.*, 2003). Its presence can often be detected early, at times within the first few months of life, even in the absence of any symptom. It will usually be isolated within the first 3 years (Burns *et al.*, 2001; Dakin *et al.*, 2002; West *et al.*, 2002; Hilliard *et al.*, 2007; Sly *et al.*, 2009; Stafler *et al.*, 2011). A prospective study has indicated that 90% of CF children aged 4 years and above presented at least 1 positive culture for PA (Li *et al.*, 2005). The early isolates of PA are generally non-mucoid and antibiotic susceptible. However, PA tends to colonise the airways of CF patients in a chronic, irreversible, fashion often associated to a change to a mucoid phenotype. At this stage, pulmonary function usually worsens and clinical symptoms become evident. Early detection of PA is crucial as there is a window of opportunity for effective eradication at this stage (Koch, 2002; Li *et al.*, 2005).

Chronic PA colonisation is associated with a lower FEV_1 in childhood (Kerem *et al.*, 1990), an accelerated rate of FEV_1 decline (Pamukcu *et al.*, 1995; Kosorok *et al.*, 2001; Emerson *et al.*, 2002), a shorter median life expectancy (CFF Registry, 1996; Emerson *et al.*, 2002) and much higher treatment costs (Baumann *et al.*, 2003). Preventing this colonisation is considered the most important challenge for the CF clinician, as it frequently determines the patient's future quality of life and long-term survival (CF Trust 2002; Koch, 2002). The current approach relies on two strategies (Frederiksen *et al.*, 1999): i) paying attention to segregate patients on bacteriological grounds in order to limit the risk of cross-infections (West *et al.*, 2002; Conway *et al.*, 2008), ii) early antibiotic treatment at the time of the first PA colonisation (Littlewood *et al.*, 1985; Valerius *et al.*, 1991; Frederiksen *et al.*, 1997; Lee *et al.*, 2004). A number of regimens have been evaluated (Stuart *et al.*, 2010) but there is no consensus about the best combination, dosage, or length of treatment course. An initial treatment protocol combining nebulised colistin with oral ciprofloxacin for 3 months is widely used. Combining this approach with intravenous antibiotics has also been reported, with a 5-year failure rate of only 12% (Douglas *et al.*, 2009). A prerequisite for this approach is a close bacteriological follow-up, with a time lapse between visits that cannot exceed 3 months. This interval is shorter (up to monthly) in many centres. An aggressive approach based on repeated BAL has not proven useful (Wainwright *et al.*, 2011). The 20% failure rate of the more commonly used approach (Frederiksen *et al.*, 1997; Lee *et al.*, 2004; Tacetti *et al.*, 2004) underlines the necessity to develop other intervention modalities.

It is paradoxical that prophylactic antibiotic therapy directed against PA has only been the subject of 1 retrospective study (Heinzl *et al.*, 2002) while prophylaxis against *Staphylococcus aureus*, whose threat is yet much easier to manage, has been investigated and hotly debated. The Austrian study was in fact very encouraging but the same group reported that long-term gentamicin inhalation in CF children was associated with reversible raised urinary N-acetyl-beta-D-glucosaminidase (NAG) activity, consistent with subtle subclinical renal tubular damage (Ring *et al.*, 1998). Tobramycin and amikacin however have lower renal toxicity than gentamicin and long-term use of high doses of inhaled tobramycin (TOBI) are now considered safe (Prober *et al.*, 2000). There are several theoretical arguments that make long-term inhaled prophylactic antibiotic therapy attractive (Lebecque *et al.*, 2008). Based on the use of low doses of Tobramycin or Amikacin, this approach has progressively been put into place at our centre over the past 20 years, and has probably contributed, along with other factors, to a distinctly low rate of chronic colonisation rate by PA in patients under 18 years of age (<5% for more than 10 years, according to Lee's definition) (Lee *et al.*, 2003).

5.3.2 Challenge 2: Maintain adequate nutrition

The poorer prognosis associated with being relatively underweight has long been recognized in CF children (Kraemer *et al.*, 1978). An overall parallelism exists between respiratory function and nutritional status progress over time (Zemel *et al.*, 2000; Steinkamp *et al.*, 2002; Konstan *et al.*, 2003; Milla, 2004; Pedreira *et al.*, 2005). While severe pulmonary disease seriously compromises the maintenance of a satisfactory nutritional status, proof of the opposite has also been demonstrated: maintaining a good nutritional status promotes respiratory function preservation. Evidence of the possible influence of maintaining a good nutritional status was first suggested by a comparison of the CF centres of Boston and Toronto (Corey *et al.*, 1988). In Toronto, CF patients had better respiratory function and were better fed, and the main difference in management appeared to be the lack of fat restriction in the Canadian hospital. Maintaining an adequate nutritional status has become a priority of CF care.

5.3.3 Many other challenges...

Early detection and adequate management of poor clinical course find their place here, along with appropriate management of complications, particularly those linked to an accelerated rate of FEV_1 decline as in ABPA (Kraemer *et al.*, 2006), diabetes (Milla *et al.*, 2000), gastro-esophageal reflux (Levy *et al.*, 1986), colonisation by *Burkolderia cenocepacia* (Ledson *et al.*, 2002; Courtney *et al.*, 2004) non-mucoid strains in particular (Zlosnik *et al.*, 2011), or by MRSA (Dasenbrook *et al.*, 2008). In the same vein it is worth insisting on the vulnerable period spanning from pre-adolescence to adolescence (Konstan *et al.*, 2007). The rate of FEV_1 decline is faster at that time, and the various reasons for which this is considered a risk period should especially mobilise the attention and energy of the care management teams (Segal, 2008). In the context of CF, ABPA diagnosis is often delicate, (de Almeida *et al.*, 2006; Thia *et al.*, 2009) as many features overlap with those of infective exacerbations in CF, but it is important: failing to recognize ABPA can lead to irreversible lesions, whereas overtreatment exposes the patient to deleterious side-effects of systemic corticosteroids.

The prevention of cross-infections is a daily preoccupation that predetermines the detailed organisation of the CF centres. One of the major challenges is to limit *Burkholderia cepacia complex* (BCC) infections. The prognostic significance of colonisation by *B. cenocepacia* is particularly dreaded, as its presence is associated to an accelerated rate of FEV_1 decline and a clinical picture that is often fatal (*cepacia* syndrome) (Isles *et al.*, 1984) and can affect patients up to then in very good health. In addition, *B. cenocepacia* is a cause for increased mortality following lung transplantation (Aris *et al.*, 2001; Boussaud *et al.*, 2008). Other germs of the BCC group such as B. *multivorans* or B. *dolosa* have a less gloomy effect on prognosis but have exceptionally also been associated to the occurrence of a *cepacia* syndrome (Zahariadis *et al.*, 2003; Blackburn *et al.*, 2004; Kalish *et al.*, 2006).

Several other essential factors are involved in global care management. There is no equivalent long-term illness to CF today in terms of the heavy burden of its symptomatic treatment. In a recent US study, adult patients - of whom only half had performed airway clearance - reported a mean time spent on treatment activities of 108 minutes per day (Sawicki *et al.*, 2009). Though very difficult to assess (Modi *et al.*, 2006), treatment adherence is undoubtedly a key issue in CF (Eakin et al, 2011) and requires permanent assessment and support (Pendleton, 2000). There is no magic recipe, but this subject has to be bridged at every consultation, in an open manner, with empathy and as part of a 'therapeutic alliance' (Lask, 1994; Cohen-Cymberknoh *et al.*, 2011). Another objective is to be able to propose psychological and/or social support in response to specific situations, either linked to the disease or impacting on treatment in real life.

5.3.4 Flags or indications for treatment intensification

Several clinical or biological markers have been associated with poorer outcome. Their main interest is that they can point to the need for reconsidering and optimizing symptomatic treatment. Some of these associations may appear simple common sense but the reality is often more complex: in-depth statistical analysis can reveal multiple independent factors and it is important to bear in mind that a statistically significant association is not equivalent to the demonstration of a causality link. For instance, a recent Canadian study showed that adult patients with CF who experienced at least 3 pulmonary exacerbations per year over a 3-year follow-up period were clearly high-risk patients, who warranted timely consideration for lung transplantation (de Boer *et al.*, 2011). However, such patients were more likely to be female and diabetic, two risk factors linked to poorer outcome. In addition, while frequent pulmonary exacerbations may predispose a patient to lung transplantation, patients on the list for lung transplants may be more aggressively treated, thereby appearing to have more exacerbations. Raised serum IgG levels (Wallwork *et al.*, 1974; Matthews *et al.*, 1980; Wheeler *et al.*, 1984; Proesmans *et al.*, 2011) and the presence of localized auscultation anomalies (Konstan *et al.*, 2007) also belong to the list of 'flags' for treatment intensification.

6. Environmental factors

6.1 Socioeconomic status

As for all chronic diseases, CF prognosis is more sombre in patients of poor socio-economic status (SES). In 1986, there were 113 deaths registered of CF patients in the UK. Median age of death was 17 years overall, but it was above 20 for patients whose parents had a non-manual job whereas it was below 10 for the others (Britton *et al.*, 1989). In a study of CF patients in the United States, the adjusted risk of death for indigent patients who qualified for Medicaid was 3.65 times higher than for those not receiving Medicaid. The average FEV_1 of Medicaid patients was less by 9.2% predicted than that of non-Medicaid patients, a difference which slightly increased by 0.54% per year of age (Schechter *et al.*, 1998). In a CFF study of 23,817 white patients diagnosed before the age of 18 years, a strong association was found between the median household income and the mortality rate. At 6 years of age, the absolute differences in mean FEV_1 and weight percentiles from the lowest to the highest income category were already very significant and they persisted into adulthood (O'Connor *et al.*, 2003). Furthermore, this study also clearly showed that the relationship between outcome and SES was incremental, rather than dichotomous and only affecting the most indigent. Though access to health insurance is much better in many European countries than in the US, the overall costs of CF treatment and follow-up are so high that patients with low SES are particularly at risk of inadequate resources and poor adherence. A better understanding of SES-related disparities and its causes is necessary to clarify the respective roles of a link between poverty and other environmental factors, health behaviours and limited access to optimal care. Low SES has recently been associated with lower health-related quality of life in CF patients and parents. After accounting for the effects of disease severity and SES, a negative effect of membership to a racial or ethnic minority on social and emotional functioning was also evident (Quittner *et al.*, 2010).

6.2 Exposure to smoking

Exposure to passive or active smoking has deleterious effects in healthy subjects and in patients with respiratory diseases. An accelerated rate of FEV_1 decline with age is documented in healthy adult smokers. Functional repercussions of passive smoking were assessed in a large study concerning 812 CF patients (Collaco *et al.*, 2008). Over a fifth of them (188, i.e. 23%) were exposed to passive smoking. At the age of 20, the mean FEV_1 of exposed patients was, independently of SES, 8% lower than that of non-exposed patients. This effect was even more pronounced in patients who were not homozygous for the *F508del* mutation, and was twice higher in patients who were also carriers of an unfavourable genotype with respect to the *TGFß₁* modifier gene. Deleterious effects of active smoking should a priori be more severe but have not been investigated specifically in the context of CF. Exposure to smoking is a major environmental factor and screening for it should become routine practice in CF care as several pharmacological and non-pharmacological smoking cessation aids have proven their efficacy, the best results being obtained by combining modalities and tailoring therapy (Laniado-Laborin, 2010).

6.3 Other environmental factors

In a CF registry study, exposure to ozone and annual average exposure to particulate air pollution were both associated with an increased likelihood of pulmonary exacerbations. Exposure to particulate matter with an aerodynamic diameter of 2.5 µm or less was also associated with a decline in lung function (Goss *et al.*, 2004). Though environmental factors are not considered the main pathogenic factors in ABPA, experts have suggested that it may be worth examining the patient's environment in refractory cases (Stevens *et al.*, 2003). Altough the mechanisms are unclear, recent published evidence supports a link between climatic conditions (ambient temperature) and lung function in CF (Collaco et al., 2011). According to the authors, a hypothetical 18 year old white male with CF (Height: 175cm) with an FEV1 of 73.5% percent living in a cold climate would be expected to have an FEV1 of 66.1% had he resided in a 17 degree (Celsius) warmer climate.

Recreational use of marijuana is common in many countries. In a study of 173 adults, this drug was used by 20% of patients (Stern et al., 1987). In the general population, such use has been associated with pulmonary manifestations (bronchitis, pneumothorax, apical bullae) (Tetrault et al., 2007; Han et al., 2010; Gao et al., 2010) that could overlap clinical and radiological signs of CF, making it challenging to suspect them. Further studies seem warranted in this field.

7. Genetic factors

7.1 CFTR genotype

Depending on their repercussions on the synthesis of the CF Transmembrane conductance Regulator (CFTR) protein, mutations of the CF gene are usually classified into 5 groups (Welsh et al., 1993). Mutations of classes I, II and III lead to the total or near-total absence of functional CFTR protein, whereas those of classes IV or V are associated to residual function of the CFTR protein, corresponding to a small % of normal activity. Pancreatic insufficiency is present in over 95% of patients carrying 2 class I, II or III mutations, whereas it is only rarely observed in patients carrying at least 1 class IV or V mutation (CF genotype-phenotype consortium, 1993; Koch et al., 2001). Diabetes and severe hepatic involvement are 2 important CF complications that usually only occur in patients with exocrine pancreatic insufficiency. A recent study of 505 patients registered in Israel's databases did not observe a single case amongst 139 pancreatic sufficient patients (Augarten et al., 2008). The relationship between CFTR genotype and the severity of the pulmonary involvement is much looser. On the whole, the genotype of patients carrying 2 mutations of class I, II or III is still considered high risk and is associated to earlier mortality than genotypes including at least 1 mutation of class IV or V ('low risk' genotypes) (Mc Kone et al., 2006). Similarly, although their phenotype can be extremely variable, an overall more favourable prognosis has been associated to some mutations of class IV or V. Amongst the latter, there are mutations A455E (Gan et al., 1995), 3849 +10kbC->T (Highsmith et al., 1994; Duguéperoux et al., 2005), 2789+5G->A (Duguéperoux et al., 2005), D1152H (Musaffi et al., 2006; Burgel et al., 2010), R334W (Antinolo et al., 1997), 3272-26A->G (Amaral et al., 2001). The penetrance of the R117H mutation has convincingly been shown to be very low (Thauvin-Robinet et al., 2009) and is modulated by the polypyrimidine variant in the intron 8 acceptor splice site (T7 or T5) in cis with R117H. However, FEV_1 at a given age can be extremely variable in patients sharing a same CFTR genotype and this is observed in patients homozygous for the F508del mutation as well as in patients carrying a "milder" genotype (Gan et al., 1995). In practice, the link between CFTR genotype and severity of lung disease is not tight, making CFTR genotype most often of little value in predicting the prognosis at the individual level.

7.2 Modifier genes

Every clinician has in mind extreme examples of the heterogeneity of functional respiratory progress in CF patients, including amongst those that are homozygous for the F508del mutation. Though poorly compliant, chronically colonized by PA since adolescence and diabetic for 10 years, one 40 year-old patient keeps his FEV_1 above 80% of the predicted value whereas a young lady, with an optimal follow-up since birth and only occasionally *Aspergillus fumigatus* in sputum experiences a rapid functional decline from age 12 and requires a lung transplantation at 20. Environmental factors may play a role but admittedly such patients have to be either 'protected' for one or 'condemned' for the other, by particular allele combinations of modifier genes probably modulating the immune and inflammatory response in the lungs.

Family-based studies and especially comparisons of monozygous and dizygous twin pairs have proven fruitful in identifying and assessing the contribution of modifier genes in CF disease. Many studies in this field have yielded conflicting results and it is now realized that the repeatability of SNP–phenotype association studies with positive findings was low when less than 500 participants were included (Boyle, 2007). More recent studies are more powerful and use more sophisticated tools including whole-genome methods. Quite convincing evidence is now available that variants of at least 3 genes can be associated with lung disease severity in CF (Cutting, 2010): i) *MBL2*-deficient (10q) genotype: in normal subjects, mannose binding lectin (MBL) aids the phagocytosis of bacteria and deficiency in MBL seems to predispose to early infection with PA in CF ii) Increased *TGFß₁* (19q) expression (Drumm *et al.*, 2005): this gene, which also modulates the risk for asthma and chronic obstructive pulmonary disease, encodes a cytokine playing a role in the regulation of inflammation and tissue remodelling iii) Increased *EDNRA* (4q) expression: Endothelin is a proinflammatory peptide and smooth muscle agonist which is increased in CF airways. Deleterious effects could be related to an impact on smooth muscle tone in the airways and/or vasculature (Darrah *et al.*, 2010). More recently, two loci causing variations in CF lung disease severity have been identified on chromosomes 11p and 20q respectively (Wright *et al.*, 2011). Variation in *TCF7L2* (10q) was reported to increase the risk of diabetes about threefold and even more in patients without previous treatment with systemic steroids (Blackman *et al.*, 2009). Variants of other genes are suspected to increase the risk of liver cirrhosis (Bartlett *et al.*, 2009) or meconium ileus. Further progress in the identification of modifier genes should result in an increased ability to predict severity of CF disease, and hopefully be accompanied by new perspectives for therapeutic intervention.

8. Conclusions

For patients, their relatives and also their carers, facing CF is often compared to running a long-distance race. It is also a team race, where no-one can let go. In terms of life expectancy, prognosis of the disease has been improving continuously since 40 years. However, it is almost always impossible to predict CF prognosis at the individual level. The quality of an early global care management is an essential prognostic determinant. Further progress in symptomatic CF treatment remains necessary, especially towards better prevention of respiratory involvement in early-diagnosed newborns and in the field of immunosuppression in lung transplantation. The discovery of a cure for the respiratory disease in CF would be a real breakthrough. A pharmacological approach tailored to the class mutations of the CFTR gene appears currently the most encouraging route in this direction.

Meanwhile, the essence of the carer's role today remains founded on these two maxims: 'Do not abandon the marathon' and 'Always try to do better'.

9. References

Abbott, J., Hart, A., Havermans T. *et al.* (2011). Measuring health-related quality of life in clinical trials in cystic fibrosis. *J Cyst Fibros*. Vol. 10, Suppl 2, pp 82-85.

Accurso, F., Sontag M. & Wagener J. (2005). Complications associated with symptomatic diagnosis in infants with cystic fibrosis. *J Pediatr*. Vol. 147, Suppl. 3, pp 37-41.

Accurso F., Rowe S., Clancy J. *et al.* (2010). Effect of VX-770 in persons with cystic fibrosis and the G551D-CFTR mutation. *N Engl J Med*. Vol. 363, No 21, pp 1191-2003.

Amaral, M., Pacheco P, Beck S. *et al.* (2001). Cystic fibrosis patients with the 3272-26A>G splicing mutation have milder disease than F508del homozygotes: a large European study. *J Med Genet*. Vol. 38, No 11, pp 777-783.

Amaral, M. (2011). Targeting CFTR: how to treat cystic fibrosis by CFTR-repairing therapies. *Curr Drug Targets* Vol. 12, No 5, pp 683-693.

Antinolo G., Borrego S, Gili M. *et al.* (1997). Genotype-phenotype relationship in 12 patients carrying cystic fibrosis mutation R334W. *J Med Genet*. Vol. 34, No 2, pp 89-91.

Aris R., Routh J, LiPuma J. *et al.* (2001). Lung transplantation for cystic fibrosis patients with Burkholderia cepacia complex. Survival linked to genomovar type. *Am J Respir Crit Care Med*. Vol. 164, No 11, pp 2102-2106.

Augarten A., Ben Tov A., Madgar I. *et al.* (2008). The changing face of the exocrine pancreas in cystic fibrosis: the correlation between pancreatic status, pancreatitis and cystic fibrosis genotype. *Eur J Gastroenterol Hepatol*. Vol. 20, No 3, pp 164-168.

Balaguer A. & González de Dios J. (2008). Home intravenous antibiotics for cystic fibrosis. *Cochrane Database Syst Rev*. CD001917.

Bartlett J., Friedman K, Ling S. *et al.* (2009). Genetic modifiers of liver disease in cystic fibrosis. *JAMA*. Vol. 302, No 10, pp 1076-1083.

Bauernfeind A., Marks M. & Strandvik B. (1996). Cystic fibrosis pulmonary infections: lessons from around the world. Birkhauser Verlag AG, Basel. ISBN-13: 978-3764350277

Baumann U., Stocklossa C., Greiner W. *et al.* (2003). Cost of care and clinical condition in paediatric cystic fibrosis patients. *J Cyst Fibros*. Vol. 2, No 2, pp 84-90.

Baussano I., Tardivo I., Belleza-Fontana R. *et al.* (2006). Neonatal screening for cystic fibrosis does not affect time to first infection with Pseudomonas aeruginosa. *Pediatrics*. Vol. 118, No 3, pp 888-895.

Berge M, Wiel E, Tiddens H. *et al.* (2003). DNase in stable cystic fibrosis infants: a pilot study. *J Cyst Fibros*. Vol. 2, No 4, pp 183-188.

Blackburn L., Brownlee K., Conway S. *et al.* (2004). 'Cepacia syndrome' with Burkholderia multivorans, 9 years after initial colonization. *J Cyst Fibros*. Vol. 3, No 2, pp 133-134.

Blackman S., Hsu S, Ritter S *et al.* (2009). A susceptibility gene for type 2 diabetes confers substantial risk for diabetes complicating cystic fibrosis. *Diabetologia* Vol. 52, No 9, pp 1858-1865.

Borowitz D., Robinson K., Rosenfeld M. *et al.* (2009). Cystic Fibrosis Foundation evidence-based guidelines for management of infants with cystic fibrosis. *J Pediatr*. Vol. 155, Suppl. 6, pp 73-93.

Boussaud V., Guillemain R, Grenet D *et al.* (2008). Clinical outcome following lung transplantation in patients with cystic fibrosis colonised with Burkholderia cepacia complex: results from two French centres. *Thorax*. Vol. 63, No 8, pp 732-737.

Borsje P, deJongste J, Mouton J *et al*. (2000). Aerosol therapy in cystic fibrosis: a survey of 54 CF centers. *Pediatr Pulmonol*. Vol. 30, No 5, pp 368-376.

Boyle M. (2007). Strategies for identifying modifier genes in cystic fibrosis. *Proc Am Thorac Soc*. Vol 4, No 1, pp 52-57.

Briggs T., Bryant M. & Smyth R. (2006). Controlled clinical trials in cystic fibrosis--are we doing better? *J Cyst Fibros*. Vol. 5, No 1, pp 3-8.

Britton J. (1989). Effects of social class, sex, and region of residence on age at death from cystic fibrosis. *BMJ*. Vol. 298, pp 483-7.

Britton L., Thrasher S. & Guttierez H. (2008). Creating a culture of improvement: experience of a pediatric cystic fibrosis center. *J Nurs Care Qual*. Vol. 23, No 2, pp 115-120.

Burgel P, Fajac I, Hubert D. *et al*. (2010). Non-classic cystic fibrosis associated with D1152H CFTR mutation. *Clin Genet*. Vol. 77, No 4, pp 355-64.

Burns J., Gibson R, McNamara S. *et al*. (2001). Longitudinal assessment of Pseudomonas aeruginosa in young children with cystic fibrosis. *J Infect Dis*. Vol. 183, No 3, pp 444-452.

Bush A. & Götz M. (2006). Cystic fibrosis. *Eur Respir Mon*. Vol. 37, pp 234–290.

Buzzetti R., Salvatore D., Baldo E. *et al*. (2009). An overview of international literature from cystic fibrosis registries: 1. Mortality and survival studies in cystic fibrosis. *J Cyst Fibros*. Vol. 8, No 4, pp 229-237.

Canadian CF Registry (2008), Available from http://www.fibrosekystique.ca/en/index.php

Castellani C., Southern K, Browlee K. *et al*. (2009). European best practice guidelines for cystic fibrosis neonatal screening. *J Cyst Fibros*. Vol. 8, No 3, pp 153-173.

CF Genotype-Phenotype Consortium (1993). Correlation between genotype and phenotype in patients with cystic fibrosis. *N Engl J Med*. Vol. 329, No 18, pp 1308-1313.

CFF Registry (1996), Cystic Fibrosis Foundation Patient Registry 1996 Annual Data Report. Bethesda, Maryland

CFF Registry (2000), Cystic Fibrosis Foundation Patient Registry 2000 Annual Data Report. Bethesda, Maryland

CFF Registry (2007), Cystic Fibrosis Foundation Patient Registry 2007 Annual Data Report. Bethesda, Maryland

CFF Registry (2008), Cystic Fibrosis Foundation Patient Registry 2008 Annual Data Report. Bethesda, Maryland Available from http://www.cff.org/research/ClinicalResearch/PatientRegistryRport/

CF Trust (2002). Nutritional management in cystic fibrosis.

CF Trust (2004). Pseudomonas aeruginosa infection in people with Cystic Fibrosis. Suggestions for Prevention and Infection Control.

CF Trust (2009). Antibiotic Treatment for Cystic Fibrosis.

CF Trust (2010). Laboratory Standards for Processing Microbiological Samples from People with Cystic Fibrosis.

Cheng K., Smyth R, Motley J. *et al*. (2000). Randomized controlled trials in cystic fibrosis (1966-1997) categorized by time, design, and intervention. *Pediatr Pulmonol*. Vol. 29, No 1, pp 1-7.

Cohen-Cymberknoh M., Shoseyov D. & Kerem E. (2011). Managing cystic fibrosis: strategies that increase life expectancy and improve quality of life. *Am J Respir Crit Care Med*. Vol. 183, no 11, pp 1463-1471.

Collaco J., Vanscoy L., Bremer L. *et al.* (2008). Interactions between secondhand smoke and genes that affect cystic fibrosis lung disease. *JAMA.* Vol. 299, No 4, pp 417-424.

Collaco J., McGready J., Green D. *et al.* (2011). Effect of temperature on cystic fibrosis lung disease and infections: a replicated cohort study. *PLoS One.* Vol. 6, No 11, e27784.

Collins C., MacDonald-Wicks L., Rowe S. *et al.* (1999). Normal growth in cystic fibrosis associated with a specialised centre. *Arch Dis Child.* Vol. 81, No 3, pp 241-246.

Colombo C. & Littlewood J. (2011). The implementation of standards of care in Europe: state of the art. *J Cyst Fibros.* Vol. 10, Suppl. 2, pp 7-15.

Comeau A., Accurso F., White T. *et al.* (2007). Guidelines for implementation of cystic fibrosis newborn screening programs: Cystic Fibrosis Foundation workshop report. *Pediatrics.* Vol. 119, No 2, pp e495-518.

Conway S. (2008). Segregation is good for patients with cystic fibrosis. *J R Soc Med.* Vol. 101, Suppl. 1, pp 31-35.

Corey M., Mc Laughlin F, Williams M. *et al.* A comparison of survival, growth, and pulmonary function in patients with cystic fibrosis in Boston and Toronto. *J Clin Epidemiol.* Vol. 41, No 6, pp 583-591.

Courtney J., Dunbar K, Mc Dowell A. *et al.* (2004). Clinical outcome of Burkholderia cepacia complex infection in cystic fibrosis adults. *J Cyst Fibros.* Vol. 3, No 2, pp 93-98.

Crozier D. (1974). Cystic fibrosis: a not-so-fatal disease. *Pediatr Clin North Am.* Vol. 21, No 4, pp 935-950.

Cutting G. (2010). Modifier genes in Mendelian disorders: the example of cystic fibrosis. *Ann N Y Acad Sci.* No. 1214, pp 57-69.

Dakin C., Numa A, Wang H. *et al.* (2002). Inflammation, infection, and pulmonary function in infants and young children with cystic fibrosis. *Am J Respir Crit Care Med.* Vol. 165, no 7, pp 904-910.

Darrah R., Mc Kone E., O'Connor C. *et al.* (2010). EDNRA variants associate with smooth muscle mRNA levels, cell proliferation rates, and cystic fibrosis pulmonary disease severity. *Physiol Genomics.* Vol. 41, No 1, pp 71-77.

Dasenbrook E., Merlo C., Diener-West *et al.* (2008). Persistent methicillin-resistant Staphylococcus aureus and rate of FEV1 decline in cystic fibrosis. *Am J Respir Crit Care Med.* Vol. 178, No 8, pp 814-821.

David T. (2001). Elusiveness of cystic-fibrosis treatment. *Lancet.* Vol. 357, p 633.

Davis P. (2006). Cystic fibrosis since 1938. *Am J Respir Crit Care Med.* Vol. 173, No 5, pp 475-482.

Davis S., Brody A., Emond M. *et al.* (2007). Endpoints for clinical trials in young children with cystic fibrosis. *Proc Am Thorac Soc.* Vol 4, No 4, pp 418-430.

de Almeida M., Bussamra M. & Rodrigues J. (2006). Allergic bronchopulmonary aspergillosis in paediatric cystic fibrosis patients. *Paediatr Respir Rev.* Vol. 7, No 1, pp 67-72.

De Boeck K., Vermeulen F., Wanyama S. *et al.* (2011). Inhaled corticosteroids and lower lung function decline in young children with cystic fibrosis. *Eur Respir J.* Vol. 37, No 5, pp 1091-1095.

de Boer K., Vandemheen K., Tullis E. *et al.* (2011). Exacerbation frequency and clinical outcomes in adult patients with cystic fibrosis. *Thorax* Vol. 66, No 8, pp 680-685.

Dodge J., Lewis P., Stanton M *et al.* (2007). Cystic fibrosis mortality and survival in the UK: 1947-2003. *Eur Respir J.* Vol. 29, No 3, pp 522-526.

Döring G., Conway S., Heijerman H. *et al.* (2000). Antibiotic therapy against Pseudomonas aeruginosa in cystic fibrosis: a European consensus. *Eur Respir J.* Vol. 16, No 4, pp 749-767.

Döring G., Hoiby N & Consensus study group. (2004). Early intervention and prevention of lung disease in cystic fibrosis: a European consensus. *J Cyst Fibros.* Vol. 3, no 2, pp 67-91.

Douglas T., Brennan S., Gard S. *et al.* (2009). Acquisition and eradication of P. aeruginosa in young children with cystic fibrosis. *Eur Respir J.* Vol. 33, no 2, pp 305-311.

Driever, M. (2002). Are evidenced-based practice and best practice the same? *West J Nurs Res.* Vol. 24, No 5, pp 591-597.

Drumm M., Konstan M., Schluchter M. *et al.* (2005). Genetic modifiers of lung disease in cystic fibrosis. N Engl J Med. Vol. 353, No 14, pp 1443-1453.

Duguépéroux I. & De Braekeleer M. (2005). The CFTR 3849+10kbC->T and 2789+5G->A alleles are associated with a mild CF phenotype. *Eur Respir J.* Vol. 25, No 3, pp 468-473.

Eakin M., Bilderback A., Boyle M. *et al.* (2011). Longitudinal association between medication adherence and lung health in people with cystic fibrosis. *J Cyst Fibros.* Vol. 10, No 4, pp 258-64. ISSN 1569-1993

Edenborough F., Borgo G., Knoop C. eta l. (2008). Guidelines for the management of pregnancy in women with cystic fibrosis. *J Cyst Fibros.* Vol. 7, Suppl. 1, pp 2-32.

Elborn J., Shale D. & Britton J. (1991). Cystic fibrosis: current survival and population estimates to the year 2000. *Thorax* Vol. 46, No 12, pp 881-885.

Emerson J., Rosenfeld M., McNamara S. *et al.* (2002). Pseudomonas aeruginosa and other predictors of mortality and morbidity in young children with cystic fibrosis. *Pediatr Pulmonol.* Vol. 34, No 2, pp 91-100.

Farrell P., Li Z., Kosorok M *et al.* (2003). Bronchopulmonary disease in children with cystic fibrosis after early or delayed diagnosis. *Am J Respir Crit Care Med.* Vol. 168, No 9, pp 1100-1108.

Farrell P., Rosenstein B., White T. *et al.* (2008). Guidelines for diagnosis of cystic fibrosis in newborns through older adults: Cystic Fibrosis Foundation consensus report. *J Pediatr.* Vol. 153, No 2, pp 4-14.

Ferris T. & Torchiana D. Public release of clinical outcomes data – Online CABG report cards. *N Engl J Med* 363: 1593-5.

Flume P., Mogayzel P., Robinson K. *et al.* (2010). Cystic fibrosis pulmonary guidelines: pulmonary complications: hemoptysis and pneumothorax. *Am J Respir Crit Care Med.* Vol. 182, No 3, pp 298-306.

Frederiksen B., Koch C. & Hoiby N. (1997). Antibiotic treatment at time of initial colonisation with Pseudomonas aeruginosa postpones chronic infection and prevents deterioration in pulmonary function in patients with cystic fibrosis. *Pediatr Pulmonol.* Vol. 23, No 5, pp 330–335.

Frederiksen B., Koch C. & Hoiby N. (1999) Changing epidemiology of Pseudomonas aeruginosa infection in Danish cystic fibrosis patients (1974-1995). *Pediatr Pulmonol.* Vol. 28, No 3, pp 159-166.

Gan K., Veeze H., van den Ouweland *et al.* (1995). A cystic fibrosis mutation associated with mild lung disease. *N Engl J Med.* Vol. 333, No 2, pp 95-99.

Gao Z., Wood-Baker R., Harle R. *et al.* (2010). "Bong lung" in cystic fibrosis: a case report. *J Med Case Reports.* Vol. 4, p 371.

Gibson R., Burns J. & Ramsey B. (2003). Pathophysiology and management of pulmonary infections in cystic fibrosis. *Am J Respir Crit Care Med.* Vol. 168, No 8, pp 918-951.

Goss C., Newsom S., Schildcrout J. *et al.* (2004). Effect of ambient air pollution on pulmonary exacerbations and lung function in cystic fibrosis. *Am J Respir Crit Care Med.* Vol. 169, No 7, pp 816-821.

Han B., Gfroerer J. & Colliver J. (2010). Associations between duration of illicit drug use and health conditions: results from the 2005-2007 national surveys on drug use and health. *Ann Epidemiol.* Vol. 20, No 4, pp 289-297.

Hankinson J., Odencrantz J., Fedan K. (1999). Spirometric reference values from a sample of the general U.S. population. *Am J Respir Crit Care Med.* Vol. 159, No 1, pp 79–87.

Hansen C., Pressler T., Koch C. *et al.* (2005). Long-term azitromycin treatment of cystic fibrosis patients with chronic Pseudomonas aeruginosa infection; an observational cohort study. *J Cyst Fibros.* Vol. 4, No 1, pp 35-40.

Heinzl B., Eber E, Oberwaldner B. *et al.* (2002). Effects of inhaled gentamicin prophylaxis on acquisition of Pseudomonas aeruginosa in children with cystic fibrosis: a pilot study. *Pediatr Pulmonol.* Vol. 33, No 1, pp 32-37.

Highsmith W., Burch L, Zhou Z. *et al.* (1994). A novel mutation in the cystic fibrosis gene in patients with pulmonary disease but normal sweat chloride concentrations. *N Engl J Med.* Vol. 331, No 15, pp 974-980.

Hill D., Martin A., Davidson G. *et al.* (1985). Survival of cystic fibrosis patients in South Australia. Evidence that cystic fibrosis centre care leads to better survival. *Med J Aust.* Vol. 143, No 6, pp 230-232.

Hilliard T., Sukhani S. Francis J. *et al.* (2007). Bronchoscopy following diagnosis with cystic fibrosis. *Arch Dis Child.* Vol. 92, No 10, pp 898-899.

Høiby N., Frederiksen B. & Pressler T. (2005). Eradication of early Pseudomonas aeruginosa infection. *J Cyst Fibros.* Vol. 4, Suppl. 2, pp 49-54.

Isles, A., McLusky I., Corey M. *et al.* (1984). Pseudomonas cepacia infection in cystic fibrosis: an emerging problem. *J Pediatr.* Vol. 104, No 2, pp 206-210.

Jackson A., Daly L., Kelleher C. *et al.* (2011). Validation and use of a parametric model for projecting cystic fibrosis survivorship beyond observed data: a birth cohort analysis. *Thorax.* Vol. 66, No 8, pp 674-679.

Johansen H., Nir M., Hoiby N. *et al.* (1991). Severity of cystic fibrosis in patients homozygous and heterozygous for delta F508 mutation. *Lancet.* Vol. 337, pp 631-634.

Johnson C., Butler S., Konstan M. *et al.* (2003). Factors influencing outcomes in cystic fibrosis: a center-based analysis. *Chest.* Vol. 123, No 1, pp 20-27.

Kalish L., Waltz D., Dovey M. *et al.* (2006). Impact of Burkholderia dolosa on lung function and survival in cystic fibrosis. *Am J Respir Crit Care Med.* Vol. 173, No 4, pp 421-425.

Kerem E., Corey M., Gold R. *et al.* (1990). Pulmonary function and clinical course in patients with cystic fibrosis after pulmonary colonization with Pseudomonas aeruginosa. *J Pediatr.* Vol. 116, No 5, pp 714-719.

Kerem E., Corey M., Kerem B. *et al.* (1990). The relation between genotype and phenotype in cystic fibrosis--analysis of the most common mutation (delta F508). *N Engl J Med.* Vol. 323, No 22, pp 1517-1522.

Kerem E., resiman J., Corey M. *et al.* (1992). Prediction of mortality in patients with cystic fibrosis. *N Engl J Med*. Vol. 326, No 18, pp 1187-1191.

Kerem E., Conway S., Elborn S. *et al.* (2005). Consensus Committee. Standards of care for patients with cystic fibrosis: a European consensus. *J Cyst Fibros*. Vol. 4, No 1, pp 7-26.

Khan T., Wagener J., Bost T. *et al.* (1995). Early pulmonary inflammation in infants with cystic fibrosis. *Am J Respir Crit Care Med*. Vol. 151, No 4, pp 1075-1082.

Koch C., Cuppens H., Rainisio M. *et al.* (2001). European Epidemiologic Registry of Cystic Fibrosis (ERCF): comparison of major disease manifestations between patients with different classes of mutations. *Pediatr Pulmonol*. Vol. 31, No 1, pp 1-12.

Koch C. (2002). Early infection and progression of cystic fibrosis lung disease. *Pediatr Pulmonol*. Vol. 34, No 3, pp 232-236.

Konstan M., Byard P. Hoppel C. *et al.* (1995). Effect of high-dose ibuprofen in patients with cystic fibrosis. *N Engl J Med*. Vol. 332, No 13, pp 848-854.

Konstan M., Butler S., Whol M. *et al.* (2003). Growth and nutritional indexes in early life predict pulmonary function in cystic fibrosis. *J Pediatr*. Vol. 142, No 6, pp 624 –630.

Konstan M., Scluchter M., Xue W. *et al.* (2007). Clinical use of Ibuprofen is associated with slower FEV1 decline in children with cystic fibrosis. *Am J Respir Crit Care Med*. Vol. 176, No 11, pp 1084-1089.

Konstan M., Morgan W., Butler S. *et al.* (2007). Risk factors for rate of decline in forced expiratory volume in one second in children and adolescents with cystic fibrosis. *J Pediatr*. Vol. 151, No 2, pp 134-139.

Konstan M., VanDevanter D., Rasouliyan L. *Et al.* (2010). Trends in the use of routine therapies in cystic fibrosis: 1995-2005. *Pediatr Pulmonol*. Vol. 45, No 12, pp 1167-1172.

Konstan M., Wagener J., Pasta D. *et al.* (2011). Clinical use of dornase alpha is associated with a slower rate of FEV1 decline in cystic fibrosis. *Pediatr Pulmonol*. Vol. 46, No 6, pp 545-553.

Kosorok M., Zeng L, West S. *et al.* (2001). Acceleration of lung disease in children with cystic fibrosis after Pseudomonas aeruginosa acquisition. *Pediatr Pulmonol*. Vol. 32, No 4, pp 277-287.

Kraemer R., Rüdeberg A., Hadorn B. *et al.* (1978). Relative underweight in cystic fibrosis and its prognostic value. *Acta Paediatr Scand*. Vol. 67, No 1, pp 33-37.

Kraemer R., Deloséa N., Ballinari P. *et al.* (2006). Effect of allergic bronchopulmonary aspergillosis on lung function in children with cystic fibrosis. *Am J Respir Crit Care Med*. Vol. 174, No 11, pp 1211-1220.

Kraynack N. & McBride J. (2009). Improving care at cystic fibrosis centers through quality improvement. *Semin Respir Crit Care Med*. Vol. 30, No 5, pp 547-558.

Kraynack N., Gothard M., Falletta L. *et al.* (2011). Approach to treating cystic fibrosis pulmonary exacerbations varies widely across us CF care centers. *Pediatr Pulmonol*. Apr 4. doi: 10.1002/ppul.21442. [Epub ahead of print]

Lai H. & Shoff S. (2008). Classification of malnutrition in cystic fibrosis: implications for evaluating and benchmarking clinical practice performance. *Am J Clin Nutr*. Vol. 88, No 1, pp 161-166.

Laniado-Laborin R (2010). Smoking cessation intervention: an evidence-based approach. *Postgrad Med*. Vol. 122, No 2, pp 74-82.

Lask B. (1994). Non-adherence to treatment in cystic fibrosis. *J R Soc Med*. Vol. 87, Suppl. 21, pp 25-27.

Lau E., Morarty C., Ogle R. *Et al.* (2010). Pregnancy and cystic fibrosis. *Paediatr Respir Rev*. Vol. 11, No 2, pp 90-94.

Leal T., Reychler G., Mailleux P. *et al.* (2007). A specific database for providing local and national level of integration of clinical data in cystic fibrosis. *J Cyst Fibros*. Vol. 6, No 3, pp 187-193.

Lebecque P., Leal T., Zylberberg K. *et al.* (2006). Towards zero prevalence of chronic Pseudomonas aeruginosa infection in children with cystic fibrosis. *J Cyst Fibros*. Vol. 5, No 4, pp 237-244.

Lebecque P., Leonard A., De Boeck K. *et al.* (2009). Early referral to cystic fibrosis specialist centre impacts on respiratory outcome. *J Cyst Fibros*. Vol. 8, No 1, pp 26-30.

Lebecque P, De Boeck K., Wanyama S. *et al.* (2010). CF Registries – plea for annual reports focusing on patients homozygous for the F508del mutation. *J Cyst Fibros*. Vol. 9, Suppl. 1, p 114 (A).

Ledson M., Gallagher M., Jackson M. *et al.* (2002). Outcome of Burkholderia cepacia colonisation in an adult cystic fibrosis centre. *Thorax*. Vol. 57, No 2, pp 142-145.

Lee T., Brownlee K., Conway S. *et al.* (2003). Evaluation of a new definition for chronic Pseudomonas aeruginosa infection in cystic fibrosis patients. *J Cyst Fibros*. Vol. 2, No 1, pp 29-34.

Lee T., Brownlee K., Denton M. *et al.* (2004). Reduction in prevalence of chronic Pseudomonas aeruginosa infection at a regional pediatric cystic fibrosis center. *Pediatr Pulmonol*. Vol. 37, No 2, pp 104-110.

Levy L., Durie P., Pencharz P. *et al.* (1986). Prognostic factors associated with patient survival during nutritional rehabilitation in malnourished children and adolescents with cystic fibrosis. *J Pediatr Gastroenterol Nutr* Vol. 5, No 1, pp 97–102.

Li Z., Kosorok M., Farrell P. *et al.* (2005). Longitudinal development of mucoid Pseudomonas aeruginosa infection and lung disease progression in children with cystic fibrosis. *JAMA*. Vol. 293, No 5, pp 581-588.

Liou T., Adler F., Fitzsimmons S. *et al.* (2001). Predictive 5-year survivorship model of cystic fibrosis. *Am J Epidemiol*. Vol. 153, No 4, pp 345-352.

Littlewood J., Miller M., Ghoneim A. *et al.* (1985). Nebulised colomycin for early pseudomonas colonisation in cystic fibrosis. *Lancet*. Vol. 1, p 865.

Littlewood J. (2000). Good care for people with cystic fibrosis. *Paediatr Respir Rev*. Vol. 1, No 2, pp 179-189.

Littlewood J. (2005). European cystic fibrosis society consensus on standards – a roadmap to "best care". *J Cyst Fibros*. Vol. 4, No 1, pp 1-5.

Mahadeva R., Webb K., Westerbeek R. *et al.* (1998). Clinical outcome in relation to care in centres specialising in cystic fibrosis: cross sectional study. *BMJ* Vol. 316, pp 1771-1775.

Matthews W., Williams M, Oliphint B. *et al.* (1980). Hypogammaglobulinemia in Patients with Cystic Fibrosis. *N Engl J Med*. Vol. 302, No 5, pp 245-249

McKone E., Goss C. & Aitken M. (2006). CFTR genotype as a predictor of prognosis in cystic fibrosis. *Chest*. Vol. 130, No 5, pp 1441-1447.

Mehta G., Macek M., Mehta A. *et al.* (2010). Cystic fibrosis across Europe: EuroCareCF analysis of demographic data from 35 countries. *J Cyst Fibros.* Vol. 9, Suppl. 2, pp 5-21.

Mérelle M., Schouten J, Gerritsen J. *et al.* (2001). Influence of neonatal screening and centralized treatment on long-term clinical outcome and survival of CF patients. *Eur Respir J.* Vol. 18, No 2, pp 306-315.

Miles A., Louglin M. & Polychronis A. (2008). Evidence-based healthcare, clinical knowledge and the rise of personalised medicine. *J Eval Clin Pract.* Vol. 14, No 5, pp 621-649.

Miles A. & Loughlin M. (2011). Models in the balance: evidence-based medicine versus evidence-informed individualized care. *J Eval Clin Pract.* Vol. 17, No 4, pp 531-536.

Milla C., Warwick W. & Moran A. (2000). Trends in pulmonary function in patients with cystic fibrosis correlate with the degree of glucose intolerance at baseline. *Am J Respir Crit Care Med.* Vol. 162, No 3 Pt 1, pp 891-895.

Milla C. (2004). Association of nutritional status and pulmonary function in children with cystic fibrosis. *Curr Opin Pulm Med* Vol. 10, No 6, pp 505–509.

Modi A., Lim C., Yu N. *et al.* (2006). A multi-method assessment of treatment adherence for children with cystic fibrosis. *J Cyst Fibros.* Vol 5, No 3, pp 177-185.

Moran A., Dunitz J. & Nathan B. *et al.* 2009. Cystic fibrosis–related diabetes: current trends in prevalence, incidence, and mortality. *Diabetes Care.* Vol. 32, No 9, pp 1626–1631

Moran A., Becker D., Casella S. *et al.* (2010). Epidemiology, pathophysiology, and prognostic implications of cystic fibrosis-related diabetes: a technical review. *Diabetes Care.* Vol. 33, No 12, pp 2677-2683.

Mott L., Gangell C., Murray C. *et al.* (2009). Bronchiectasis in an asymptomatic infant with cystic fibrosis diagnosed following newborn screening. *J Cyst Fibros.* Vol. 8, No 4, pp 285-287.

Mussaffi H., Prais D., Mei-Zahav M. *et al.* (2006). Cystic fibrosis mutations with widely variable phenotype: the D1152H example. *Pediatr Pulmonol.* Vol. 41, No 3, pp 250-254.

Nick J., Chacon C., Brayshaw S. *et al.* (2010). Effects of gender and age at diagnosis on disease progression in long-term survivors of cystic fibrosis. *Am J Respir Crit Care Med.* Vol. 182, No 5, pp 614-626.

Nielsen O., Thomsen B., Green A. *et al.* (1988). Cystic fibrosis in Denmark 1945 to 1985. An analysis of incidence, mortality and influence of centralized treatment on survival. *Acta Paediatr Scand.* Vol. 77, No 6, pp 836-841.

O'Connor G., Quinton H., Kneeland T. *et al.* (2003). Median household income and mortality rate in cystic fibrosis. *Pediatrics.* Vol. 111, No 4 Pt 1, pp e333-339.

Olesen H., Pressler T., Hjelte L. *et al.* (2010). Gender differences in the Scandinavian cystic fibrosis population. *Pediatr Pulmonol.* Vol. 45, No 10, pp 959-965.

Padman R., McColley S., Miller D. *et al.* (2007). Infant care patterns at epidemiologic study of cystic fibrosis sites that achieve superior childhood lung function. *Pediatrics.* Vol. 119, no 3, pp e531-537.

Padman R., Werk L., Ramirez-Garnica G. *et al.* (2008). Association between practice patterns and body mass index percentile in infants and young children with cystic fibrosis. *J Cyst Fibros.* Vol. 7, No 5, pp 385-390.

Pamukcu A., Bush A. & Buchdahl R. (1995). Effects of pseudomonas aeruginosa colonization on lung function and anthropometric variables in children with cystic fibrosis. *Pediatr Pulmonol.* Vol. 19, No 1, pp 10-15.

Pedreira C., Robert R., Dalton V. *et al.* (2005). Association of body composition and lung function in children with cystic fibrosis. *Pediatr Pulmonol.* Vol. 39, no 3, pp 276-280.

Pendleton D. The compliance conundrum in cystic fibrosis. *J R Soc Med.* Vol. 93, Suppl. 38, pp 9-13.

Prober C., Walson P. & Jones J. (2000). Technical report: precautions regarding the use of aerosolized antibiotics. Committee on Infectious Diseases and Committee on Drugs. *Pediatrics.* Vol. 106, No 6, p E89.

Proesmans M., Els C., Vermeulen F. *et al.* (2011). Change in IgG and evolution of lung function in children with cystic fibrosis. *J Cyst Fibros.* Vol. 10, No 2, pp 128-131.

Que C., Cullinan P. & Geddes D. (2006). Improving rate of decline of FEV1 in young adults with cystic fibrosis. *Thorax.* Vol. 61, No 2, pp 155-157.

Quinton, H. (2004). Using data to identify opportunities for change and to monitor progress. *Pediatr Pulmonol.* Vol. 38, Suppl. 27, pp 124-125.

Quinton H. & O'Connor G. (2007). Current issues in quality improvement in cystic fibrosis. *Clin Chest Med.* Vol. 28, No 2,pp 459-472.

Quittner A., Schechter M, Rasouliyan L. *et al.* (2010). Impact of socioeconomic status, race, and ethnicity on quality of life in patients with cystic fibrosis in the United States. *Chest.* Vol. 137, No 3, pp 642-650.

Quon B. & Goss C. (2011). A story of success: continuous quality improvement in cystic fibrosis care in the USA. *Thorax.* Aug 3. [Epub ahead of print]

Ranganathan S., Dezateux C., Bush A. *et al.* (2001). Airway function in infants newly diagnosed with cystic fibrosis. *Lancet.* Vol. 358, pp 1964-1965.

Ring E., Eber E., Erwa W. *et al.* (1998). Uinary N-acetyl-beta-D-glucosaminidase activity in patients with cystic fibrosis on long-term gentamicin inhalation. *Arch Dis Child.* Vol. 78, No 6, pp 540-543.

Rogan M. & Stoltz D. (2011). Cystic fibrosis transmembrane conductance regulator intracellular processing, trafficking, and opportunities for mutation-specific treatment. *Chest* Vol. 139, No 6, pp 1480-1490.

Rosenbluth D., Wilson K., Ferkol T. *et al.* (2004). Lung function decline in cystic fibrosis patients and timing for lung transplantation referral. *Chest* Vol. 126, No 2, pp 412-419.

Rosenfeld M., Davis R., Fitzsimmons S. *et al.* (1997). Gender gap in cystic fibrosis mortality. *Am J Epidemiol.* Vol. 145, no 9, pp 794-803.

Rosenfeld M., Emerson J., Mc Namara S. *et al.* (2010). Baseline characteristics and factors associated with nutritional and pulmonary status at enrollment in the cystic fibrosis EPIC observational cohort. *Pediatr Pulmonol.* Vol. 45, No 9, pp 934-944.

Saarni S. & Gylling H. (2004). Evidence based medicine guidelines: a solution to rationing or politics disguised as science? *J Med Ethics.* Vol. 30, No 2, pp 171-175.

Saiman L. & Siegel J. (2003). Infection control recommendations for patients with cystic fibrosis: Microbiology, important pathogens, and infection control practices to prevent patient-to-patient transmission. *Am J Infect Control.* Vol. 31, Suppl. 3, pp 1-62.

Sawicki G., Sellers D. & Robinson W. (2009). High treatment burden in adults with cystic fibrosis: challenges to disease self-management. *J Cyst Fibros.* Vol. 8, No 2, pp 91-96.

Schechter M., Shelton B., Margolis P. *et al.* (2001). The association of socioeconomic status with outcomes in cystic fibrosis patients in the United States. *Am J Respir Crit Care Med.* Vol. 163, No 6, pp 1331-1337

Schechter M. (2002). Demographic and center-related characteristics associated with low weight in pediatric CF patients. *Pediatr Pulmonol.* Vol. 34, Suppl. 24, p 331 (A)

Schechter, M. (2004). Key strategies for improving care. *Pediatr Pulmonol.* Vol. 38, Suppl. 27, pp 120-121.

Schechter M. & Margolis P. (2005). Improving subspecialty healthcare: lessons from cystic fibrosis. *J Pediatr.* Vol. 147, No 3, pp 295-301.

Schechter M. & Guttierez H. (2010). Improving the quality of care for patients with cystic fibrosis. *Curr Opin Pediatr.* Vol. 22, No 3, pp 296-301.

Schluchter M., Konstan M., Davis P. (2002). Jointly modelling the relationship between survival and pulmonary function in cystic fibrosis patients. *Stat Med.* Vol. 21, No 9, pp 1271-1287.

Segal, T. (2008). Adolescence: what the cystic fibrosis team needs to know. *J R Soc Med.* Vol. 101, Suppl 1, pp 15-27.

Sermet-Gaudelus I., Mayell S., Southern K. *et al.* (2010). Guidelines on the early management of infants diagnosed with cystic fibrosis following newborn screening. *J Cyst Fibros.* Vol. 9, No 5, pp 323-329.

Shahar E. (2008). Does anyone know the road from a randomized trial to personalized medicine? A review of 'Treating Individuals. From Randomized Trials to Personalised Medicine' *J Eval Clin Pract.* Vol. 14, No 5, pp 726-731.

Sims E., McCormick J., Mehta G. *et al.* (2005). Neonatal screening for cystic fibrosis is beneficial even in the context of modern treatment. *J Pediatr.* Vol. 147, Suppl. 3, pp 42-46.

Sims E., Clark A., McCormick J. *et al.* (2007). Cystic fibrosis diagnosed after 2 months of age leads to worse outcomes and requires more therapy. *Pediatrics.* Vol. 119, No 1, pp 19-28.

Sinaasappel M., Stern M., Littlewood J. *et al.* (2002). Nutrition in patients with cystic fibrosis: a European Consensus. *J Cyst Fibros.* Vol. 1, No 2, pp 51-75.

Siret D., Bretaudeau G., Branger B. *et al.* (2003). Comparing the clinical evolution of cystic fibrosis screened neonatally to that of cystic fibrosis diagnosed from clinical symptoms: a 10-year retrospective study in a French region (Brittany). *Pediatr Pulmonol.* Vol. 35, No 5, pp 342-349.

Sly P., Brennan S., Gangell C. *et al.* (2009). Lung disease at diagnosis in infants with cystic fibrosis detected by newborn screening. *Am J Respir Crit Care Med.* Vol. 180, No 2, pp 146-152.

Smyth A., O'Hea U., Williams G. *et al.* Passive smoking and impaired lung function in cystic fibrosis. *Arch Dis Child.* Vol. 71, No 4, pp 353-354.

Stafler P., Davies J., Balfour-Lynn I. *et al.* (2011). Bronchoscopy in cystic fibrosis infants diagnosed by newborn screening. *Pediatr Pulmonol.* Vol. 46, No 7, pp 696-700.

Stallings V., Stark L, Robinson K. *et al.* (2008). Evidence-based practice recommendations for nutrition-related management of children and adults with cystic fibrosis and pancreatic insufficiency: results of a systematic review. *J Am Diet Assoc*. Vol. 108, No 5, pp 832-839.

Steinkamp G. & Wiedemann B. (2002). Relationship between nutritional status and lung function in cystic fibrosis: cross sectional and longitudinal analyses from the German CF quality assurance (CFQA) project. *Thorax*. Vol. 57, No 7, pp 596-601.

Stern R., Byard P., Tomashefski J. *et al.* (1987). Recreational use of psychoactive drugs by patients with cystic fibrosis. J Pediatr. Vol. 111, no 2, pp 293-299.

Stern M., Wiedemann B., Wenzlaff P. *et al.* (2008). From registry to quality management: the German Cystic Fibrosis Quality Assessment project 1995 2006. *Eur Respir* J. Vol. 31, No 1, pp 29-35.

Stern M., Niemann M., Wiedemann B. *et al.* (2011). Benchmarking improves quality in cystic fibrosis care: a pilot project involving 12 centres. *Int J Qual Health Care*. Vol. 23, No 3, pp 349-356.

Stevens D., Moss R., Kurup V. *et al.* (2003). Allergic bronchopulmonary aspergillosis in cystic fibrosis--state of the art: Cystic Fibrosis Foundation Consensus Conference. *Clin Infect Dis*. Vol. 37, Suppl. 3, pp 225-264.

Stick S., Brennan S., Murray C. *et al.* (2009). Bronchiectasis in infants and preschool children diagnosed with cystic fibrosis after newborn screening. *J Pediatr*. Vol. 155, No 5, pp 623-628.e1

Stuart B., Lin J. & Mogayzel P. (2010). Early eradication of Pseudomonas aeruginosa in patients with cystic fibrosis. *Paediatr Respir Rev*. Vol. 11, No 3, pp 177-184.

Taccetti G., Festini F., Campana S. *et al.* (2004). Neonatal screening for cystic fibrosis and Pseudomonas aeruginosa acquisition. *J Pediatr*. Vol. 145, No 3, p 421.

Tetrault J., Krothers K., Moore B. *et al.* (2007). Effects of marijuana smoking on pulmonary function and respiratory complications: a systematic review. *Arch Intern Med*. Vol. 167, No 3, pp 221-228.

Thauvin-Robinet C., Munck A., Huet F. *et al.* (2009). The very low penetrance of cystic fibrosis for the R117H mutation: a reappraisal for genetic counselling and newborn screening. *J Med Genet*. Vol. 46, No 11, pp 752-758.

Thia L. & Balfour-Lynn I. (2009). Diagnosing allergic bronchopulmonary aspergillosis in children with cystic fibrosis. *Paediatr Respir Rev*. Vol. 10, No 1, pp 37-42.

Tiddens H. (2009). Quality improvement in your CF centre: taking care of care. *J Cyst Fibros*. Vol. 8, Suppl. 1, pp 2-5.

UK CF Registry (2008), Available from http://www.cftrust.org.uk/aboutcf/publications/cfregistryreports/

Treacy K., Elborn S., Rendall J. *et al.* (2008). Copying letters to patients with cystic fibrosis (CF): letter content and patient perceptions of benefit. *J Cyst Fibros*. Vol. 7, No 6, pp 511-514.

van Koolwijk L., Uiterwaal C., van der Laag J. *et al.* (2002). Treatment of children with cystic fibrosis: central, local or both? *Acta Paediatr*. Vol. 91, No 9, pp 972-977.

Valerius N., Koch C. & Høiby N. (1991). Prevention of chronic Pseudomonas aeruginosa colonisation in cystic fibrosis by early treatment. *Lancet*. Vol. 338, pp 725-726.

van der Ent C. (2008). Quality assessment: is the truth in the outcome? *Eur Respir J*. Vol. 31, No 1, pp 6-7.

Verma A., Dodd M., Haworth C. *et al.* (2000). Holidays and cystic fibrosis. *J R Soc. Med*. Vol. 93, Suppl. 38, pp 20-26.

Verma N., Bush A. & Buchdahl R. (2005). Is there still a gender gap in cystic fibrosis? *Chest.* Vol. 128, no 4, pp 2824-2834.

Wainwright C., Vidmar S., Armstrong D. *et al.* (2011). Effect of bronchoalveolar lavage-directed therapy on Pseudomonas aeruginosa infection and structural lung injury in children with cystic fibrosis: a randomized trial. *JAMA.* Vol. 306, No 2, pp 163-171.

Walters S., Britton J. & Hodson M. (1994). Hospital care for adults with cystic fibrosis: an overview and comparison between special cystic fibrosis clinics and general clinics using a patient questionnaire. *Thorax* Vol. 49, No 4, pp 300-306.

Wallwork J., Brenchley P, Mc Carthy J. *et al.* (1974). Some aspects of immunity in patients with cystic fibrosis. *Clin Exp Immunol.* Vol. 18, No 3, pp 303-320.

Wang X., Dockery D., Wypij D. *et al.* (1993). Pulmonary function between 6 and 18 years of age. *Pediatr Pulmonol* Vol. 15, No 2, pp 75-88.

Welsh M. & Smyth A. (1993). Molecular mechanisms of CFTR chloride channel dysfunction in CF. *Cell.* Vol. 73, No 7, pp 1251-1254.

West S., Zeng L., Lee B. *et al.* (2002). Respiratory infections with Pseudomonas aeruginosa in children with cystic fibrosis: early detection by serology and assessment of risk factors. *JAMA.* Vol. 287, No 22, pp 2958-2967.

Wheeler W., Williams M., Matthews W. *et al.* (1984). Progression of cystic fibrosis lung disease as a function of serum immunoglobulin G levels: a 5-year longitudinal study. *J Pediatr.* Vol. 104, no 5, pp 695-699.

Wolfenden L., Schechter M. (2009). Genetic and non-genetic determinants of outcomes in cystic fibrosis. *Paediatr Respir Rev.* Vol. 10, No 1, pp 32-36.

Wright F., Strug L, Doshi V. *et al.* (2011). Genome-wide association and linkage identify modifier loci of lung disease severity in cystic fibrosis at 11p13 and 20q13.2. *Nat Genet.* Vol. 43, No 6, pp 539-546.

Yankaskas J., Marshall B, Ebeling M. *et al.* (2004). Cystic fibrosis adult care: consensus conference report. *Chest.* Vol. 125, Suppl. 1, pp 1-39.

Zahariadis G., Lewy M. & Burns J. (2003). Cepacia-like syndrome caused by Burkholderia multivorans. *Can J Infect Dis.* Vol. 14, No 2, pp 123-125.

Zemanick E., Harris J., Conway S. *et al.* (2010). Measuring and improving respiratory outcomes in cystic fibrosis lung disease: opportunities and challenges to therapy. *J Cyst Fibros.* Vol. 9, No 1, pp 1-16.

Zemel B., Jawad A., Fitzsimmons S. *et al.* (2000). Longitudinal relationship among growth, nutritional status, and pulmonary function in children with cystic fibrosis: analysis of the Cystic Fibrosis Foundation National CF Patient Registry. *J Pediatr.* Vol. 137, no 3, pp 374-380.

Zlosnik J., Costa P., Brant R. *et al.* (2011). Mucoid and Nonmucoid Burkholderia cepacia Complex Bacteria in Cystic Fibrosis Infections. *Am J Respir Crit Care Med.* Vol. 183, No 1, pp 67-72.

Zolin A. (2010). Differences in disease severity of F508del homozygotes across European countries. *J Cyst Fibros.* Vol. 9, Suppl. 1, p 110 (A)

2

Cystic Fibrosis and Infertility

Maria do Carmo Pimentel Batitucci,
Angela Maria Spagnol Perrone and Giselle Villa Flor Brunoro
Federal University of Espírito Santo
Brazil

1. Introduction

Cystic fibrosis (CF) – or mucoviscidosis – is a common autosomal recessive inherited disease, affecting the whole body and causing progressive deficiencies. The name 'cystic fibrosis' refers to the characteristic scarring (fibrosis) and formation of cysts in the pancreas. The first anatomical and pathological description of the disorder was done by Landsteiner in 1905. In 1936, Fanconi et al. identified it as an autonomous illness, and in 1994 Farber et al. named it mucoviscidosis, due to the thick and viscous mucus secreted by the exocrine glands. It is accounted for by several clinical manifestations. Respiratory impairment is the most serious symptom (resulting from chronic infection in the lungs) and, though it is treatable, it is resistant to antibiotics and other medication. The large number of other symptoms include sinusitis, inadequate growth, diarrhoea and infertility, each of which is an effect of CF in other parts of the body. The mutated gene is transmitted by father and mother – although it may be that neither of them manifest the disease – and it is accounted for by the change in carrying ions through the membranes of the cells (Quinton et al., 1983). This compromises the function of the exocrine glands that produce thicker and hard-eliminating substances (mucus, sweat or pancreatic enzymes).

In 1953, Di Sant'Agnase et al. noted an increased sodium chloride rate eliminated through the sweat of patients with CF. Gibson and Cooke (1958) standardised the sweat test, which has become an important tool in the diagnosis of the disease. In 1958, Shwachman and Kulczucki designed a disease-severity assessment system. In 1985, the position of the CFTR gene was determined on the long arm of chromosome 7, q31 band, by restriction fragment linked polymorphism (Knowlton et al., 1985), and, in 1989, the full-length gene was sequenced (Collins, 1992).

The clinical manifestations of CF are primarily due to the obstruction of the ducts of organs (such as the lung and the pancreas) by thick, viscous secretions, changes in electrolytic concentrations, and the presence of abnormal contents. The primary cellular defect consists of a decreased or else absent expression of the CF transmembrane conductance regulator (CFTR) protein, which causes changes in chloride secretion. This protein is present in all endodermal and mesodermal cells, and it has been found in sweat glands, organs of the digestive system, and the airways' epithelium layer (Bargon et al., 1999). The primary defect causes dehydration of the airways, leading to an increased viscosity of mucus in the intercellular environment, and it predisposes the body to chronic bacterial infections

(Tummler et al., 1999). At birth, the lung is histologically normal, and the pathophysiological changes evolve with aging (Shwachman et al., 1970). CF leads to pulmonary bronchiectasis and atelectasis, compromising the bronchi and bronchioles and so causing pulmonary emphysema. The pancreas is the organ that presents the largest functional and structural changes (Rozov et al., 1991). The blockage of glandular ducts leads to malnutrition syndrome, biliary liver cirrhosis, intestinal obstruction, and gastroesophageal reflux. In newborn infants, the presence of ileum-meconium can mark the first manifestation of CF (Feingold et al., 1999). Exocrine insufficiency of the pancreas occurs in 95% of cases (Mousia-Arvanitakis, 1999) and results in a decrease or the absence of lipolytic, proteolytic and amylolytic enzymes in the pancreatic juice, leading to chronic diarrhoea with bulky, greasy and fetid faeces. As a result, malnutrition becomes evident, owing to the loss of calories and proteins through poor digestion (Reis e Damasceno, 1998). The blockage can also affect the biliary ducts – the thick bile leads to difficulties of drainage, and there may be a full blockage of the ducts which may evolve into cirrhosis (Kopel, 1992).

Advances in genetic engineering and the development of transgenic animals during the last decade of the twentieth century, in conjunction with the prospect of early diagnosis, has contributed to the provision of proper and effective treatments that can increase the quality of life of patients with CF.

1.1 Incidence

The incidence of CF varies according to ethnicity, ranging from 1 CF individual per 2,000 to 5,000 Caucasian live births in Europe, the United States and Canada, 1 CF individual per 15,000 African Americans, and from 1 CF individual per 40,000 live births in Finland (Brunechy, 1972). In Brazil, the estimated incidence for the southern region is closer to that of Central Europe's Caucasian population, whereas for other regions it reduces to 1 per 10,000 live births. This is despite the fact that there are variations in the frequency of mutations in different geographic regions, which would probably reflect a different prevalence of the disease (Raskum et al., 1993). In the US and in European countries, early diagnosis – before the first year of life – allows affected children to be promptly treated and monitored with regard to the variables that directly influence the prognosis of the disease, such as the follow-up of the weight and height curve, and the presence of upper airway colonisation by pathogens (which is closely related to worse prognosis).

In Brazil, since 2001, and with the approval of the National Newborn Screening Program and its introduction by the laboratory of the Ecumenical Foundation for Exceptional Protection (FEPE-PR, Portuguese acronym), CF screening has been implemented in the State of Parana. Before the establishment of the National Newborn Screening Program for CF, the data showed that the average age receiving a diagnosis of the disease ranged at around 1.6 years (Santos et al., 2005).

1.2 Genetics

The isolation of the CFTR is a result of many years of study on the part of numerous research groups. Situated in long arm of the chromosome 7, at band q31.3 (Heng et al., 1993), with 250 Kb, the region codifier of the CFTR consists in 27 exons. Most of the exons are far from one another by between 50 and 250 base pairs, except for exon 13 which has 723 base pairs of the genomic DNA. The CFTR protein has a molecular weight of 168,138 Da and it belongs to a transmembrane chloride ion channel superfamily protein, with 1,480 amino acids (Harris, 1992) present in apical membranes of those cells lining the surface of the gland tubes and the airways.

About 1,500 mutations have already been identified in the CFTR: the most frequent mutation is F508del, which is found in 30% of patients with CF (Zielenski, 2000). This mutation is caused by the deletion of three base pairs corresponding to the codon that translates a residue phenylalanine at position 508 of the CFTR polypeptide chain (Morral, 1994). Depending on ethnic groups in different geographic locations the relative frequency of this mutation vary among individuals affected by CF. In Northern Europe and North America, it reaches 70-90%; however it is less frequent in Southern Europe, where less of 50% of the CF chromosomes have this mutation (Morral et al., 1994).

The G542X mutation is considered to be the second most frequent mutation, and it accounts for 3.4% of alleles in CF (Tsui, 1992). At a molecular level, it leads to a replacement of nucleotides, which results in a stop codon at position 542 of the polypeptide chain, and thus the translation product is a non-functional peptide that will be degraded. According to the geographic location, the frequency of this mutation varies among the CF individuals. It may be found in the compound heterozygous with the ΔF508 mutation. Raskin et al. (1993) have noted the frequency of the G542X mutation in 5% of the Brazilian population.

The G551D mutation affects 2.4% of the chromosomes of the population of individuals with CF – in general – and it leads to a replacement of guanine for adenine in nucleotide 1784 and, as with the G542X mutation, it also is located in exon 11. In Brazil, it presents a frequency of 1% (Raskin et al., 1993). Other, less frequent, mutations include: W1282X, N1303K, R553X, R1162X, and R334W (with their incidence varying according to population). Table 1 shows the molecular changes, and consequences of the more common mutations in the cystic fibrosis gene (Tsui, 1992).

1.3 Treatment

Approximately 50% of affected individuals are diagnosed in the age range from zero to six years but this percentage goes to 90% for those aged zero to eight years. Since reinforced nutrition is associated with a better prognosis, the screening of newborn infants is indicated. CF is one of most studied genetic diseases under the new therapy approaches, such as gene therapy which aims to restore the CFTR function. Clinical trials of gene therapy have been performed with viral vectors and cationic lipids. Despite advances in our knowledge of the disease, there is no specific treatment for CF yet. Due to its multi-systemic and chronic character, its treatment should be performed in reference centres and with a multidisciplinary team. Patients responding well to the treatment showed a median survival which has been increasing year to year, from over two years in 1950 up to between thirty and forty years today (Ribeiro et al., 2002). It is necessary to establish a strong and uninterrupted treatment program which is addressed to the prophylaxis of infections and complications. It should be started as soon as possible and it should be individualised, taking into account its severity and the organs affected. Early treatment decreases the evolution of the pulmonary lesions, improves prognosis, and increases the chances of survival.

NAME	MUTATION	CONSEQUENCE
ΔF508	Deletion of 3pb between 1652 and 1655 of the exon 10	Deletion of Phe in codon 508
G542X	G→T in nt 1756 of exon 11	Gly→ stop code in codon 542
G551D	G→A in nt 1784 in exon 11	Gly→ Asp in codon 551
W1282X	G→A in nt 3978 of exon 20	Trp→ stop code in codon 1282
3905insT	Insertion of T after the nt 3905 of exon 20	Change the reading chart.
N1303K	C→G in nt 4041 of exon 21	Asn→Lys in codon 1303
3849+10kbC → T	C→T in a Eco RI fragment at the attachment 5′ of intron 19	ABERRANTE excision
R553X	C→T in nt 1789 of exon 11	Arg→ stop code in codon 553
621+1G→T	G→T in nt 1 of attachment 5′ of intron 4	Excision mutation
1717-1G→A	G→A in nt 1 of attachment 3′ of intron 10	Excision mutation
1078delT	Deletion of T in nt 1078 of exon 7	Change reading chart
2789+5G→A	G→A in nt 5 of end 5′ of intron 14b	Excision mutation
3849+4ᴬ→G	A→G in nt 4 of end 5′ of intron 19	Excision mutation
711+1G→T	G→T in nt 1 of attachment 5′ of intron 5	Excision mutation
R1162X	C→T in nt 3616 of exon 19	Arg→ stop code in codon 1162
1898+1G→A	G→A in nt 1 of attachment 5′ of intron 5	Excision mutation
R117H	G→A in nt 482 of exon 4	Arg→His in codon 117
3659delC	Deletion of C in nt 3659 of exon 19	Change the reading chart
G85E	G→A in nt 386 of exon 3	Gly→Glu in codon 85
2184delA	Deletion of A in nt 2184 of exon 13	Change the reading chart
Δ1507	Deletion of 3pb between nt 1648 and 1653 of exon 10	Deletion of IIe at codon 506 or excision mutation
R347P	G→C in nt 1772 of exon 7	Arg→Pro in codon 347
R560T	G→C in nt 1811 of exon 11	Art→Thr in codon 560 or excision mutation
A455E	C→A in nt 1496 of exon 9	Ala→Glu in codon 455
R334W	C→T in nt 1132 of exon 7	Arg→Trp in codon 334
S549R(T→G)	T→G in nt 1779 of exon 11	Ser→Arg in codon 549
Q493X	C→T in nt 1609 of exon 10	Gln→ stop code in codon 493
S549N	G→A in nt 1778 of exon 11	Ser→Asn in codon 549

Table 1. Table obtained from Tsui (1992).

Pseudomonas aeruginosa has been found in more than 80% of teenagers with CF (Dubouix et al., 2003). Once established in the airways, the *Pseudomonas aeruginosa* infection is not eradicated by antibiotics, which only reduce the number of the colonies of bacteria. In order to treat CF, antibiotics can be administered through oral, intravenous or inhalation routes – the choice of which route should be made according to demand, prophylaxis and maintenance.

Ribeiro et al. (2002) defined the main objective of the treatment of CF, namely: the continued education of patients and their relatives concerning the disease; prophylaxis of the infections with a full vaccination program; early detection and control of pulmonary infection; respiratory physiotherapy and the improvement of bronchial blockage; the correction of pancreatic insufficiency; nutritional support with guidelines for diet and vitamin supplementation; monitoring the progress of the disease and any complications; family genetic counselling; finally, the provision of any information to patients and relatives concerning any advances in knowledge of CF.

1.4 Genetic counselling

Genetic counselling is essential in order to improve the understanding of the medical, psychological and familial implications of the disease. This process consists of the following steps: the interpretation of the familial medical history so as to assess the possibility of any occurrence or recurrence of the disease; the provision of education on heredity, genetic tests, the management of the disease, prevention, resources and research; the offer of counselling so as to properly inform the patient of the risks of having an affected child and its future life chances (Resta et al., 2006). Thus, counselling involves confirmation of the diagnosis, the estimated risk of recurrence, the provision of information about the disease, offers of support, and assistance with the acceptance of the diagnosis. It also suggests the provision of proper treatment and the offer of alternatives for prevention, such as pre-natal diagnosis and pre-implantation diagnosis. The first step for effective genetic counselling is the confirmation of the diagnosis of the affected individual (Harper, 2000). The definitive diagnosis of the disease is done with clinical features and the increased concentration of electrolytes (chloride and sodium) in sweat. The presence of the disease may be supposed from an altered neonatal screening, before the onset of symptoms. The CF hereditary pattern is autosomal recessive (i.e. in order to manifest the disease, the individual should present a mutation in two of the alleles of the CFTR). Therefore, both of the parents of the affected individual are carriers (heterozygous), and the risk of the recurrence of a CF child at birth is 25%. The individual with CF may show the same mutation in both of the alleles (homozygous for certain mutations) or else different mutations in each of the alleles (compound heterozygous). Healthy individuals carrying the mutation in only one of the alleles are called heterozygous (Saraiva-Pereira et al., 2011).

With the increase in the life expectancy of CF patients, many women carrying the disease have had pregnancies, whereas the affected men had shown infertility secondary to the obstructive azoospermia; nonetheless they may also have children because of assisted reproduction techniques. The risk of a CF individual having affected children depends upon her/his partner – if the partner is a carrier of the disease, that risk is 50%. The frequency of carriers for CF within the general population varies according to ethnic origin. In Caucasian populations, the frequency of heterozygous varies from 1/25 to 1/30 individuals (Saraiva-Pereira et al. 2011). The main difficulties for the genetic counselling of CF are those cases in which clinical confirmation is uncertain or else those cases in which is not possible to detect carriers within the family.

2. CF and infertility

2.1 Clinical features of infertility in CF

CF is a genetic disorder caused by mutations in the Cystic Fibrosis Transmembrane Regulator (CFTR) gene (Kerem et al., 1989; Riordan et al., 1989; Rommens et al., 1989). The CFTR is an anion channel regulated by cAMP-dependent phosphorylation, and it is expressed in the apical membrane of epithelial cells of a wide variety of tissues, including the reproductive tracts. The physiological role of CFTR in reproduction and its involvement in the pathogenesis of reproductive diseases remains largely unknown (Chan et al., 2009). The CF disorder is characterised by altered chloride and the bicarbonate transport of secretory epithelial cells (Chan et al., 2006; Li et al., 2010; Quinton, 1990, 1999).

Approximately 97% CF men are sterile due to the congenital bilateral absence of the vas deferens (CBAVD) and obstructive azoospermia (Wong, 1998). It has been suggested that the absence of vas deferens might be related to the requirement of the CFTR function at the embryonic stage (Li et al., 2010). It was demonstrated that the expression of the CFTR is developmentally regulated: cultured epithelial cells from the human foetal vas deferens have been shown to express the CFTR (Harris et al., 1991). Therefore, it is conceivable that fluid secretion by the Wolffian duct is required for the normal development of vas deferens. When secretion is impaired in CF individuals, normal development might be interrupted and so lead to vas agenesis (Wong, 1998).

Clinically, CF patients present a spectrum of genital phenotypes ranging from normal fertility to severely unpaired spermatogenesis and CBAVD (Xu et al., 2007). The diagnosis of CBAVD is based on the presence of azoospermia in subjects with normal or small size testes, non-palpable vas deferens, the characteristic ultrasonography view, and changes in the physical and biochemical properties of ejaculate (Jarzabek et al., 2004). Male CF patients' semen is characterised by azoospermia, low volume, low or normal viscosity, and increased turbidity. Testicular specimens show active spermatogenesis, although 50% of the spermatozoa have malformed heads. The pre-meiotic spermatogonia in CF patients appear to be morphologically normal, whereas the post-meiotic spermatogenic stages show malformation or the impairment of nuclear division (Denning et al., 1968). Testicular biopsies of post-pubertal men with CF have shown abnormal histological findings, such as pathological spermatogenesis and an increased number of dysmorphic spermatozoa (Mak et al., 2000).

The investigation of CFTR expression in male reproductive tissues showed that CFTR was present in the epididymis and vas deferens throughout post-natal life. High levels of CFTR expression were found in the head of the epididymis, but a variable expression was seen in distal epididymis. No CFTR was detected in the human testis. Accordingly, it was suggested that the anomalies in spermatozoa described in CF adult patients may result from epididymal dysfunction (Tizzano et al., 1994). Primary cultures of rat epididymal epithelial cells demonstrated the functional expression of CFTR and its involvement in the regulation of chloride secretion and fluid formation in the epididymis (Wong, 1998). Under basal conditions, the epididymis generally reabsorbs fluid to concentrate sperm. However, the observation that neurohormonal factors stimulate CFTR-mediated chloride secretion by epididymal epithelia (Wong, 1998) suggests that epididymal fluid secretion may be stimulated so as to create the optimal fluid environment for sperm maturation, storage, and even transport during ejaculation (Chan et al., 2009). Approximately 18 % of non-clinical CF men with infertility due to a reduction of sperm quality, and 15 % men with azoospermia, have at least one mutation in the CFTR. The frequency of mutations in infertile males presents a significantly higher than expected 4 % of the CF carrier frequency within the population. This increased frequency of CFTR mutations in healthy men with reduced sperm quality, and in men with azoospermia without CBAVD, suggests that the CFTR protein might be involved in the process of spermatogenesis or sperm maturation, over and above playing a critical role in the development of the epididymal glands and the vas deferens (Van der Ven et al., 1996).

In order to fertilise eggs, mammalian sperm must acquire fertilising potential in the female reproductive tract through a process known as capacitation. Sperm capacitation is a prerequisite for the acrosome reaction, which is an exocytotic event releasing hydrolytic enzymes from the acrosome so as to enable spermatozoa to penetrate the egg investments and its plasma membrane (Jarzabek et al., 2004; Xu et al., 2007). Capacitation is associated with the elevation of intracellular pH and the hyperpolarisation of the sperm plasma membrane (Meizel & Deamer, 1978; Zeng et al., 1995). These events depend on extracellular bicarbonate, which activates adenylyl cyclase pathway producing cyclic adenosine monophosphate (cAMP) and various downstream cellular events (such as protein tyrosine phosphorylation) and results in sperm capacitation (Demarco et al., 2003; Xu et al., 2007).

As has been shown, CFTR secretes bicarbonate in the uterus and sperm, and its impairment leads to reduced sperm capacitation and the fertilising capacity of sperm (Wang et al., 2003; Xu et al., 2007). The interaction of the CFTR protein with its inhibitor or antibody significantly reduces sperm capacitation and associated bicarbonate-dependent events, including increases in intracellular pH, cAMP production, and membrane hyperpolarisation. The fertilising capacity of the sperm obtained from heterozygous CFTR mutant mice is also significantly lower compared with the wild-type. These findings suggest that sperm CFTR may be involved in the transport of bicarbonate important for sperm capacitation, and that CFTR mutations causing impaired CFTR function may lead to a reduced sperm fertilising capacity and male infertility other than CBAVD (Xu et al., 2007). A recent study showed that human sperm capacitation as facilitated by progesterone and acrossome reactions induced by recombinant human zona pellucida 3 peptides (rhuZP3) were both significantly inhibited by a CFTR inhibitor. In a group of fertile men, the percentage of spermatozoa expressing CFTR was significantly higher than that of the healthy and infertile men's group. In addition, the study showed that the presence of a CFTR inhibitor markedly depresses intracellular cAMP levels, sperm hyperactivation and the sperm penetration of zona-free hamster eggs (Li et al., 2010). Moreover, when spermatozoa from CF patients with CBAVD are used for intracytoplasmic sperm injection, fertilisation rates are not reduced, suggesting a specific defect in zona pellucid penetration or membrane fusion capacity in these spermatozoa (Silber et al., 1994; Li et al., 2010). CFTR appears to have a profound role in regulating sperm function (Chan et al., 2009).

In CF female patients, the cause of reduced fertility remains obscure. CFTR is expressed throughout the female reproductive tract in the cervix, oviduct, ovary, and uterus (Chan et al., 2002; Tizzano et al., 1994). CF has been associated with menstrual irregularities, including amenorrhea, irregular cycles, anovulation, smaller uteri, and delayed puberty (Johannesson et al., 1998; Stead et al., 1987). The absence of obvious anatomical abnormalities in the female reproductive tract – except for thick and tenacious cervical mucus with altered water and electrolyte content (Kopito et al., 1973) – has led to the general belief that abnormal mucus contributes to the reduced fertility of CF women by acting as a barrier to sperm passage (Chan et al., 2009). However, repeated and unsuccessful attempts with intrauterine insemination were also reported (Epelboin et al., 2001; Rodgers et al., 2000), suggesting that further abnormalities (such as inadequate fluid control throughout the rest of the reproductive tract) could also contribute to infertility in humans (Hodges et al., 2008).

As already noted, CFTR plays a crucial role in mediating uterine bicarbonate secretion and sperm capacitation, leading to the thought that CFTR bicarbonate secretion dysfunction might induce an impaired sperm fertilising capacity and reduced fertility in CF women. In a mouse sperm-endometrial epithelial cell co-culture system, it was demonstrated that endometrial epithelial cells possess a CFTR-mediated bicarbonate transport mechanism. A substantial decrease in apical fluid bicarbonate contents was observed after treatment with both blockers of CFTR and antisense oligonucleotides against CFTR when compared with the control. These results are consistent with the CFTR's mediating uterine bicarbonate secretion, and they indicate that defective CFTR might lead to impaired bicarbonate secretion in the uterus. *In vitro* fertilisation assays on zona-intact mouse eggs further demonstrated that the number of two-cell embryos obtained with sperm capacitated in a conditioned medium from CFTR antisense-treated endometrial cells was significantly reduced as compared with that obtained from sense-treated controls. Sperm capacitation and egg-fertilising ability depend – critically – on CFTR and bicarbonate content and defective CFTR-mediated bicarbonate secretion, and the lower fertilising capacity of sperm might also account for lower CF female fertility (Chan et al., 2009; Wang et al., 2003).

CFTR expression in the uterus is regulated by ovarian hormones with increasing expression in response to estrogen and decreasing expression in response to progesterone; this is a pattern that correlates with cyclic changes in uterine fluid (Zheng et al., 2004). Hormone changes have been observed in CF female adolescents, who displayed reduced estradiol and FSH levels (Reiter et al., 1981), and CF female adults, who displayed increased testosterone and reduced estradiol and progesterone levels, compared with age-matched controls (Johannesson et al., 1998). Interestingly, through observations in rodent uterus, CFTR was found to be co-expressed with the epithelial sodium channel (ENaC) in an out-of-phase fashion. With the maturation of ovarian follicles and the estrogen secretion phase, CFTR is highly expressed and ENaC is poorly expressed. Inversely, with corpus luteum activity and progesterone secretion, low CFTR expression and high ENaC expression are observed (Chan et al., 2002). This may explain maximal fluid secretion during the early phase of the oestrous cycle, when the level of oestrogen is at its highest. Similarly, at dioestrus, the attenuated fluid production with down-regulation of CFTR and increased reabsorption by up-regulation of ENaC may account for the disappearance of uterine fluid. These cyclic changes in CFTR and ENaC expression which result in uterine fluid volume variation have physiological significance. Maximal CFTR expression and – therefore – high uterine fluid production may lubricate the cervical and vaginal lumen for sperm movement towards the oviduct as well as sperm capacitation. Equally, low CFTR expression and – consequently – reduced fluid volume may enhance close contact on the endometrial surface, facilitating embryo implantation. Dynamic changes in the fluid microenvironment, particularly the fluid volume, in the female reproductive tract are dictated by CFTR expression, which is normally regulated by ovarian hormones throughout the cycle and accommodating various reproductive events. The impairment of CFTR expression may lead to the disturbance of the fluid environment, resulting in various pathological conditions and infertility (Chan et al., 2007; Chan et al., 2009).

Interestingly, abnormalities in the reproductive endocrine axis have been viewed as an indirect consequence of CF, though they have been largely ignored as possible contributors to observed female infertility (Stead et al., 1987). CFTR expression was found in the areas of the rat hypothalamus (thalamus and amygdale) which are involved in the regulation of sexual maturation and reproduction. CFTR might increase the acidification of synaptic vesicles, and thus play an important role in the central regulation of sexual maturation and fertility (Johannesson et al., 1997b). Delayed pubertal increments of serum gonadotropin and sex hormone levels in CF patients suggest a late maturation of the reproductive system (Reiter et al., 1981). Anovulatory women showed significantly lower luteal oestradiol and progesterone, but higher total testosterone concentrations when compared to healthy controls and the ovulatory CF women (Johannesson et al., 1998). In a mouse model, increased FSH levels were found in CFTR mutant females as a result of a decreased number of ovulatory follicles, leading to less estradiol production and a lack of feedback inhibition of FSH secretion. CF female mice exposed to exogenous hormones showed a correction of organ size and ovulation. These findings suggests that the CF reproductive organs can respond to gonadotropins, but that an impaired hypothalamic-pituitary-gonadal (HPG) axis may be a direct cause of reduced fertility in women with CF (Hodges et al., 2008; Johannesson et al., 1997b).

In CF women, late puberty and amenorrhea are common clinical findings due to the deficit in their nutritional status. It has also been suggested that the lack of ovulation is a consequence of malnutrition and catabolism. Clinically, the anovulatory women presented more profound essential fatty acid deficiency (EFAD) and hypersecretion of insulin during an oral glucose tolerance test compared to the ovulatory women (Johannesson et al., 1998). However, it was shown that menarcheal age was also delayed in CF females in good clinical and nutritional condition. Homozygous patients for the most common mutation – F508del – and those with a pathological glucose tolerance test (OGTT) showed the most delay in menarcheal age (Johannesson et al., 1997a). This may be explained by the fact that ovarian cells express insulin receptors that mediate gonadal steroid production. Experimental data has shown that insulin has a gonadotropic effect through different mechanisms, such as a direct effect on steroidogenic enzymes, the modulation of FSH or LH receptor number, synergism with FSH and LH, and nonspecific enhancement of cell viability (Porestky & Kalin, 1987). Insulin appears to be necessary for the ovary to reach its full steroidogenic potential. The difference observed in the insulin pattern in the pathological OGTT group might alter ovarian function and thereby cause further delay in sexual maturation (Johannesson et al., 1998). Polycystic ovaries were also described in CF women (Stead et al., 1987).

CFTR mutations were previously associated with Congenital Absence of Uterus and Vagina (CAUV). CF mutations might affect the normal embryological development of the Müllerian ducts. During the seventh week of gestation, the cranial end of the Müllerian duct is immediately adjacent to the Wolffian duct, and both ducts share a common basement membrane. The Wolffian duct then guides the caudal growth of the Müllerian ducts. By the ninth week of gestation, the Müllerian duct reaches the caudal end of the adjacent Wolffian duct. At this time, these ductal systems separate from each other, form separate basement membranes, and continue to develop independently (Ludwig, 1998). The interdependency of these two systems suggests that the same genetic factors may control the early development of both systems. Failure of the development of the Müllerian duct causes CAUV in females. The incidence of most common CFTR mutations found in patients with CAUV (8%) is twice that which is found in the general population (4%), but much less than the incidence of CFTR mutations in men with CBAVD (80%). This suggests that it is unlikely for CFTR mutations to cause CAUV in females as they cause CBAVD in some males. As such, the effect of the abnormal CFTR protein product on the Wolffian duct must occur at a time when the development of the Müllerian duct is no longer dependent on the Wolffian duct (Timmreck et al., 2003).

CF female patients have such pregnancy complications as premature labour and delivery and increased maternal and prenatal mortality due to severe maternal pulmonary infection and maternal weight loss (Cohen et al., 1980; Kent & Farquharson, 1993). However, the risk of the deterioration of health during pregnancy for females with CF is considered to be small, if good medical care is provided and if women are in a stable and good clinical condition (FitzSimmons et al., 1996).

There remain many unanswered questions as to the cause of infertility in CF, and the exact role of CFTR in reproductive physiology and the contribution of CFTR dysfunction to infertility in both sexes is far from understood (Chan et al., 2009).

2.2 CFTR mutations closely related to CF infertility

Infertility, or at least subfertility, in males with CF was first suspected in the 1960s (Denning et al., 1968; Radpour et al., 2008). Depending upon their molecular consequences, CFTR mutations may result in either a typical CF or else an atypical (often monosymptomatic) CF, such as congenital absence of the vas deferens (bi- or unilateral), bilateral ejaculatory duct obstruction, or bilateral obstructions within the epididymis (Jarzabek et al., 2004). Approximately 80% of CF male patients present CBAVD, a Wolffian duct anomaly (Radpour et al., 2008). Male infertility due to CBAVD has been shown to be commonly linked to CFTR mutations, and it is considered to be a genital form of CF or a CFTR-associated disease with incomplete CF expression (Dequeker et al., 2009; Kanavakis et al., 1998; Rave-Harel et al., 1997). Men with CBAVD are apparently healthy, with relatively normal lung and pancreatic functions. CBAVD appears to be a heterogeneous genetic condition, with many cases being mild forms of CF (DeBraekeleer and Férec, 1996).

Extensive studies have shown that patients with isolated CBAVD carry two CFTR mutations, usually in compound heterozygosity (Chillón et al., 1995; Claustres et al., 2000). Of isolated CBAVD patients, where the mutation is found on both CFTR, about 88% carry one severe mutation and one mild mutation, whilst the remaining 12% carry mild mutations on both CFTR (Claustres et al., 2000). This is in contrast to classical clinically CF patients, where about 88% of the CF patients carry severe mutations on both CFTR, whilst about 11% carry a severe mutation on one CFTR and a mild mutation on their second one (Claustres et al., 2000; Radpour et al., 2008). The most frequent CFTR mutation conferring a mild phenotype found in CBAVD patients is the 5T polymorphism (Chillón et al., 1995), which is an allele found at the polymorphic Tn locus in intron 8 of the CFTR, and which can be found as a stretch of 5, 7, or 9 thymidine residues at this locus. Less efficient splicing will occur when a lower number of thymidines are found, resulting in CFTR transcripts that lack exon 9 sequences (Chu et al., 1993; Radpour et al., 2008). Men with the 5T variant in the non-coding region of the gene will produce an abnormally low level of CFTR protein in the epididymis. However, there may be sufficient proteins for the prevention of disease in other organs (such as the lung and the gastrointestinal glands) normally affected by CF, which might explain why the lung and pancreas are normal in CBAVD, but the epididymis is not (DeBraekeleer and Férec, 1996; Jarzabek et al., 2004; Wong, 1998). The analysis of the level of correctly spliced RNA transcribed from the 5T allele in different tissues (nasal and epididymal epithelium) and its correlation with CF disease expression, has shown that in infertile males with normal lung function the level of correctly spliced transcripts found in the nasal epithelium was higher than the level found in the epididymal epithelium. It indicates that there is variability in the efficiency of the splicing mechanism both between different individuals and between different organs of the same individual. In many human monogenic diseases, high variability in disease expression is found among patients carrying the same genetic defect (Levy et al., 2010; Rave-Harel et al., 1997). The molecular basis for this variability has been suggested to be allelic heterogeneity, additional genetic loci, and/or environmental factors. Accordingly, allelic variants of genes involved in the splicing regulation might contribute to the different efficiencies of alternative splicing found amongst different individuals (Rave-Harel et al., 1997).

CFTR mutations may represent one of the most common abnormalities associated with male infertility, especially with CBAVD but also with obstructive azoospermia (Kanavakis et al., 1998). A screening of the entirety of the *CFTR* in males with CUAVD (congenital unilateral absence of vas deferens), CBAVD and obstructive azoospermia of the vas deferens, has shown that almost 64% of patients carry two *CFTR* mutations. The most frequent mutations observed amongst those patients were F508del (44.7%), T5 allele (36.2%), and R117H (19.1%) (Jézéquel et al., 2000). In a large French cohort study, the most frequent allele mutations identified in CBAVD male patients were F508del (21.7%), the 5T allele (16.3%) and R117H (4.4%), followed by D1152H (1.19%) and D443Y (0.93%). Two CFTR mutations (including the 5T allele) were present in 47.7% and one mutation in 24.6% of CBAVD patients, while no mutation was reported in the remaining 27.7%. Approximately 43.5% of patients with CBAVD carried one F508del allele, and 31.7% had at least one 5T allele. Altogether, at least one CFTR mutation was identified in 72.25% individuals with CBAVD (Claustres et al., 2000). In an Italian multicentric study, a molecular screening of the most common CFTR mutations in infertile couples was performed. CFTR mutations were detected in 4.6% of subjects, a percentage that overlaps with the general population carrier frequency. However, it was found a mutation-frequency of over 37% amongst CBAVD individuals and of 6% in males with non-obstructive azoospermia (Stuppia et al., 2005). In another study, the carrier status of CBAVD patients for the F508del mutation was screened and 57% were found to be carriers. Amongst these patients, 25% were later found to have compound heterozygotes for the F508del and R117H mutations (Williams et al., 1993). A study of the entire coding region of the CFTR of CBAVD patients found that 28.6% have mutations in both copies of the CFTR, 42.8% had one CFTR mutation, whilst in the remaining 28.6% no CFTR mutations were found (Kanavakis et al., 1998). These figures give an average of an eleven-fold increase of the carrier frequency compared to the population data on CFTR mutations in CBAVD patients. (Uzun et al., 2005). Amongst cases of obstructive azoospermia, 30% had one CFTR mutation whilst in the remaining 70% no mutations were found – this indicates an association between cases of obstructive azoospermia without CBAVD with CFTR mutations. The frequency of the IVS8(5T) allele was 14.3% for the CBAVD cases, which was three-fold higher than for normal chromosomes (Kanavakis et al., 1998). Similarly, another extensive analysis of the CFTR in CBAVD patients revealed that 42% of subjects were carriers of one CFTR allele and that 24% were compound heterozygous for CFTR alleles. The presence of only one CF allele in approximately 42% of CBAVD patients implies some role on the part of CF in CBAVD, although additional factors or genes are necessary for the development of CBAVD in those patients (Mercier et al., 1995; Van der Ven et al., 1996; Williams et al., 1993). The CFTR mutations commonly associated with male infertility are F508del, R117H, and the IVS8 (5T) polymorphism, each of which exhibit diverse frequencies among different cohorts (Van der Ven et al., 1996). Since the spectrum of CFTR mutations is markedly different amongst populations, the ethnic background of the patients should be taken into account so as to ensure that the most prevalent mutations appropriate to that particular population are included in the screening panel (DeBraekeleer & Férec, 1996). Altogether, the mutation-frequencies in infertile male patients are significantly higher than the expected carrier-frequencies in the general population (Van der Ven et al., 1996).

There are only a few studies on female CFTR mutation-frequency in the literature. It is generally assumed that fertility is reduced in CF women, although not as dramatically as in men. It was already proposed that CFTR mutations do not appear to be involved in female infertility (Morea et al., 2005) and CAUV condition (Radpour et al., 2008). The most common CFTR mutations – including the 5T allele – were tested in isolated CAUV female patients. These mutations were only found in 8% of the subjects, suggesting that it is unlikely that CFTR mutations cause CAUV in females (Timmreck et al., 2003). In a recent study, 24 women with altered fertility were screened for the F508del mutation. Amongst them, 37.5% showed reduced fertility without a known cause, 20.8% presented reduced fertility due to polycystic ovarian syndrome (although two of them demonstrated malformations of the reproductive tract), 37.5% had been pregnant previously although most of them had spontaneous abortions, and 8.3% presented early menopause. It was found that one patient who was a F508del mutation carrier and who had had an early menopause had also had a previous abortion. Unexpectedly – considering that Brazilian population is greatly mixed – the carrier frequency for the most common mutation in CF amongst infertile Brazilian women was similar to that of Caucasian populations. It was proposed that there are common clinical features between women with altered fertility and with CF women, and that CF mutations may be more frequent than expected amongst patients with fertility issues (Brunoro et al., 2010). Large cohort studies on CFTR mutation-frequency among infertile women are needed.

2.3 Considerations for CF mutation screening tests

According to the CF Mutation Database, around 20 mutations have individual worldwide frequencies greater than 0.1%, and can thus be considered to be common mutations (Lay-son et al., 2011). These common mutations vary by geographic and/or ethnic origin. Latin American countries have a high ethnic admixture and they show a wide distribution of 89 different mutations. Most of these mutations are frequent in Spain, Italy, and Portugal, and so is consistent with the origin of the European settlers. A few mutations found among Africans are also present in those countries which were part of the slave trade. This may be the result of the miscegenation of these populations. New mutations were also found which possibly originated in America (Pérez et al., 2007). As in most countries, F508del was the most common mutation detected, but in a lower proportion than the average frequency of 45–46% published for Latin-American countries (Keyeux et al., 2003; Pérez et al., 2007; Zielenski & Tsui, 1995), and the reported worldwide frequency of 66% (Lay-son et al., 2010; Zielenski & Tsui, 1995). The G542X mutation is the second most frequent mutation in Latin America, with a total frequency of 5.07%. N1303K, W1282X and R1162X are the next most frequent mutations, with variations from 0.59% to 3.95%. The frequency of the rest of the mutations varies from one country to another, but their overall frequencies are less than 1%, and could be considered to be rare in Latin America (Pérez et al., 2007). The carrier-rate and mutation-frequencies vary widely in different populations, and so screening tests with high detection-rates for CFTR mutations have to consider the population's ethnicity (Pieri et al., 2007).

There is increasing evidence that CFTR mutations may contribute etiologically to certain monosymptomatic disorders. Infertile men with isolate obstructive azoospermia may have mutations in the CFTR, many of which are rare in classical CF and not evaluated in most routine mutation screening. It was demonstrated that the routine mutation panel has failed to identify CFTR mutations and the IVS8-5T allele in 46% of CBAVD groups, 50% of CUAVD groups, and 79% of idiopathic epididymal obstruction groups. These results demonstrate that routine testing for CFTR mutations for infertile men may miss mild or rare gene alterations. The DNA sequence method detects more CFTR mutations than common mutation panels. This represents a significant problem because advances in assisted reproduction have allowed infertile male patients to conceive, raising the concern of transmitting – when present – pathogenic CFTR mutations onto progeny. The importance of accurate CFTR mutation detection in men with obstructive azoospermia and their partners has already been highlighted (Danzinger et al., 2004; Mak et al., 1999). Today, screening for a panel of CFTR mutations is offered to infertile men prior to in vitro fertilisation (IVF) or *intra cytoplasmic sperm injection* (ICSI), and includes only the most common mutations found amongst the CF patients of European and North American origin. The atypical CBAVD phenotype, however, is caused by milder mutations, most of them very rare or even not yet described, and thus not included in the panel of CF mutations usually screened. It was proposed that only an extensive CFTR screening can detect rare mutations that are not found by conventional screenings and commercial tests, and can thus improve the diagnosis and care of CF and CAVD as well as the prevention of new cases through the use of reproductive technologies (Pieri et al., 2007).

However, genetic testing should only be performed in the context of appropriate genetic counselling and laboratories should work in close association with clinical geneticists and reference laboratories so as to ensure that pertinent tests are performed and that proper information is provided to patients. There is no standard or preferred method, but laboratories should be aware of the limitations of their chosen method and they should know which mutations are not identified, whether the techniques are commercially available or else being developed within the laboratory. This means that individual laboratories should choose a method which is suited to their experience, workload, and scope of testing. In addition to the screen for frequent mutations, a complementary panel may be required to test population-specific mutations with a frequency above 1%. The knowledge of the ethnic or geographic origins of patients and their parents and grandparents is therefore important in order to determine the analysis to be performed (Dequeker et al., 2009). The knowledge of geographic or ethnic variations in the local population mutation-frequency is crucial so as to properly achieve effective genetic counselling and improve the cost-effectiveness of screening and diagnostic tests (Lay-son et al., 2011).

2.4 Ethical implications of genetic testing

According to the Patient Registry 2009 of the CF Foundation, USA there are growing numbers of CF adults 18 years of age and over. The percentage of CF patients aged 18 years or older has risen from 30% in 1990 to over 47% in 2009. It also have indicated that the median age of survival of patients with CF has risen from 27 years in 1985 to almost 36 years in 2009, leading to greater concern for the disease management of CF adults (Cystic Fibrosis Foundation Patient registry 2009: Annual data report, 2011). Coupled with an improved life expectancy, adult CF patients are more likely to seek independence from their families and pursue typical adult activities, such as attending college, entering serious relationships and pursuing careers (Modi et al., 2010). Issues related to sexual maturation, fertility, pregnancy and contraception have thus become important in the comprehensive care of CF patients (Tizzano et al., 1994). Fertility bears centrally to reproductive decision-making, determining whether natural conception is even an option or whether adoption or assisted reproductive technology must be considered (Hull & Kass, 2000). Along with the wish to conceive, CF parents and physicians confront major ethical issues regarding abortions, the premature termination of pregnancies, and possible arrangements in the event of morbidity or maternal mortality which should all be discussed prior to pregnancy (Barak et al., 2005).

There are still many paediatric CF clinics that continue to care for patients up to 18 years of age. Several studies have suggested that teenage patients and their parents have unmet information needs regarding the patient's sexual health. Usually, unplanned sex tends to be done without protection. An important priority for the CF team is to try to ensure that women with CF are aware of the risks of unplanned pregnancy. Collaboration between the family planning clinician and the teenager's CF physician is recommended (Roberts & Green, 2005). As such, reproductive counselling and reproductive health issues must be carefully addressed to CF adult patients (Hull & Kass, 2000; Sawyer, 1996). CF healthcare providers are an important source of information, and early discussion of sexual and reproductive health is indicated in paediatric settings for the adolescent patients, since a very high interest in future parenting is expressed by CF men. It has been suggested that there should be greater emphasis on infertility, semen analysis, and the prevention of sexually transmitted infections, backed with a greater focus on reproductive options within adult healthcare services (Sawyer et al., 2005).

In the 1980s, it was thought to be too risky for a woman with CF to get pregnant and that it was impossible for a man with CF to father a child. Nowadays, improvements in the nutrition and lung function of these patients make it possible for CF women to have a healthy pregnancy and baby. In 2009, the Patient Registry reported that 226 women with CF were pregnant. Successful outcomes can be achieved for both the CF mother and the child with careful patient assessment, combined with the integration of a multidisciplinary team, composed of the CF physician, the fertility specialist and the obstetrician (CF Foundation Patient registry 2009: Annual data report, 2011). Close follow-up of the maternal and foetal condition, along with careful monitoring of ventilation, immunology, diabetes, glucose tolerance and nutrition is important since all these parameters may be adversely affected in a CF pregnancy (Barak et al., 2005; Rodgers et al., 2000).

For CF men, advances in fertility medicine have given them the option to father children (CF Foundation Patient registry 2009: Annual data report, 2011). The use of assisted reproductive techniques (such as testicular micro-aspiration and intracytoplasmic sperm injection (ICSI)) has enabled testicular spermatozoa to fertilise ova without the need to be capacitated, or to undergo acrosome reaction or else penetrate and fuse it with the egg (Wong, 1998). A report on CF men that have undergone ICSI coupled with IVF showed that 62% of the couples successfully achieved pregnancy (McCallum et al., 2000). A group of CF azoospermia males were submitted to ICSI and 63% of the couples had clinical pregnancy (Hubert et al., 2006). However, before such measures are taken, genetic screening and counselling for the men and their partners should be mandatory in safeguarding their offspring from the risk of clinical CF (DeBraekeleer and Férec, 1996). Moreover, CF men should be informed about their own health and any long-term issues (such as the likelihood of premature death) and this information should be clearly shared with their partner (Hubert et al., 2006). In the case of CBAVD patients – a genital form of CF – most carry a severe CF-causing CFTR mutation and, therefore, have a 0.5% chance of transmitting the CFTR mutation to the child. Assuming a risk of 1/25 of the partner being a CF carrier, and that a carrier has a chance of 0.5% of transmitting the mutant CFTR to the child, the combined risk of CBAVD couples of having a CF child is 1/100 when compared with a risk of 1/2500 amongst general population (Radpour et al., 2008). The detection of a CFTR mutation in CF male patients and their spouses is crucial, since the presence of a CFTR mutation would present a high-risk situation whereas its absence would present a low-risk situation (DeBraekeleer and Férec, 1996). In cases of oligozoospermia, it is also ideal to screen both partners. It was also recommended that – if resources are stretched – amongst couples with a CBAVD male only the female needs to be routinely CF screened because, if she is negative, then the couple's residual risk of having a CF or CBAVD child will be reduced to 1:960 (Lewis-Jones et al., 2000). The reproductive options for the majority of CF men who are infertile include not having children, adoption, in vitro fertilisation with donor sperm, and microscopic epididymal sperm aspiration (MESA) coupled with in vitro fertilisation. There is also a complementary option, namely pre-implantation genetic diagnosis (PGD). PGD refers to the genetic testing of embryos created through IVF for the purpose of selecting embryos that would lead to the birth of a child unaffected by a detectable genetic defect. The notion of preventing a disease by preventing the birth of an individual with that disease is controversial. The CFF has no official position on this practice, and this type of decision is a personal choice to be made by the individual together with his/her physician (Davis et al., 2010).

3. Conclusion

The National Institutes of Health, USA recommends genetic counselling for any couple attempting assisted reproductive techniques where the man has CF or obstructive azoospermia and is positive for a CFTR mutation. It is important to analyse the clinical genetic conditions of the families by evaluating the full family history, by documenting the pregnancy and foetal, neonatal, and paediatric loss of life, as well as by cytogenetic studies of the couple and analysis for CFTR mutations. At this time, it is debatable whether it is better to perform the screening for mutations in the full gene or whether it is better to screening for typical local mutations of a population. It is also subject of debate if it is better to perform the screening for mutations in CF affected individuals only or also in their partner. All these choices have ethical and social implications and there may be better resolution with new population studies focused on the frequency of mutations in CF individuals with infertility. CF is now a disease of the adult population with many adult-specific issues. As such, adult CF patients must be treated by a well-trained interdisciplinary team of adult-care providers within the environment of the CF care network.

4. References

Barak, A., Dulitzki, M., Efrati, O., Augarten, A., Szeinberg, A., Reichert, N., Modan, D., Weiss, B., Miller, M., Katzanelson, D. & Yahav, Y. Pregnancies and outcome in women with cystic fibrosis. Isr Med Assoc J, Vol. 7, No. 2 (February 2005), pp. 95-98.

Bargon, J., Stein, J., Dietrich, C.F., Muller, U., Caspary,W.F., & Wagner, T.O. (1999). Gastrointestinal complications of adult patients with cystic fibrosis. J Gastroenterol, Vol. 37, No. 8, PP.739-749.

Brunoro, G.V., Wolfgramm, E.V., Louro, I.D., Degasperi, I.I., Busatto, V.C., Perrone, A.M., Batitucci, M.C. (2010). Cystic fibrosis Δf508 mutation screening in Brazilian women with altered fertility. Mol Biol Rep, November 2010, pp.1-4.

Brunecki, Z. The incidence and genetics of cystic fibrosis. (1972) J. Med. Genet., Vol. 9, pp. 33-37, 1972.

Chan, L. N., Tsang, L.L., Rowlands, D.K., Rochelle, L.G., Boucher, R.C., Liu, C.Q. & Chan, H.C. (2002). Distribution and regulation of ENaC subunit and CFTR mRNA expression in murine female reproductive tract. J. Membr Biol, Vol. 185, No. 2, pp. 165–176.

Chan, H.C., Shi, Q.X., Zhou, C.X., Wang, X.F., Xu, W.M., Chen, W.Y., Chen, A.J., Ni, Y. & Yuan, Y.Y. (2006). Critical role of CFTR in uterine bicarbonate secretion and the fertilizing capacity of sperm. Mol Cell Endocrinol, Vol. 250, pp.106–113.

Chan, H.C., He, Q., Ajonuma, L.C. & Wang, X.F. (2007). Epithelial ion channels in the regulation of female reproductive tract fluid microenvironment: implications in fertility and infertility. Sheng Li Xue Bao, Vol. 59, No. 4 (August 2007), pp. 495-504.

Chan, H.C., Ruan, Y.C., He, Q., Chen, M.H., Chen, H., Xu, W.M., Chen, W.Y., Xie, C., Zhang, X.H. & Zhou, Z. (2009). The cystic fibrosis transmembrane conductance regulator in reproductive health and disease. J Physiol, Vol. 587, No. 10 (May 2009), pp. 2187-95.

Chillón, M., Casals, T., Mercier, B., Bassas, L., Lissens, W., Silber, S., Rommey, M.-C., Ruiz-Romero, J., Verlingue, C., Claustres, M., Nunes, V., Férec, C., & Estivill, X. (1995). Mutations in the cystic fibrosis gene in patients with congenital absence of the vas deferens. N. Engl. J. Med, Vol. 332, No. 22 (June 1995), pp. 1475–1480.

Chu, C.S., Trapnell, B.C., Curristin, S., Cutting, G.R. & Crystal, R.G. (1993). Genetic basis of variable exon 9 skipping in cystic fibrosis transmembrane conductance regulator mRNA. Nat Genet, Vol. 3, No. 2 (February 1993), pp. 151-156.

Claustres, M., Guittard, C., Bozon, D., Chevalier, F., Verlingue, C., Ferec, C., Girodon, E., Cazeneuve, C., Bienvenu, T., Lalau, G., Dumur, V., Feldmann, D., Bieth, E., Blayau, M., Clavel, C., Creveaux, I., Malinge, M.C., Monnier, N., Malzac, P., Mittre, H., Chomel, J.C., Bonnefont, J.P., Iron, A., Chery, M. & Georges, M.D. (2000). Spectrum of CFTR mutations in cystic fibrosis and in congenital absence of the vas deferens in France. Hum Mutat, Vol. 16, No. 2, pp. 143-56.

Cohen, L.F., Di Sant'Agnese, P.A. & Friedlander, J. (1980). Cystic fibrosis and pregnancy. A national survey. Lancet, Vol. 2, No. 8199 (October 1980), pp. 842–844.

Collins. F.S. (1992) Cystic Fibrosis. Molecular biology and therapeutic implications . Science, Vol. 256, pp. 774-779.

Cystic Fibrosis Foundation. (2011). Cystic Fibrosis Foundation Patient Registry 2009: Annual data report. 24.07.2011, Available from http://www.cff.org/LivingWithCF/QualityImprovement/PatientRegistry Report.

Danziger, K.L., Black, L.D., Keiles, S.B., Kammesheidt, A. & Turek, P.J. (2004). Improved detection of cystic fibrosis mutations in infertility patients with DNA sequence analysis. Hum Reprod, Vol. 19, No. 3 (March 2004), pp. 540-546.

Davis, L.B., Champion, S.J., Fair, S.O., Baker, V.L., Garber, A.M. (2010). A cost-benefit analysis of preimplantationpre-implantation genetic diagnosis for carrier couples of cystic fibrosis. Fertil Steril, Vol. 93, No. 6, pp. 1793-1804.

DeBraekeleer, M. & Férec, C. (1996). Mutations in the cystic fibrosis gene in men with congenital bilateral absence of the vas deferens. Mol. Hum. Reprod, Vol. 2, No. 9 (September 1996), pp. 669–677.

Demarco, I.A., Espinosa, F., Edwards, J., Sosnik, J., Vega-Beltra´ n, J.L., Hockensmith, J.W., Kopf, G.S., Darszon, A. & Visconti, P.E. (2003). Involvement of a Na^+/HCO_3^- Cotransporter in Mouse Sperm Capacitation. J Biol Chem, Vol. 278, No. 9 (February 2003), pp. 7001-7009.

Denning, C.R., Sommers, S.C., & Quigley, H.J. (1968). Infertility in male patients with cystic fibrosis. Pediatrics, Vol. 41, No. 1 (January 1968), pp. 7-17.

Dequeker, E., Stuhrmann, M., Morris, M.A., Casals, T., Castellani, C., Claustres, M., Cuppens, H., Des Georges, M., Ferec, C., Macek, M., Pignatti, P.F., Scheffer, H., Schwartz, M., Witt, M., Schwarz, M. & Girodon, E. (2009). Best practice guidelines for molecular genetic diagnosis of cystic fibrosis and CFTR-related disorders-- updated European recommendations. Eur J Hum Genet, Vol. 17, No. 1 (January 2009), pp. 51-65.

DI Sant'Agnese, P.A.,Darling, R.C., Perera, G.A. & Schea, E. (1953). Abnormal electrolyte composition of sweat in fibrosis of the pancreas. Pediatrics, pp. 12:549.

Dubouix ,A., Campanac, C., Fauvel, J., Simon, M.F., Salles, J.P., Roques, C., Chap, H., Marty, N. (2003). Bactericidal properties of group IIa secreted phospholipase A(2) against *Pseudomonas aeruginosa* clinical isolates. *J Med Microbiol*, Vol. 52, No. 12 (December 2003), pp. 1039-1045.

Epelboin, S., Hubert, D., Patrat, C., Abirached, F., Bienvenu, T. & Lepercq, J. (2001). Management of assisted reproductive technologies in women with cystic fibrosis. *Fertil Steril*, Vol. 76, No. 6 (December 2001), pp. 1280–1281.

Fanconi, G., Uehlinger, E. & Knauer, C. (1936). Das Coeliakie-Syndrom bei angeborenem zystichem pâncreas fibromatose and bronkiektasen. *Wien Med Wochenschr*, Vol. 86, pp 753-756.

Farber, S. (1944). Pancreatic function and disease and early life. *Arch Pathol*, pp 37:238.

Feingoud, J. & Guilloud,-Bataille, M. (1999). Genetic comparisonsof patients with fibrosis cystic with or without meconium ileus. *Ann Genet*, Vol. 42, No. 3, pp. 147-150.

FitzSimmons, S.C., Fitzpatrick, S., Thompson, B., *Aitkin, M., Fiel, S., Winnie, G. & Hilman, B.* (1996). A longitudinal study of the effects of pregnancy on 325 women with cystic fibrosis. *Pediatr. Pulm.*, Vol. 13, pp. 99–101.

Gibson, L.E. & Cooke, R.E. (1959). A test for concentration of electrolytes in sweat in cystic fibrosis of the pancreas utilizing pilocarpine by iontophoresis. *Pediatrics*, Vol. 23, pp. 545-549.

Harper, P. (2000). *Practical Genetic Counselling.* 5th edition. Ed. Butterworth-Henemann. Cambridge.

Harris, A., Chalkley, G.C., Lankester, S.A. & Coleman, L.S. (1991). Expression of the Cystic Fibrosis gene in human development. *Development*, Vol. 113, No. 1 (September 1991), pp. 305-310.

Harris, A.(1992). Cystic fibrosis gene. *Brit. Med. Bull.* Vol. 48, pp. 736-753.

Heng, H.H.Q., Shi, X.M., Tsui, L.C. (1993). Fluorescence in situ hybridization mapping of the cystic fibrosis transmembrane conductance regulator (CFTR) gene to 7q31.3. *Cytogenet Cell Genet*, Vol. 62, pp. 108-109.

Hodges, C.A., Palmert, M.R. & Drumm, M.L. (2008) Infertility in females with cystic fibrosis is multifactorial: evidence from mouse models. *Endocrinology*, Vol. 14, No. 6 (June 2008), pp. 2790-2797.

Hubert, D., Patrat, C., Guibert, J., Thiounn, N., Bienvenu, T., Viot, G., Jouannet, P. & Epelboin, S. (2006). Results of assisted reproductive technique in men with cystic fibrosis. Hum Reprod, Vol. 21, No. 5 (May 2006), pp. 1232-1236.

Hull, S.C. & Kass, N.E. (2000). Adults with cystic fibrosis and (in)fertility: how has the health care system responded? J Androl, Vol. 21, No. 6 (November 2000), pp. 809-813.

Jarzabek, K., Zbucka, M., Pepiński, W., Szamatowicz, J., Domitrz, J., Janica, J., Wołczyński, S. & Szamatowicz, M. (2004). Cystic fibrosis as a cause of infertility. *Reprod Biol*, Vol. 4, No. 2 (July 2004), pp. 119-29.

Jézéquel, P., Dubourg, C., Le Lannou, D., Odent, S., Le Gall, J.Y., Blayau, M., Le Treut, A. & David, V. (2000). Molecular screening of the CFTR gene in men with anomalies of the vas deferens: identification of three novel mutations. Mol Hum Reprod, Vol. 6, No. 12 (December 2000), pp. 1063-1067.

Johannesson, M., Gottlieb, C. & Hjelte, L. (1997a). Delayed puberty in girls with cystic fibrosis despite good clinical status. *Pediatrics*, Vol. 99, No. 1 (January 1997), pp. 29–34.

Johannesson, M., Bogdanovic, N., Nordqvist, A.C., Hjelte, L. & Schalling, M. (1997b). Cystic fibrosis mRNA expression in rat brain: cerebral cortex and medial preoptic area. *Neuroreport*, Vol. 8, No. 2 (January 1997), pp. 535–539.

Johannesson, M., Landgren, B.M., Csemiczky, G., Hjelte, L. & Gottlieb, C. (1998). Female patients with cystic fibrosis suffer from reproductive endocrinological disorders despite good clinical status. *Human Reproduction*, Vol.13, No.8, pp.2092–2097.

Kanavakis, E., Tzetis, M., Antoniadi, T., Pistofidis, G., Milligos, S. & Kattamis, C. (1998). Cystic fibrosis mutation screening in CBAVD patients and men with obstructive azoospermia or severe oligozoospermia. Mol Hum Reprod, Vol. 4, No. 4 (April 1998), pp. 333-337.

Kent, N.E. & Farquharson, D.F. (1993). Cystic fibrosis in pregnancy. *Can Med Assoc J*, Vol. 149, No. 6 (September 1993), pp. 809–813.

Kerem, B.-S., Rommens, J.M., Buchanan, J.A., Markiewicz, D., Cox, T.K., Chakravarti, A., Buchwald, M. & Tsui, L.-C. (1989). Identification of the cystic fibrosis gene: genetic analysis. *Science*, Vol. 245, pp. 1073–1080.

Keyeux, G., Rodas, C., Bienvenu, T., Garavito, P., Vidaud, D., Sanchez, D., Kaplan, J.C. & Aristizábal, G. (2003). CFTR mutations in patients from Colombia: implications for local and regional molecular diagnosis programs. *Hum Mutat*, Vol. 22, No. 3 (September 2003), pp. 259.

Knowton, R.G., Cohen-Haguenauer, O. ,Van Cong, N. (1985). A polymorphic DNA marker linked to Cystic Fibrosis is located on chromosome 7. *Nature*, pp. 318: 380-382.

Kopito, L.E., Kosasky, H.J. & Shwachman, H. (1973). Water and electrolytes in cervical mucus from patients with cystic fibrosis. *Fertil Steril*, Vol. 24, No. 7 (July 1973), pp. 512–516.

Kopel, F. (1972). Gastrointestinal manifestations of cystic fibrosis. *Gastroenterology*, Vol. 62, pp.483-491.

Landsteiner, K. (1905). Darmverschluss durch eingedicktes meconium. *Zentrabl allg Path*, Vol. 6, pp. 903.

Lay-Son, G., Puga, A., Astudillo, P. & Repetto, G.M.; Collaborative Group of the Chilean National Cystic Fibrosis Program. (2011). Cystic fibrosis in Chilean patients: Analysis of 36 common CFTR gene mutations. J Cyst Fibros, Vol. 10, No. 1 (January 2011), pp. 66-70.

Levy, H., Cannon, C.L., Asher, D., García, C., Cleveland, R.H., Pier, G.B., Knowles, M.R. & Colin, A.A. (2010). Lack of correlation between pulmonary disease and cystic fibrosis transmembrane conductance regulator dysfunction in cystic fibrosis: a case report. J Med Case Reports, Vol. 4, pp. 117.

Lewis-Jones, D.I., Gazvani, M.R. & Mountford, R. (2000). Cystic fibrosis in infertility: screening before assisted reproduction: opinion. Hum Reprod, Vol. 15, No. 11 (November 2000), pp. 2415-2417.

Li, C.Y., Jiang, L.Y., Chen, W.Y., Li, K., Sheng, H.Q., Ni, Y., Lu, J.X., Xu, W.X., Zhang, S.Y. & Shi, Q.X. (2010). CFTR is essential for sperm fertilizing capacity and is correlated with sperm quality in humans. *Hum Reprod*, Vol. 25, No. 2 (February 2010), pp. 317-27.

Ludwig, K.S. (1998). The Mayer–Rokitansky–Küster syndrome, an analysis of its morphology and embryology. Part II: Embryology. *Arch Gynecol Obstet*, Vol. 262, No. 1-2, pp. 27–42.

Mak, V., Zielenski, J., Tsui, L.C., Durie, P., Zini, A., Martin, S., Longley, T.B. & Jarvi, K.A. (1999). Proportion of cystic fibrosis gene mutations not detected by routine testing in men with obstructive azoospermia. JAMA, Vol. 281, No. 23 (June 1999), pp. 2217-2224.

Mak, V., Zielenski, J., Tsui, L.C., Durie, P., Zini, A., Martin, S., Longley, T.B. & Jarvi, K.A. (2000). Cystic fibrosis gene mutations and infertile men with primary testicular failure. *Human Reproduction*, Vol. 15, pp. 436-439.

McCallum, T.J., Milunsky, J.M., Cunningham, D.L., Harris, D.H., Maher, T.A. & Oates, R.D. (2000). Fertility in men with cystic fibrosis: an update on current surgical practices and outcomes. Chest, Vol. 118, No. 4 (October 2000), pp. 1059-1062.

Meizel, S. & Deamer, D.W. (1978). The pH of the hamster sperm acrosome. *J Histochem Cytochem*, Vol. 26, pp.98–105.

Mercier, B., Verlingue, C., Lissens, W., Silber, S.J., Novelli, G., Bonduelle, M., Audrézet, M.P. & Férec, C. (1995) Is congenital bilateral absence of vas deferens a primary form of cystic fibrosis? Analyses of the CFTR gene in 67 patients. *Am. J. Hum. Genet*, Vol. 56, No. 1 (January 1995), pp. 272-277.

Modi, A.C., Quittner, A.L., & Boyle, M.P. (2010). Assessing disease disclosure in adults with cystic fibrosis: the Adult Data for Understanding Lifestyle and Transitions (ADULT) survey Disclosure of disease in adults with cystic fibrosis. *BMC Pulm Med*, Vol. 10, pp. 46.

Morea, A., Cameran, M., Rebuffi, A.G., Marzenta, D., Marangon, O., Picci, L., Zacchello, F. & Scarpa, M. (2005). Gender-sensitive association of CFTR gene mutations and 5T allele emerging from a large survey on infertility. Mol Hum Reprod, Vol. 11, No. 8 (August 2005), pp 607-614.

Morral, N., Bertranpetit, J., Estivill, X., Nunes, V., Casals, T., Gimenez, J. *et al.* (1994). The origin of the major cystic fibrosis mutation in European populations. *Nature Genet*, Vol. 7, pp. 169-175.

Mousia-Arvanitakis, J. (1999). Cystic fibrosis and the pancreas: recent scientific advances. *J Clin Gastroenterol*, Vol. 29, No. 2, pp. 138-142.

Oermann, C.M. (2000). Fertility in patients with cystic fibrosis. Chest, Vol. 118, No. 4 (October 2000), pp. 893-894.

Pérez, M.M., Luna, M.C., Pivetta, O.H. & Keyeux, G. (2007). CFTR gene analysis in Latin American CF patients: heterogeneous origin and distribution of mutations across the continent. J Cyst Fibros, Vol. 6, No. 3 (May 2007), pp. 194-208.

Pieri, P.C., Missaglia, M.T., Roque, J.A., Moreira-Filho, C.A. & Hallak, J. (2007). Novel CFTR missense mutations in Brazilian patients with congenital absence of vas deferens: counselling issues. Clinics, Vol. 62, No. 4 (August 2007), pp. 385-390.

Poretsky, L. & Kalin, M.F. (1987). The gonadotropic function of insulin. Endocr Rev, Vol. 8, No. 2 (May 1987), pp. 132-141.

Quinton, P.M. (1983). Chloride impermeability in cystic fibrosis. *Nature*, Vol 301, pp. 421-422.

Quinton, P.M. (1990). Cystic fibrosis: a disease in electrolyte transport. *FASEB J*, Vol. 4, pp. 2709-2717.

Quinton, P.M. (1999). Physiological basis of cystic fibrosis: a historical perspective. *Physiol Rev*, Vol. 79, No. 1 (January 1999), pp. S3–S22.

Radpour, R., Gourabi, H., Dizaj, A.V., Holzgreve, W. & Zhong, X.Y. (2008). Genetic investigations of CFTR mutations in congenital absence of vas deferens, uterus, and vagina as a cause of infertility. J Androl, Vol. 29, No. 5 (September 2008), pp. 506-13.

Raskin, S., Phillips III, J.A., Krishnamani, M. R. S., Jones, C., Parker, R.A. & Rozov, T. et al. DNA analysis of cystic fibrosis in Brazil by directed PCR amplification from Guthrie cards. (1993). *Am J Med Gen*, Vol. 46, pp. 665-669.

Rave-Harel, N., Kerem, E., Nissim-Rafinia, M., Madjar, I., Goshen, R., Augarten, A., Rahat, A., Hurwitz, A., Darvasi, A. & Kerem, B. (1997). The molecular basis of partial penetrance of splicing mutations in cystic fibrosis. *Am. J. Hum. Genet*, Vol. 60, No. 1 (January 1997), pp. 87-94.

Reis, F.J.C. & Damasceno, N. (1998). *Jornal de Pediatria*, Vol. 74 (Supl.1), PP. 76-94.

Ribeiro, J.D., Ribeiro, M.A.G.O., Ribeiro, A.F. (2002). *Jornal de Pediatria*, Vol. 78, Supl.2. S173.

Riordan, J.R., Rommens, J.M., Kerem, B.-S.; Alon, N., Rozmahel, R., Grzelczak, Z., Zielenski, J., Lok, S., Plavsic, N., Chou, J.-L., Drumm, M.L., Iannuzzi, M.C., Collins, F.S. & Tsui, L.-C. (1989). Identification of the cystic fibrosis gene: cloning and characterization of complementary DNA. *Science*, Vol. 245, pp. 1066-1073.

Roberts, S. & Green, P. (2005). The sexual health of adolescents with cystic fibrosis. J R Soc Med, Vol. 98, No. Suppl 45, pp. 7-16.

Rodgers, H.C., Knox, A.J., Toplis, P.J. & Thornton, S.J. (2000). Successful pregnancy and birth after IVF in a woman with cystic fibrosis. *Hum Reprod*, Vol. 15, No. 10 (October 2000), pp. 2152-2153.

Reiter, E.O., Stern. R.C. & Root, A.W. (1981). The reproductive endocrine system in cystic fibrosis. I. Basal gonadotropin and sex steroid levels. *Am J Dis Child*, Vol. 135, No. 5 (May 1981), pp. 422-426.

Resta, R., Biesecker, B.B., Bennett, R.L., Blum, S., Hahn, S.E., Strecker, M.N. &Williams, J.L. (2006). A new definition of Genetic Counselling. National Society of Genetic Counsellors' Task Force report. *J Genet Couns*. Vol. 15. No. 2, pp. 77-83.

Rommens, J.M., Iannuzzi, M.C. & Kerem, B.-S. (1989). Identification of Cystic Fibrosis gene: chromosome walking and jumping. *Science*, Vol. 245, pp.1059-1065.

Razov, T. (1991).Mucoviscidose (Fibrose Cística do pâncreas). *Revisões Pediátricas*, Projeto Áries.

Santos, G.P., Domingos, M.T., Wittig, E.O., Ried, C.A. & Rosário, N.A (2005). Neonatal cystic fibrosis screening program in the state of Paraná: evolution 30 months after implementation. *Jornal de Pediatria*, Vol. 81(3), pp. 240-244.

Saraiva-Pereira, M.L., Fitarelli-Kiehl, M. & Sanseverino, M.T.V. (2011). A Genética na Fibrose Ciística. *Rev HCPA*, Vol. 31, No. 2, pp. 160-167.

Sawyer, S.M. (1996). Reproductive and sexual health in adolescents with cystic fibrosis. *BMJ*, Vol. 313, pp. 1095-1096.

Sawyer, S.M., Farrant, B., Cerritelli, B. & Wilson, J. (2005). A survey of sexual and reproductive health in men with cystic fibrosis: new challenges for adolescent and adult services. Thorax, Vol. 60, No. 4 (April 2005, pp. 326-330.

Shwachman, H. & Kulesvecki, L.L. (1958). Long term study of 105 patients with cystic fibrosis: Studies made over a five to fourteen year period. *Am J Dis Child*, Vol. 96, pp. 6-15.

Shwachman, H., Redmond, A., Khaw, K.T.(1970). Studies in cystic fibrosis. Report of 130 patients diagnosed under 3 months of age over a 20 year period. *Pediatrics*, Vol.46, pp. 335.

Silber, S.J., Nagy, Z.P., Liu, J., Godoy, H., Devroey, P. & Van Steirteghem, A.C. (1994). Conventional in-vitro fertilization versus intracytoplasmic sperm injection for patients requiring microsurgical sperm aspiration. *Hum Reprod*, Vol. 9, No. 9 (September 1994), pp. 1705-1709.

Sokol, R.Z. (2001). Infertility in men with cystic fibrosis. *Curr Opin Pulm Med*, Vol. 7, No. 6 (November 2001), pp. 421-426.

Stead, R.J., Hodson, M.E., Batten, J.C., Adams, J. & Jacobs, H.S. (1987). Amenorrhoea in cystic fibrosis. *Clin Endocrinol*, Vol. 26, pp. 187–195.

Stuppia, L., Antonucci, I., Binni, F., Brandi, A., Grifone, N., Colosimo, A., De Santo, M., Gatta, V., Gelli, G., Guida, V., Majore, S., Calabrese, G., Palka, C., Ravani, A., Rinaldi, R., Tiboni, G.M., Ballone, E., Venturoli, A., Ferlini, A., Torrente, I., Grammatico, P., Calzolari, E. & Dallapiccola, B. (2005). Screening of mutations in the CFTR gene in 1195 couples entering assisted reproduction technique programs. Eur J Hum Genet, Vol. 13, No. 8 (August 2005), pp. 959-964.

Timmreck, L.S., Gray, M.R., Handelin, B., Allito, B., Rohlfs, E., Davis, A.J., Gidwani, G. & Reindollar, R.H. (2003). Analysis of cystic fibrosis transmembrane conductance regulator gene mutations in patients with congenital absence of the uterus and vagina. *Am J Med Genet*, Vol. 120A, No. 1 (July 2003), pp. 72–76.

Tizzano, E.F., Silver, M.M., Chitayat, D., Benichou, J.C. & Buchwald, M. (1994). Differential cellular expression of cystic fibrosis transmembrane regulator in human reproductive tissues. Clues for the infertility in patients with cystic fibrosis. *Am J Pathol*, Vol. 144, pp. 906–914.

Tummler, B., & Kiewitz, C. Cystic fibrosis: an inherited susceptibility to bacterial respiratory infections.(1999). *Mol Med Today*, Vol. 5, No. 8, pp. 351-358.

Uzun, S., Gökçe, S. & Wagner, K. (2005). Cystic fibrosis transmembrane conductance regulator gene mutations in infertile males with congenital bilateral absence of the vas deferens. Tohoku J Exp Med, Vol. 207, No. 4 (December 2005), pp. 279-285.

Van der Ven, K., Messer, L., Van der Ven, H., Jeyendran, R.S. & Ober, C. (1996). Cystic fibrosis mutation screening in healthy men with reduced sperm quality. *Hum Reprod*, Vol. 11, No. 3, pp. 513-517.

Wang, X.F., Zhou, C.X., Shi, Q.X., Yuan, Y.Y., Yu, M.K., Ajonuma, L.C., Ho, L.S., Lo, P.S., Tsang, L.S., Liu, Y., Lam, S.Y., Chan, L.N., Zhao, W.C., Chung, Y.W. & Chan, H.C. (2003). Involvement of CFTR in uterine bicarbonate secretion and the fertilizing capacity of sperm. *Nature Cell Biol* Vol. 5, No. 10 (October 2003), pp. 902–906.

Williams, C., Mayall, E.S., Williamson, R., Hirsh, A. & Cookson, H. (1993). A report on CF carrier frequency among men with infertility owing to congenital absence of the vas deferens. J Med Genet, Vol. 30, No. 11 (November 1993), pp. 973.

Wong, P.Y. (1998). CFTR gene and male fertility. Mol Hum Reprod, Vol. 4, No. 2 (February 1998), pp. 107-110.

Xu, W.M., Shi, Q.X., Chen, W.Y., Zhou, C.X., Ni, Y., Rowlands, D.K., Yi Liu, G., Zhu, H., Ma, Z.G., Wang, X.F., Chen, Z.H., Zhou, S.C., Dong, H.S., Zhang, X.H., Chung, Y.W., Yuan, Y.Y., Yang, W.X. & Chan, H.C. (2007). Cystic fibrosis transmembrane conductance regulator is vital to sperm fertilizing capacity and male fertility. *Proc Natl Acad Sci USA*, Vol. 104, No. 23, pp. 9816-9821.

Zeng, Y., Clark, E.N. & Florman, H.M (1995). Sperm membrane potential: hyperpolarisation during capacitation regulates zona pellucida-dependent acrosomal secretion. *Developmental Biology*, Vol. 171, No. 2, pp. 554-563.

Zheng, X.Y., Chen, G.A. & Wang, H.Y. (2004). Expression of cystic fibrosis transmembrane conductance regulator in human endometrium. *Hum Reprod*, Vol. 19, No. 12 (December 2004), pp. 2933– 2941.

Zielenski, J. & Tsui, L.C. (1995). Cystic fibrosis: genotypic and phenotypic variations. Annu Rev Genet, Vol. 29, pp. 777-807.

Zielenski, J. Genotype and phenotype in cystic fibrosis. (2000). *Respiration*, No. 67, pp. 117-133.

3

Radiological Features of Cystic Fibrosis

Iara Maria Sequeiros and Nabil A. Jarad
University Hospitals Bristol NHS Foundation Trust
United Kingdom

1. Introduction

With patients with cystic fibrosis (CF) living longer and reaching adulthood, conditions before not frequently encountered now play a larger role in the spectrum of CF related symptoms and complaints which continue to challenge clinicians in both outpatient and acute settings. It is in this context that the radiologist and different radiological imaging modalities can aid the clinician in order to establish an accurate diagnosis and steer appropriate treatment. In this chapter, we present a comprehensive review of common and not so common radiological features of both pulmonary and extra-pulmonary manifestations of CF.

With a huge variety of scans available at one's finger tips, or to be more precise, at the end of an electronic request form, it is vital that clinicians are familiar with the different existing imaging modalities, what information to expect from each one of them and the most appropriate scan to request to answer the specific clinical question, taking into consideration the patient's characteristics and needs- in other words, how to make best use of their Radiology Department. In this way, the required information can be obtained most rapidly and efficiently by using the correct test or tests performed in the correct order.

Chest radiographs are usually the exam of choice for the initial assessment and sequential follow-up of pulmonary disease in adult CF patients. It employs a very small dose of ionizing radiation and can be of great value in the detection of new infiltrates in acute infective exacerbations or diagnosing complications such as a pneumothorax. Plain radiography is also much used in patients complaining of acute abdominal pain, although findings can be non-specific and patients may require further imaging to characterize the abdominal pathology. An abdominal radiograph delivers a higher radiation dose and therefore should not be performed unnecessarily. Barium studies are not commonly used and it is believed that barium may cause obstruction in CF patients due to the thick intraluminal secretions. On the other hand, hypertonic oral contrast is used in some patients for the treatment of distal intestinal obstructive disease (DIOS). Air and contrast enemas continue to be used for the reduction of intussusception.

Ultrasound imaging does not carry any radiation hazard and has the added advantage of being relatively cheap and readily available. It can be useful in the chest in the assessment of pleural effusion or collection, but is most valuable for the evaluation of abdominal organs (e.g. liver, gallbladder, kidneys, spleen) and in patients with acute abdominal pain or suspected bowel pathology, such as DIOS, appendicitis or intussusception. The disadvantage of this modality is that it is completely operator dependent and sometimes images obtained are suboptimal due to patient related factors, such as obesity or overlying distended bowel gas.

Cross-sectional imaging techniques include computed tomography (CT) and magnetic resonance imaging (MRI). CT delivers high radiation – a chest CT is equivalent to over 200 chest radiographs in terms of radiation dose – and this needs to be considered, especially when dealing with young individuals such as CF patients. Chest CT imaging will be superior to plain radiograph in the assessment of initial or mild lung disease, in cases of poor clinical response when complications are suspected such as atypical mycobacteria infection and in pre-transplant evaluation. With the modern multi-detector CT scanners, the whole chest can be scanned in 10 to 20 seconds during a single breath-hold and therefore the exam is usually well tolerated even by the most breathless patient.

Much confusion is still seen when physicians request lung high resolution computed tomography (HRCT). The term high resolution implies a better quality scan, but in reality refers to 12 to 20 incremental ultra-thin 1 or 1.5mm thick image slices of the lung that are obtained at evenly spaced intervals through the chest and is indicated for the evaluation of diffuse interstitial or bronchial disease. It does not scan the whole volume of the chest and therefore is not appropriate for the assessment of lung nodules, malignancy, mediastinal lymphadenopathy or pleural disease, which are only fully imaged with a full lung volume spiral scan. HRCT increases the radiation dose delivered and should be limited to specific patients.

Abdominal CT imaging can be of great aid in the patient with acute abdominal pain in which the initial ultrasound scan was non-diagnostic. It is the scan of choice for the evaluation of the pancreas and therefore pancreatitis. MRI continues to be very expensive and not as accessible as CT. Its main indication is the assessment of hepatobiliary disease and cholangiopancreatography (MRCP). It is, as ultrasound, radiation free, but scans are sometimes prolonged and not always tolerated by those who are claustrophobic.

2. Pre-natal imaging

The use of radiological imaging in the aid of pre-natal diagnosis of CF and post-natal complications is well documented. Foetuses with CF have been associated with hyperechogenic foetal bowel detected by ultrasound during the second and third trimesters of pregnancy. Bowel is considered hyperechogenic if its echogenicity (brightness) is equal to or greater than that of the adjacent iliac bone (Al-Kouatly et al., 2001). Although this can be a normal finding, identified in 0.1-1.8% of foetuses, the risk of diagnosis of CF is greater if associated with bowel dilatation or the absence of an identifiable gallbladder (Hertzberg et al., 1996; Scotet et al., 2002).

3. The nose and sinuses

The upper airways are very frequently affected in CF, with over 75% of patients reporting some kind of sinus or nasal symptom such as nasal or sinus obstruction, nasal discharge, post-nasal drip and facial pain (Cepero et al., 1987). Sinusitis should be considered in all CF patients with nasal symptoms. A common cold is often suspected and can occur in CF patients, but when symptoms affect the CF patient only and no other member of the family, sinusitis is likely to be the cause. There is poor correlation between the severity of symptoms and imaging findings (Sakano et al., 2007). Indications for CT imaging include evaluation of the severity of the disease and pre-operative evaluation.

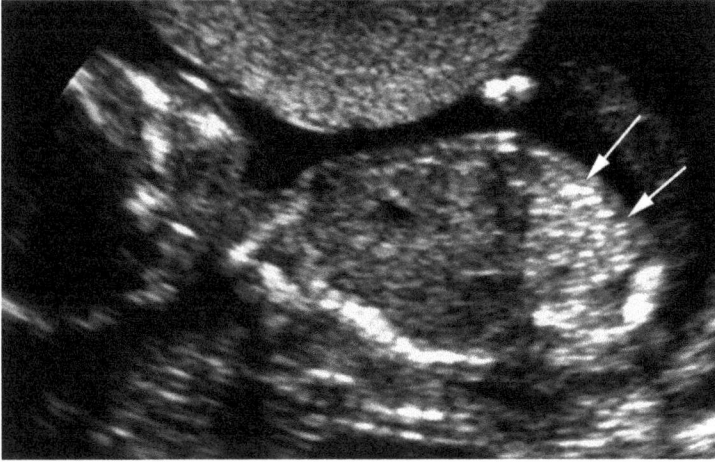

Fig. 1. Sagittal ultrasound view of a foetus with hyperechogenic bowel (arrows).

Imaging will reveal abnormalities even if not clinically manifested, such as small hypoplasic sinuses - often adult CF patients have no frontal sinus cavity - thickened nasal turbinates and thickened mucosa of the sinuses. Chronic inflammation and thickening of the mucosa of the nasal cavities and sinuses result in formation of inflammatory polyps and the accumulation of mucus in obstructed sinuses. Many patients undergo surgery to remove polyps and enlarge the outlet of obstructed sinuses, but relief tends to be temporary due to the recurrent nature of the disease.

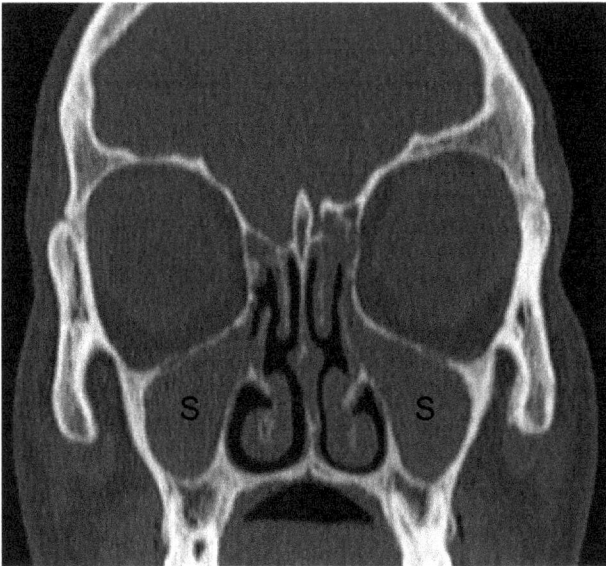

Fig. 2. Coronal CT image at the level of the nasal cavities showing complete opacification of the maxillary sinuses (S) in a case of recurrent sinusitis.

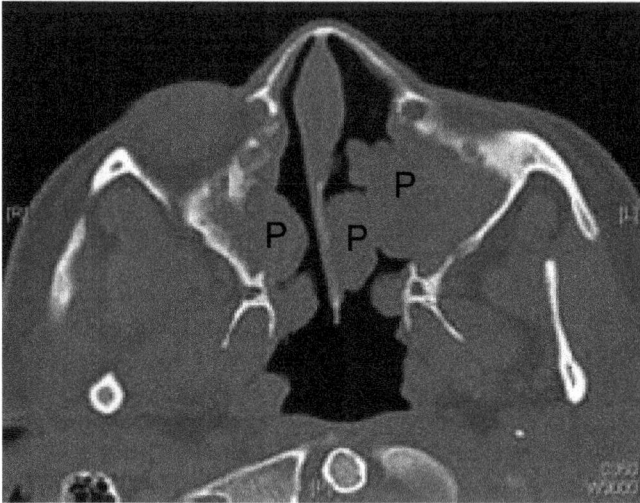

Fig. 3. Axial CT image at the level of the nasal cavities showing opacification of the maxillary sinuses and rounded densities in the nasal cavities (P) in a severe case of nasal polyposis.

4. Pulmonary manifestations

4.1 Bronchiectasis

Repeated chest infections are the hallmark of CF. These are usually associated with *Pseudomonas aeruginosa* or *Staphylococcus aureus* infection and clinically manifested by increased cough, sputum production, breathlessness and fatigue (Marshall, 2004). Classically CF initially affects the upper lobes, but severe cases will show diffuse bilateral disease affecting all of the lungs. Chest radiographs will reveal degrees of hyperinflation, dilated bronchi with thickened walls (cylindrical or cystic bronchiectasis) associated with well defined areas of air space opacification, as in lobar pneumonias, or nodules due to mucoid impaction, atelectasis, cavities and hilar lymphadenopathy. Pneumothorax is also frequently seen and can be recurrent (Hansell et al., 2005).

Chest radiographs are generally sufficient for regular clinical management and usually there is little visible radiographic change associated with clinical exacerbations. On the other hand it is now well established that CT imaging can give valuable information for the monitoring of disease progression and assessment of treatment response. Studies have shown a close relationship between HRCT findings and clinical and pulmonary functional evaluation of patients (Hansell et al., 2005). More severe cases may also show signs of right heart failure with pulmonary arterial hypertension and cor pulmonale.

4.2 Allergic bronchopulmonary aspergillosis

In patients with increased wheeze and asthma-type symptoms, and chest symptoms failing to improve despite antibiotic treatment, allergic bronchopulmonary aspergillosis (ABPA) should be suspected. Imaging can reveal transient and recurring areas of consolidation on chest radiographs, often due to atelectasis from mucoid plugging and bronchial obstruction, which subsequently improve after steroid therapy. Evaluation of ABPA in patients with CF is limited as imaging findings that are used to establish the diagnosis of ABPA in patients with asthma are common in patients with CF (Hansell et al., 2005).

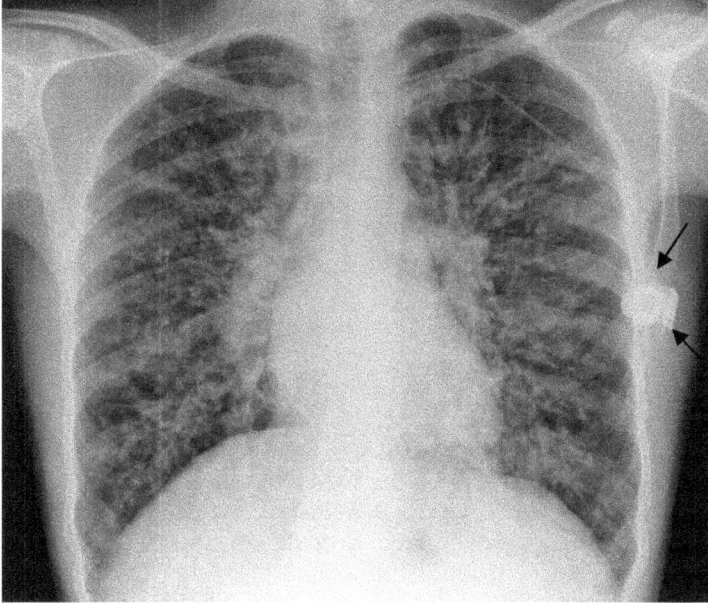

Fig. 4. Chest radiograph of a CF patient with hyperinflated lungs and severe bilateral and diffuse bronchiectasis seen as ring shadows and tram-track opacities that converge to the lung hila, which correspond to dilated thick walled bronchi. Note the port-a-cath device in the left chest wall and catheter in the distal superior vena cava used for the administration of intravenous antibiotics (arrows).

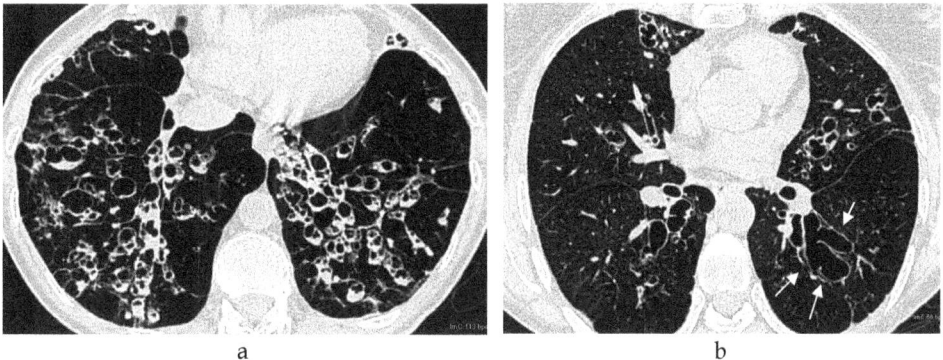

a   b

Fig. 5. Lung axial CT images demonstrating classic rounded cystic bronchiectasis throughout both lungs (fig. 5a) and varicose type bronchiectasis (arrows) (fig. 5b). The bronchi are dilated, thick walled and some contain mucus.

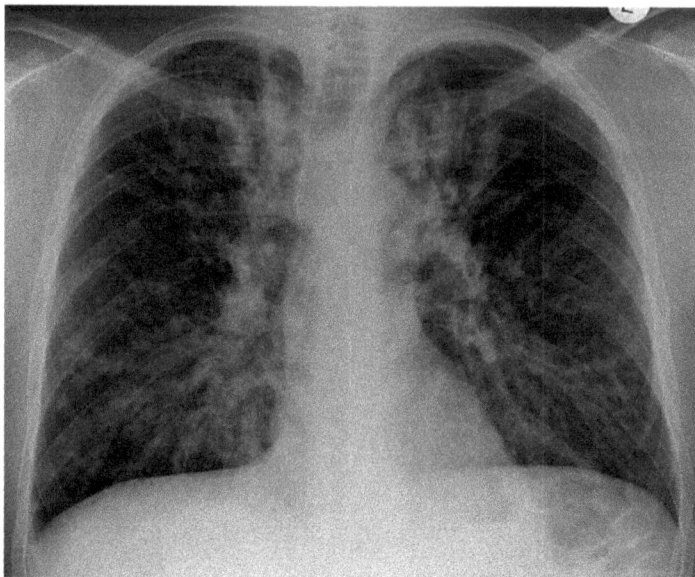

Fig. 6. Chest radiograph of CF patient with ABPA. There are bilateral widespread bronchiectasis, but the upper lobe bronchi are filled with mucus which was a new feature in comparison to previous radiographs. Clinical evaluation and elevated serum IgE and positive serum precipitins to Aspergillus confirmed the diagnosis of ABPA which improved with steroid treatment.

4.3 Non-tuberculous mycobacteria

Non-tuberculous (atypical) mycobacteria (NTBM) are increasingly isolated from CF patient's airways, although not always considered clinically significant. It is estimated that the lungs of 10% of adult CF patients are infected with NTBM. These bacteria consist of a range of organisms that differ in their virulence. Common varieties that infect CF lungs include *Mycobacterium fortuitum*, *Mycobacterium kansasii*, *Mycobacterium xenopi*, *Mycobacterium avium intracellulare* and *Mycobacterium cheloni* (*Mycobacteria abscessus*). *Mycobacterium abscessus* is especially important due to its high virulence, resistance to treatment and being one of the relative contra-indications for lung transplant.

Given the fact that chest symptoms in CF are common principally due to bronchiectatic lungs that are chronically infected with CF bacteria (mainly *P. aeruginosa*), determining the pathogenicity of NTBM is often challenging. In addition, the treatment of these bacteria is difficult with high rates of re-infection and recurrence, and long duration of treatment (12 to 18 months) that uses a combination of antibiotics often containing rifampicin, which is known to induce liver enzymes and therefore interferes with many CF drugs (antibiotics, insulin and contraceptive agents). For all these reasons, CF physicians seek confirmation of the pathogenesis of atypical mycobacteria prior to treatment. Mycobacteria is considered to play a role if the same species grows in the sputum on more than one occasion and symptoms persist after treating *P. aeruginosa*. Chest radiology using HRCT scans is therefore called upon to increase the degree of diagnostic certainty.

HRCT signs are often subtle and include one or more of the following: small centrilobular nodules and nodular changes in the periphery of the lungs, tree-in-bud opacities, new lung abscesses (Field et al., 2004; Olivier et al., 2003). Presence of one of more of these radiological signs together with chest and systemic symptoms that do not respond to anti-pseudomonas antibiotics would justify the start of treatment. Repeating the HRCT scan in 3 to 4 months after commencing the treatment is useful in showing radiological response.

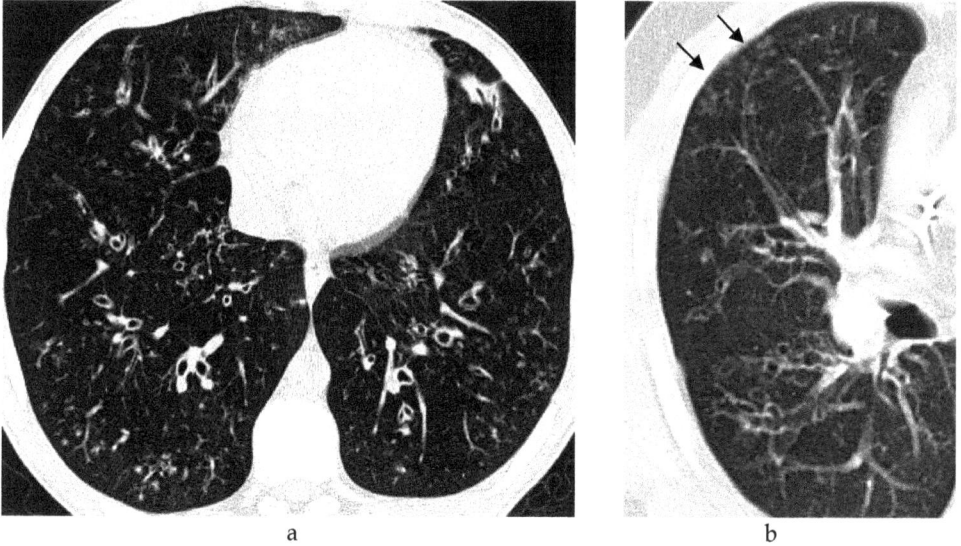

a   b

Fig. 7. Lung axial CT image showing bronchiectasis, ground-glass and tree-in-bud opacities in both lung bases associated with non-tuberculous mycobacteria infection (fig. 7a). Close-up of tree-in-bud in the right middle lobe (arrows) (fig. 7b).

5. Abdominal manifestations

5.1 The pancreas

Autolysis of the pancreas due to viscous pancreatic enzymes and obstructed pancreatic ducts is known to start during intra-uterine life (Sturgess, 1984). This leads to fibrosis, atrophy and replacement of the pancreas by fat (Sequeiros et al., 2010) which clinically results in exocrine pancreatic insufficiency and malabsorption in up to 90% of patients (Rosenstein et al., 1998).

Pancreatitis can be the first manifestation of CF and is a rare complication among patients with CF with a reported incidence of approximately 1.24%. It mainly occurs during adolescence and young adulthood and is much more common among patients with preserved pancreatic tissue (De Boeck et al., 2005) and therefore considered pancreatic sufficient (10.3% of cases), but it can also occur among patients with pancreatic insufficiency (0.5% of cases). Pancreatitis is an important differential diagnosis that should be considered in the context of a CF patient presenting with acute abdominal pain.

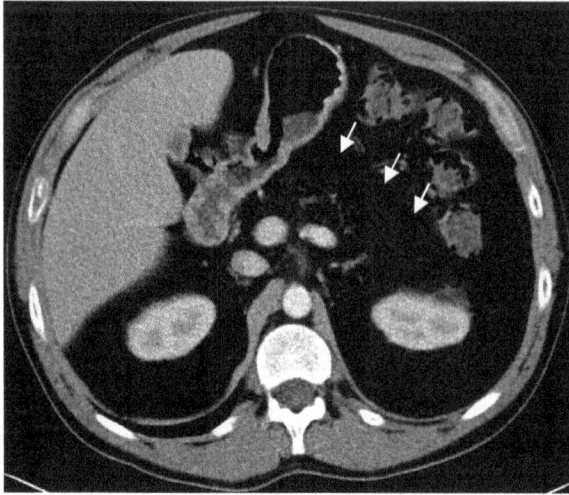

Fig. 8. Abdominal axial CT image of a CF patient at the level of the splenic vein showing the pancreas completely substituted by fat (arrows).

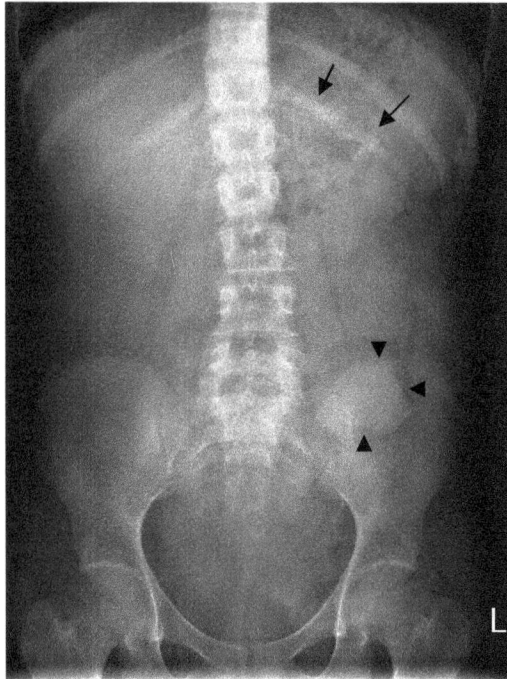

Fig. 9. Radiograph of the abdomen shows typical pancreatic calcifications secondary to CF related chronic pancreatitis in the left upper quadrant adjacent to the spine (arrows). Note the shadow in the left iliac fossa representing an ileostomy due to surgical management of previous bowel obstruction (arrow heads).

Pancreatic cysts are a relatively common finding in CF and can vary in size and number. Rarely, cysts can replace the entire pancreas in a condition called pancreatic cystosis, which can cause pain through mass effect (van Rijn et al., 2007). In such cases, surgical resection of the pancreas may be necessary.

5.2 Hepatobiliary disease

Hepatobiliary manifestations are common in CF and include fatty infiltration of the liver (steatosis), focal biliary cirrhosis with portal hypertension, microgallbladder and gallstones. Patients are more frequently asymptomatic, but liver disease is the second most common cause of death in CF (2.2% of deaths) and approximately 6-8% of individuals with CF have potentially fatal liver disease that requires liver transplantation (Genyk et al., 2001). It is thought to be a consequence of thickened secretions and abnormal bile flow within the liver causing bile duct obstruction. Signs of liver disease usually develop before or at puberty (Feigelson et al., 1993).

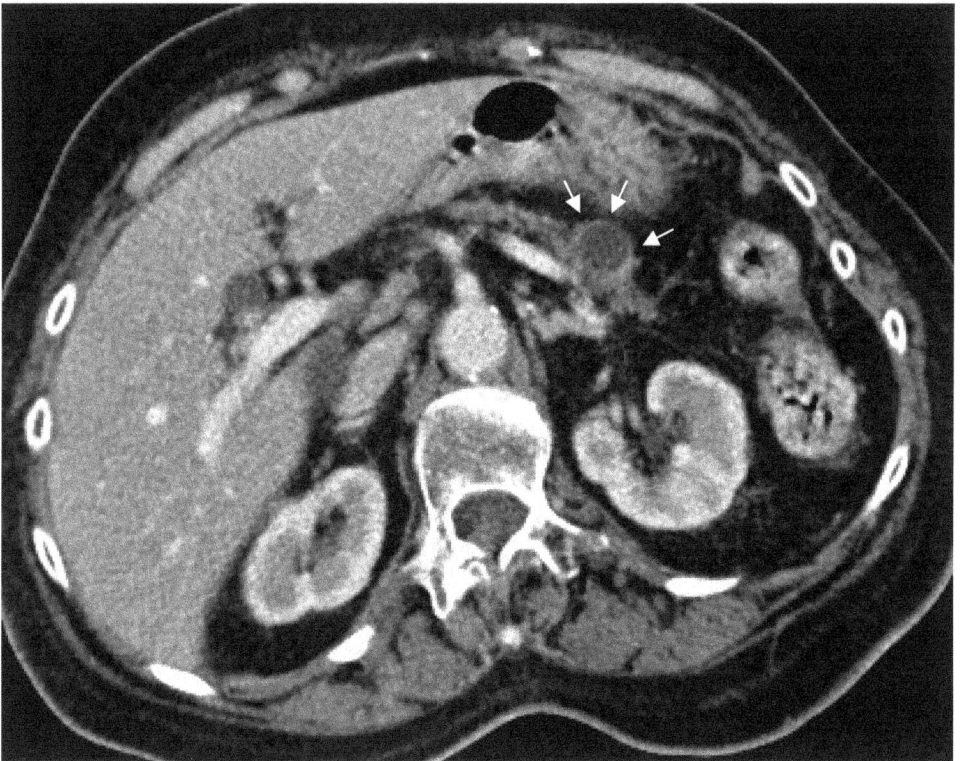

Fig. 10. Abdominal axial CT image at the level of the pancreas showing a small cyst in the tail of the pancreas (arrows).

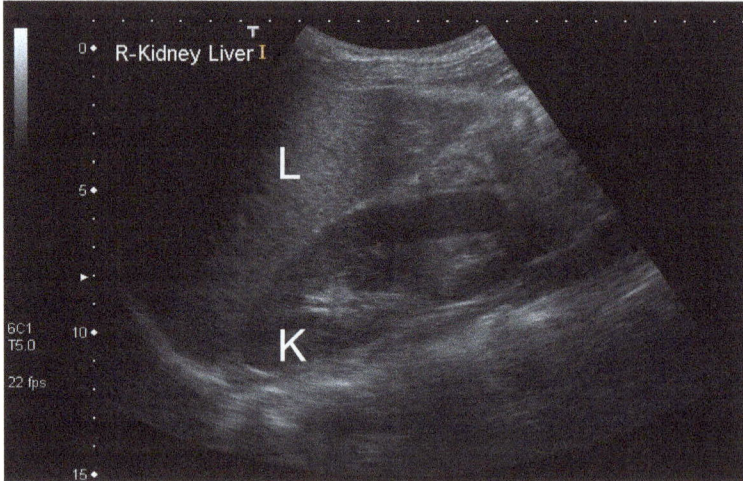

Fig. 11. Abdominal ultrasound image demonstrating echogenic (bright) liver due to diffuse fatty infiltration (L). A normal liver would look as dark as the adjacent right kidney (K).

Biliary calculi are present in 4-12% of patients. These are most commonly composed of cholesterol and thought to be a consequence of pancreatic insufficiency and the production of thick lithogenic bile (Agrons et al., 1996).

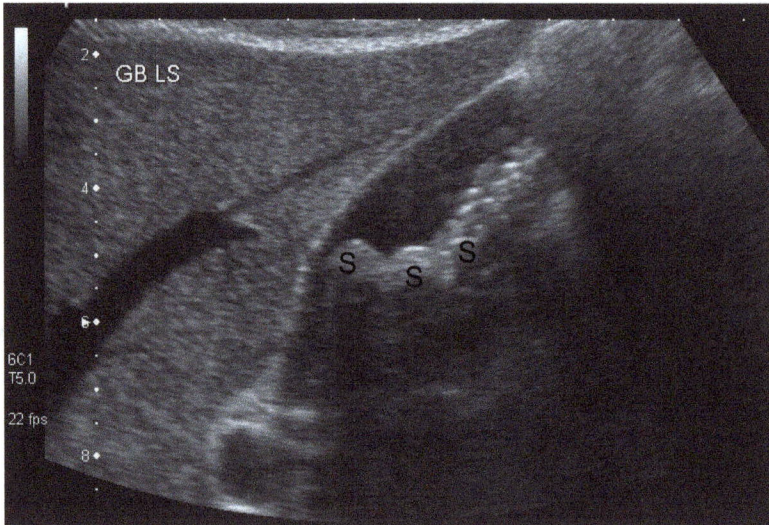

Fig. 12. Abdominal ultrasound image of a thin walled, non complicated gallbladder containing several stones (S).

Splenomegaly as a result of portal hypertension can be seen as massive enlargement of the spleen causing pain, dyspnoea and signs of hypersplenism and sometimes complicated with splenic infarcts or subcapsular haematomas.

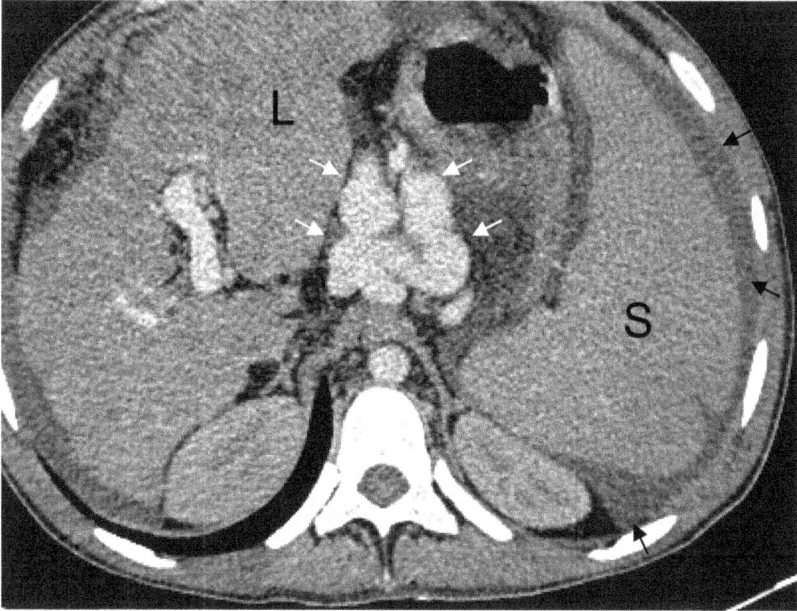

Fig. 13. Axial CT image of the abdomen showing a lobulated, macronodular cirrhotic liver (L), ascites (black arrows), splenomegaly (S) and varices (white arrows) due to portal hypertension.

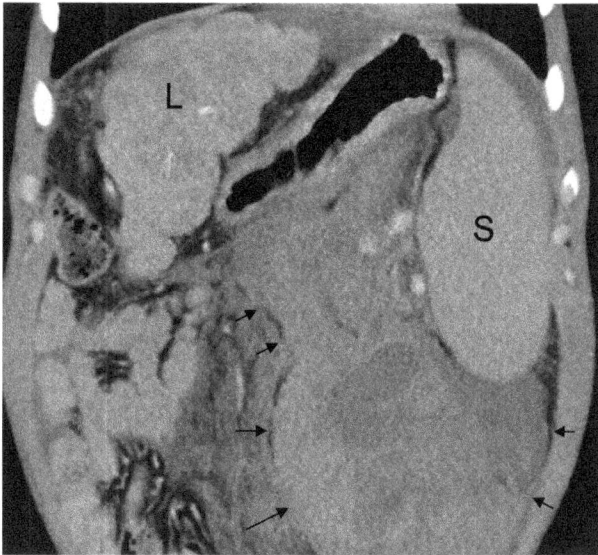

Fig. 14. Coronal CT image of the abdomen showing a large fatal spontaneous splenic haematoma (arrows) in a CF patient with severe portal hypertension and splenomegaly (S). Note the lobulated macronodular cirrhotic liver (L).

5.3 Meconium ileus

Bowel blockage of the newborn or meconium ileus is seen in 15-20% of neonates with CF and 25% of infants with meconium ileus prove to have CF (Hen et al., 1980). Meconium is composed of materials swallowed by the foetus during pregnancy, such as intestinal epithelial cells, mucus and amniotic fluid. In CF, mucus glands of the small intestine produce thick secretions and therefore the meconium sometimes becomes abnormally sticky and inspissated, causing a mechanical obstruction within the segment of the ileum. Classically, above the obstruction the bowel is greatly distended with fluid content, while below this level, the distal ileum and colon are collapsed. Soon after birth, usually in 24 to 48 hours, the newborn will present with abdominal distension and vomiting.

5.4 Distal intestinal obstructive syndrome

Distal intestinal obstructive syndrome or DIOS is the equivalent of meconium ileus in adults. It affects up to 15% of CF patients as a result of thickened intraluminal secretions, undigested food secondary to exocrine pancreatic insufficiency and impaired bowel motility (Speck & Charles, 2008). Patients complain of recurrent episodes of abdominal pain and distension, nausea and vomiting. Ultrasound imaging will reveal ditlated loops of small bowel containing "swirling" intraluminal echogenic material without forward propulsion motion in keeping with obstruction. Abdominal radiograph and CT show dilated small bowel loops with fluid levels and faecal material within the small bowel ("small bowel faeces").

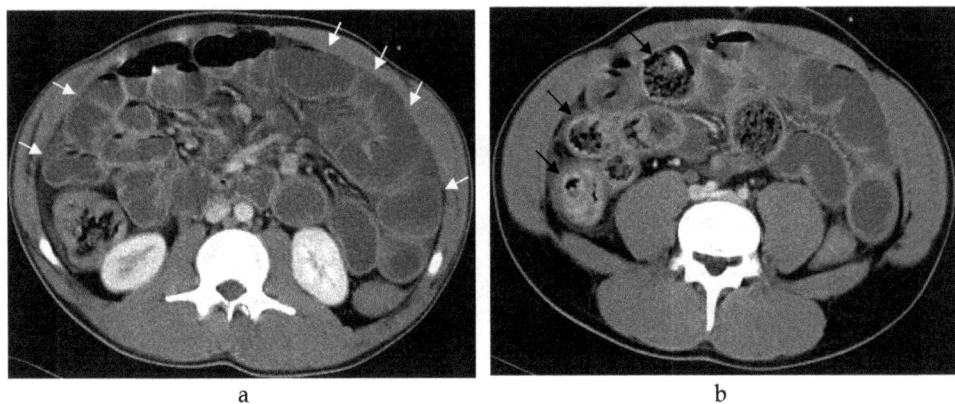

a   b

Fig. 15. Axial CT scan of the abdomen of CF patient with acute abdominal obstruction after weeks of stopping to take exocrine pancreatic enzymes. Images show dilated loops of small bowel containing fluid (white arrows) (fig. 14a) and faecal material within the distal ileum in the right iliac fossa (black arrows) (fig. 14 b) - "small bowel faeces". Surgical intervention was necessary and revealed an obstructed ileum with inspissated secretions and undigested food.

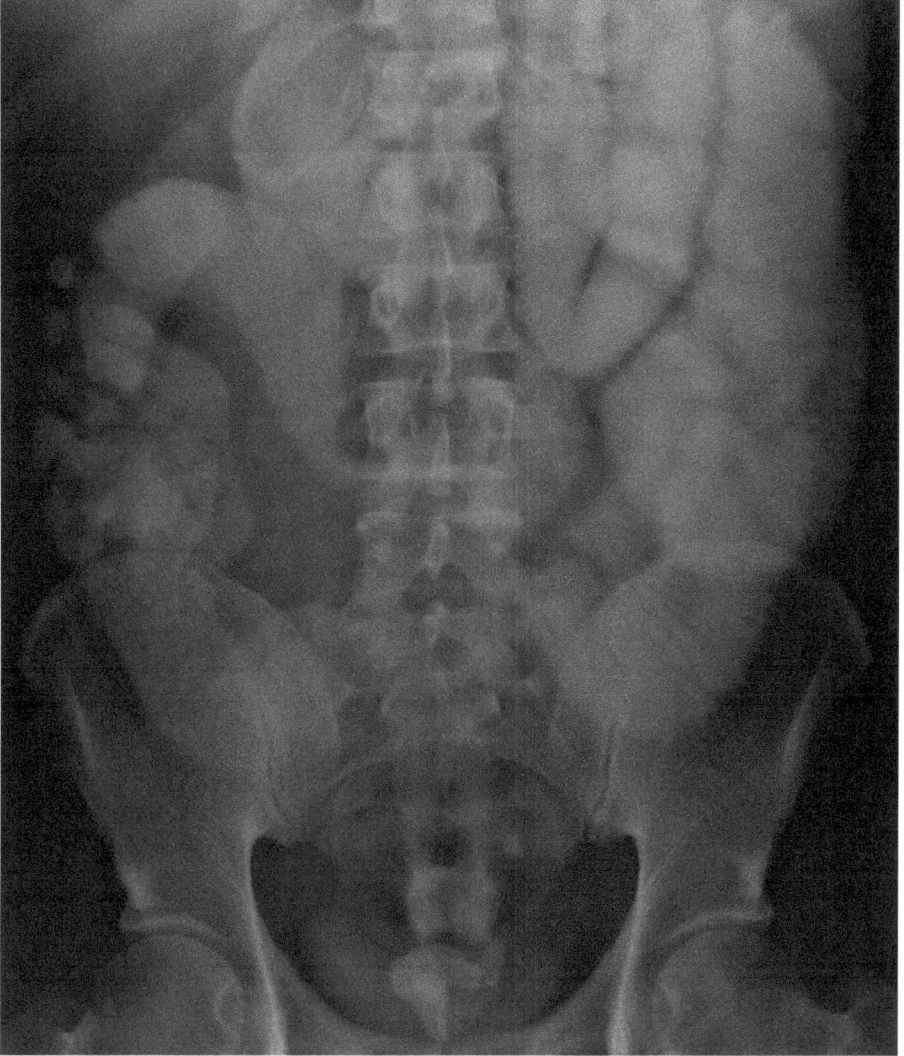

Fig. 16. CF patient with diagnosed DIOS managed clinically with hydration and oral hypertonic solution. Abdominal radiograph shows dilated loops of small bowel filled with ingested oral Gastrografin contrast agent.

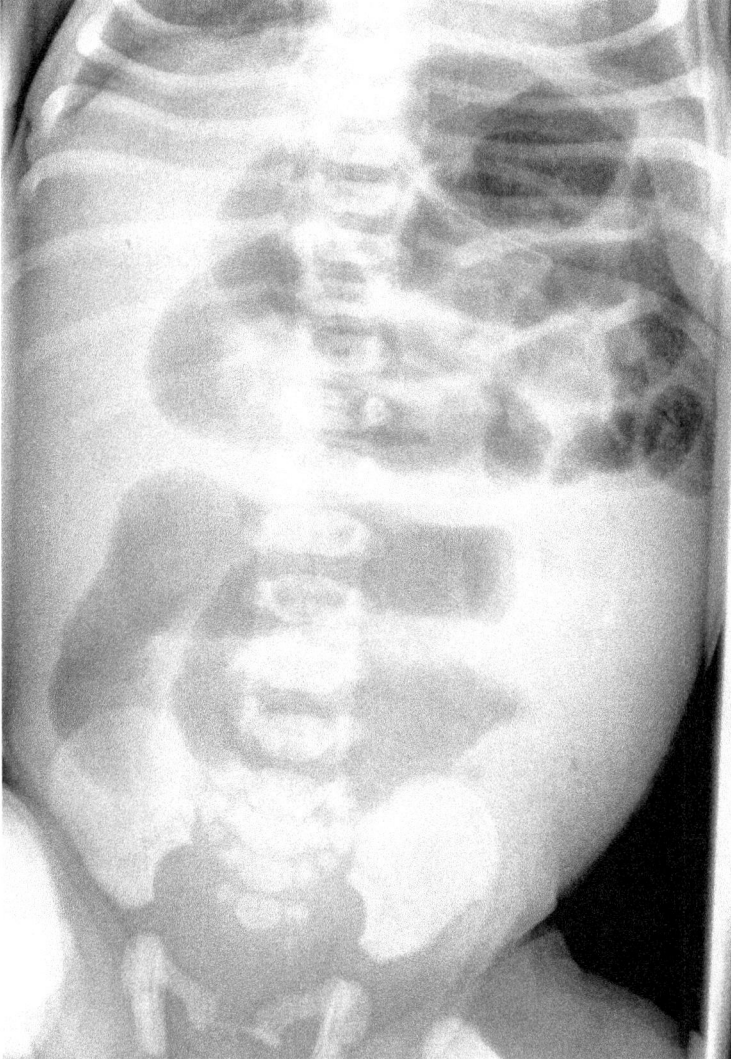

Fig. 17. Abdominal radiograph showing a pre-term infant with meconium ileus who was subsequently diagnosed with CF. He presented with marked abdominal distension at 3 days of life. There are markedly dilated loops of small bowel and no air is seen in the colon or rectum.

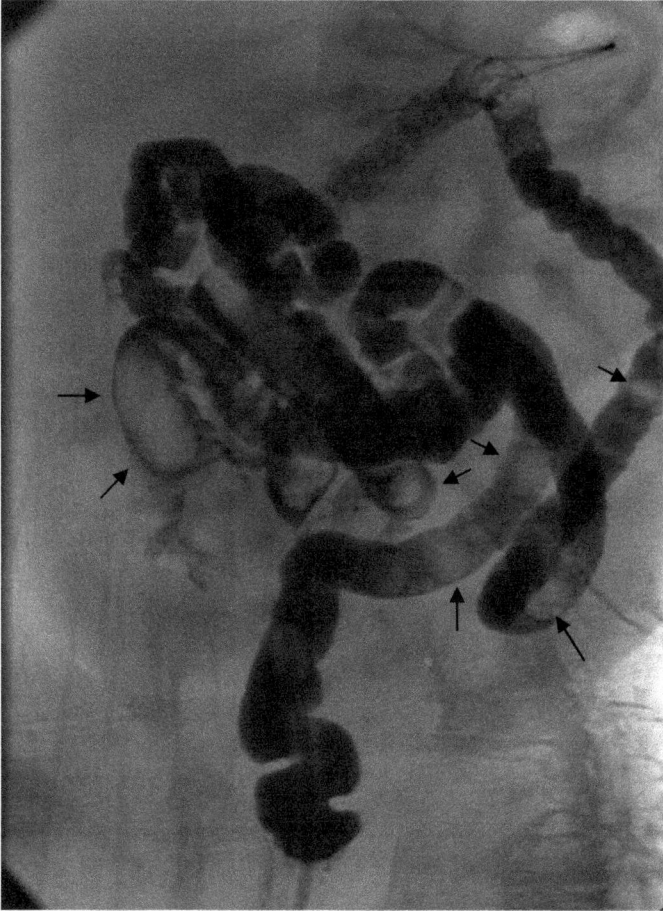

Fig. 18. Contrast enema in a neonate infant with meconium ileus. As is typical of the condition, the colon is small secondary to distal ileal obstruction and there is also small bowel dilatation. There are filling defects in the colon and terminal ileum representing meconium pellets (arrows).

5.5 Intussusception

Intussusception is more common in CF patients than in the general population and is seen in 1% of paediatric patients. It is rare in adulthood and comprises 5% of all intussusceptions and 1% of bowel obstructions (Nash et al., 2011). Intussusception can cause similar symptoms of acute abdominal pain as DIOS and is an important differential diagnosis that should be considered in acute obstruction as it may require surgical intervention, whilst DIOS is often managed non-surgically with hydration and oral hypertonic solutions (Speck & Charles, 2008). Intraluminal inspissated mucus, undigested food or enlarged lymphoid follicles can initiate an intussusception. Imaging reveals a bowel-within-bowel configuration which is pathognomonic of the condition (Gayer et al., 1998).

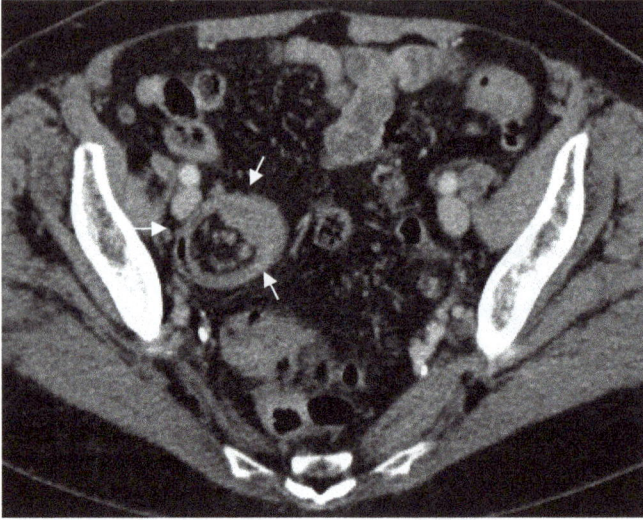

Fig. 19. Axial CT scan of the abdomen at the level of the iliac bones. Imaging reveals rounded structure with classic "bowel-within-bowel" configuration in the right iliac fossa in keeping with intussusception (arrows).

5.6 Fibrosing colonopathy

Fibrosing colonopathy is characterised clinically by right iliac fossa pain, where a thickened loop of bowel can sometimes be felt on clinical examination. It has been reported in association with children prescribed high strength pancreatic enzyme supplements, although the aetiology is not completely clear. Imaging has a limited role demonstrating non-specific large bowel wall thickening and final diagnosis is usually obtained with histology, which depicts submucosal fibrosis (Stacey et al., 1997).

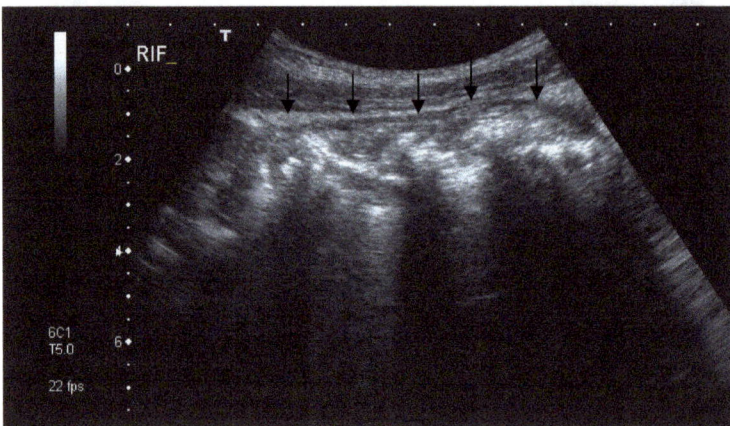

Fig. 20. Ultrasound image of the right iliac fossa showing a thick walled ascending colon (arrows) in a symptomatic CF patient.

5.7 Appendicitis

Appendicitis is relatively uncommon in CF, with a reported incidence of 1-2% compared to 7% in the general population. The cause of this is thought to be a protective effect of inspissated secretions against appendicitis (McCarthy et al., 1984). Although uncommon, it should always be considered in acute abdominal pain as a delayed diagnosis could result in subsequent rupture and abscess formation. Imaging features are similar to those seen in the general population.

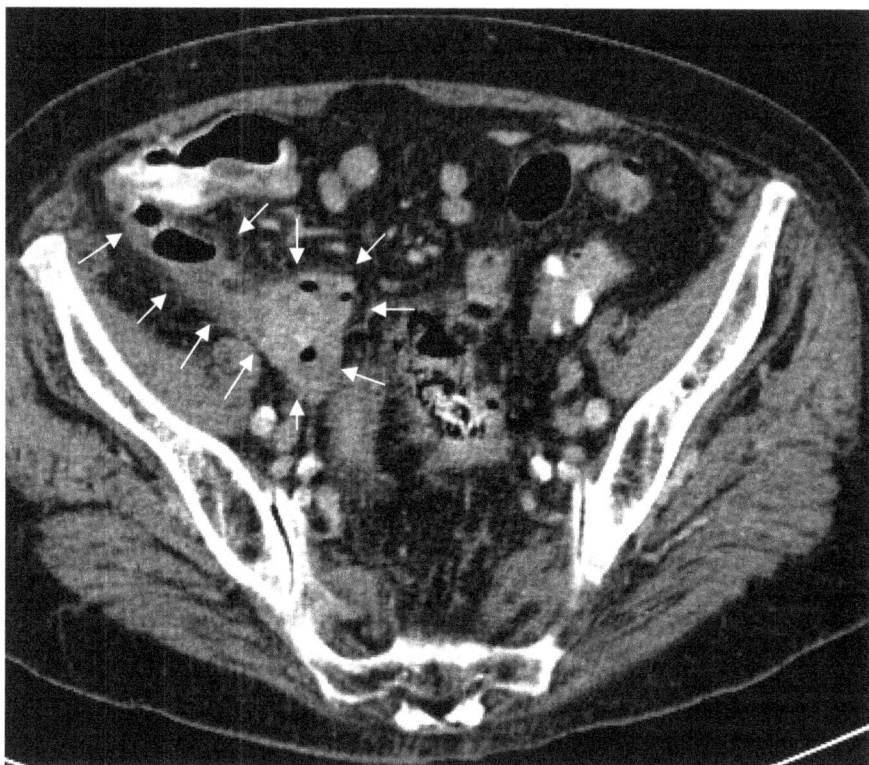

Fig. 21. Abdominal axial CT image at the level of the right iliac fossa showing a distended, thickened appendix with an associated collection (arrows) in acute appendicitis.

5.8 Nephrolithiasis

Nephrolithiasis is another important differential diagnosis of acute abdominal pain as there is a reported increased frequency of renal stone disease in CF in comparison to the general population (3-6.3% in CF patients versus 1-2% in age-matched controls) (Gibney & Goldfard, 2003). As with non CF patients, pain can affect the loin region or anywhere from the loin to the groin, and patients may also complain of haematuria and notice the voiding of tiny grains of stone. Initial assessment can be made with a CT of the kidneys, ureters and bladder (CT KUB) to confirm the diagnosis or with an ultrasound scan if obstruction and hydronephrosis is suspected in a patient with know nephrolithiasis.

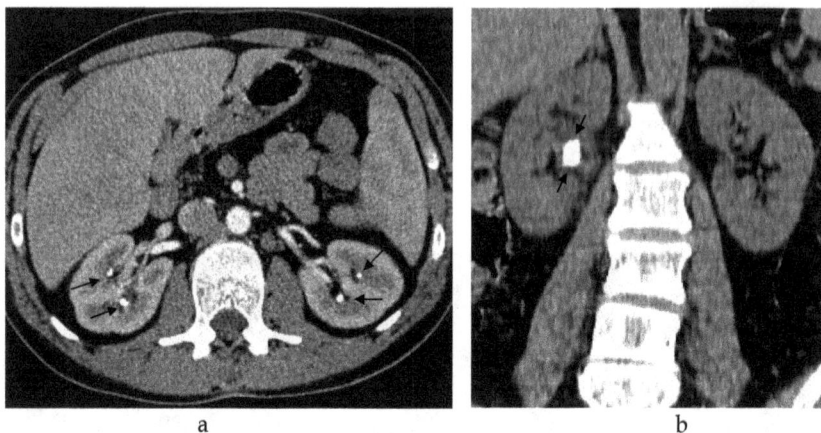

Fig. 22. Axial CT scan of the abdomen of CF patient investigated for haematuria and recurrent abdominal pain with bilateral multiple kidney stones (arrows) (fig. 22a). Coronal CT scan of another patient showing a single stone in the right renal pelvis (arrows) (fig. 22b).

6. Hypertrophic pulmonary osteoarthropathy

This condition consists of a triad of clubbing, symmetric arthritis and periosteal new bone formation. Firstly associated with brochogenic carcinoma, it is also recognised in bronchiectasis, chronic lung inflammation and infection and CF, amongst others. Finger clubbing is the result of fibroelastic proliferation in the nail bed with thickening of the skin and subcutaneous tissues of the distal end of the fingers; synovitis leads to arthralgia and stiff swollen hands; periosteal new bone formation and cortical thickening affects long bones, more frequently the radius and ulna (Martinez-Lavin et al., 1993).

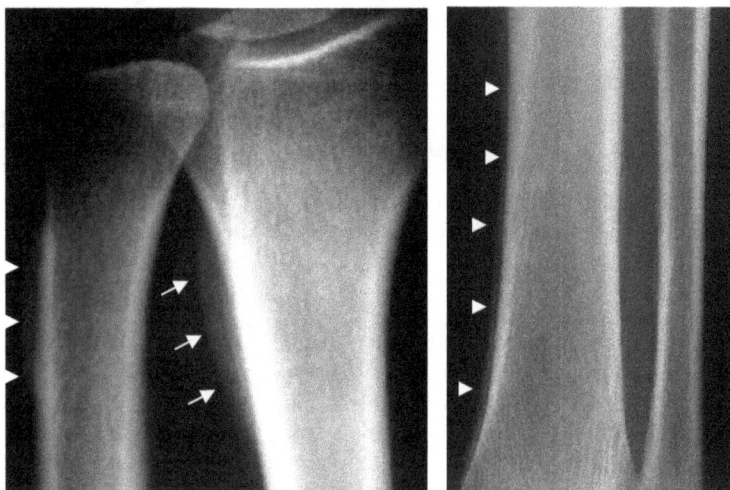

Fig. 23. Close-up radiographs of the distal long bones of the forearm and leg showing thickening of the cortical bone (arrows) as a result of chronic periostitis.

7. Conclusion

The lungs continue to account for the majority of CF complications and death, but with gastrointestinal complications becoming increasingly important and the ever growing availability of imaging facilities, clinicians and radiologists need to be aware of the larger spectrum of pathologies they might encounter and their radiological manifestations.

Imaging and close interaction between clinicians and radiologists is invaluable for the prompt and precise diagnosis of several CF related conditions. Some conditions can be diagnosed on the basis of imaging alone, avoiding unnecessary time wasting and invasive procedures, always reinforcing the necessity to maintain ionising radiation exposure to as low as reasonably achievable.

8. Acknowledgements

Dr Anthony Edey and Dr David Grier, Radiology Consultants, for kindly contributing with several images.

Kind thank you to all the cystic fibrosis patients of the Bristol Adult CF Centre for their generosity and resilience.

9. References

Agrons, GA., Corse, WR., Markowitz, RI., Suarez, ES., Perry, DR. (1996). Gastrointestinal manifestations of cystic fibrosis: radiologic-pathologic correlation. *Radiographics* 16: 871-893.

Al-Kouatly, HB., Chasen, ST., Streltzoff, J., Chervenak, FA. (2001). The clinical significance of fetal echogenic bowel. *Am J Obstet Gynecol* 185(5): 1035-1038.

Cepero, R., Smith, RJ., Catlin, FI., Bressler, KL., Furuta, GT., Shandera, KC. (1987). Cystic fibrosis - an otolaryngologic perspective. *Otolaryngol Head Neck Surg* 97(4): 356-360.

De Boeck, K., Weren, M., Proesmans, M., Kerem, E. (2005). Pancreatitis among patients with cystic fibrosis: correlation with pancreatic status and genotype. *Pediatrics* 115(4): e463-e469.

Feigelson, J., Anagnostopoulos, C., Poquet, M., Pecau, Y., Munck, A., Navarro, J. (1993). Liver cirrhosis in cystic fibrosis - therapeutic implications and long term follow up. *Arch Dis Child* 68: 653-657.

Field, SK., Fisher, D., Cowie, RL. (2004). Mycobacterium avium complex pulmonary disease in patients without HIV infection. *Chest* 126(2): 566-581.

FitzSimmons, SC., Burkhart, GA., Borowitz, D., Grand, RJ., Hammerstrom, T., Durie, PR., Lloyd-Still, JD., Lowenfels, AB. (1997). High-dose pancreatic-enzyme supplements and fibrosing colonopathy in children with cystic fibrosis. *N Engl J Med* 336: 1283-1289.

Gayer, G., Apter, S., Hofmann, C., Nass, S., Amitai, M., Zissin, R., Hertz, M. (1998). Intussusception in adults: CT diagnosis. *Clin Radiol* 53(1): 53-57.

Genyk, YS., Quiros, JA., Jabbour, N., Selby, RR., Thomas, DW. (2001). Liver transplantation in cystic fibrosis. *Curr Opin Pulm Med* 7(6): 441-447.

Gibney, EM., Goldfarb, DS. (2003) The association of nephrolithiasis with cystic fibrosis. Am J Kidney Dis 42(1): 1-11.

Hansell, DM., Armstrong, P., Lynch, DA., McAdams, HP. (2005). *Imaging of diseases of the chest, 4th edition* , Elsevier Mosby, Philadelphia.

Hen, J., Dolan, TF., Touloukian, RJ. (1980). Meconium ileus syndrome associated with cystic fibrosis and Hirschprung's disease. *Pediatrics* 66: 466-468.

Hertzberg, BS., Kliewer, MA., Maynor, C., McNally, PJ., Bowie, JD., Kay, HH., Hage, ML. (1996). Nonvisualization of the fetal gallbladder: frequency and prognostic importance. *Radiology* 199(3): 679-682.

Marshall, BC. Pulmonary exacerbation in cystic fibrosis. It's time to be explicit. (2004). *Am J Respir Crit Care Med* 169: 781-782.

Martinez-Lavin, M., Matucci-Cerinic, M., Jajic, I., Pineda, C. (1993). Hypertrophic osteoarthropathy: consensus on its definition, classification, assessment and diagnostic criteria. *J Rheumatol* 20(8): 1386-1387.

McCarthy, VP., Mischler, EH., Hubbard, VS., Chernick, MS., di Sant'Agnese, PA. (1984). Appendiceal abscess in cystic fibrosis. A diagnostic challenge. *Gastroenterology* 86(3): 564-568.

Nash, EF., Stephenson, A., Helm, EJ., Ho, T., Thippanna, CM., Ali, A., Whitehouse, JL., Honeybourne, D., Tullis, E., Durie, PR. (2011). Intussusception in adults with cystic fibrosis: a case series with review of the literature. *Dig Dis Sci* Jun 16 [Epub ahead of print].

Olivier, KN., Weber, DJ., Wallace Jr., RJ., Faiz, AR., Lee, JH., Zhang, Y., Brown-Elliot, BA., Handler, A., Wilson, RW., Schechter, MS., Edwards, LJ., Chakraborti, S., Knowles, MR., for the Nontuberculous Mycobacteria in Cystic Fibrosis Study Group. (2003). Non-tuberculous mycobacteria: multicentre prevalence study in cystic fibrosis. *Am J Respir Crit Care Med* 15: 828-834.

Rosenstein, BJ., Cutting, GR., and for the Cystic Fibrosis Foundation Consensus Panel. (1998). The diagnosis of cystic fibrosis: a consensus statement. *J Pediatr* **132**(4): 589-595.

Sakano, E., Ribeiro, AF., Barth, L., Neto, AC., Ribeiro, JD. (2007). Nasal and paranasal endoscopy computed tomography and microbiology of upper airways and the correlations with genotype and severity of cystic fibrosis. *Intl J Ped Otorhinol* 71: 41-50.

Scotet, V., De Braekeleer, M., Audrezet, MP., Quere, I., Mercier, B., Dugueperoux, I., Andrieux, J., Blayau, M., Ferec, C. (2002). Prenatal detection of cystic fibrosis by ultrasonography: a retrospective study of more than 346 000 pregnancies. *J Med Genet* 39(6): 443-448.

Speck, K., Charles, A. (2008). Distal intestinal obstructive syndrome in adults with cystic fibrosis: a surgical perspective. *Arch Surg* 143(6): 601-603.

Sequeiros, I., Hester, K., Callaway, M., Williams, A., Garland, Z., Powell, T., Wong, FS., Jarad, NA. (2010) MRI appearances of the pancreas in patients with cystic fibrosis: a comparison of pancreas volume in diabetic and non-diabetic patients. *Br J Radiol* 83: 921-926.

Sturgess, JM. (1984). Structural and developmental abnormalities of the exocrine pancreas in cystic fibrosis. *J Pediatr Gastroenterol Nutr* 3 Suppl 1:S55-66.

van Rijn, RR., Schilte, PP., Wiarda, BM., Taminiau, JA., Stoker, J. (2007). Case 113: Pancreatic cystosis. *Radiology* 243: 598-602.

4

The Cystic Fibrosis 'Gender Gap': Past Observations, Present Understanding and Future Directions

Sanjay H. Chotirmall[1], Catherine M. Greene[1],
Brian J. Harvey[2] and Noel G. McElvaney[1]
[1]*Respiratory Research Division, Department of Medicine*
[2]*Department of Molecular Medicine, Royal College of Surgeons in Ireland*
Ireland

1. Introduction

Cystic Fibrosis (CF) is a systemic disease impacting upon several organ systems. These include gastrointestinal, reproductive, endocrine and pulmonary manifestations of which the latter contributes the heaviest burden of disease morbidity, mortality and impact on quality of life. The defective protein in the disease state is the Cystic Fibrosis Transmembrane Regulator (CFTR) that normally functions as an ion channel permitting intracellular chloride escape. Regulated by cyclic adenosine monophosphate (cAMP) and localized to the apical membrane of epithelial cells, CFTR's function is diminished or absent in CF precipitating a cycle of events including sodium hyper-absorption, mucus hypersecretion, impaired mucociliary clearance and pathogenic colonization with microorganisms. This in turn leads to the clinical picture of recurrent infections, bronchiectasis and airway destruction culminating in respiratory failure and premature death (Davis et al., 1996).

Several hundred mutations of the CFTR gene have been described with a sub-group causing disease. Differing mutations impact upon CFTR channel expression, localization and activity and in some cases a combination of these important functions. Dependent on these factors, CFTR mutations have been stratified into six distinct classes for example the class II ΔF508 mutation encodes a CFTR protein that is both defectively folded and processed resulting in disease (Rowe et al., 2005). Whilst the Republic of Ireland has both the highest incidence and carrier rates of CF worldwide, ΔF508 accounts for >95% alleles identified (Farrell, 2008).

An important long-standing observation in CF remains the fact that a gender dichotomy has been described. Females have poorer survival, worse lung function and earlier colonization with *Pseudomonas aeruginosa* when compared to males without adequate explanation. The following chapter will initially outline past epidemiological observations that have been made with regard to the CF 'gender gap' followed by our present understanding of potential explanations for these gender differences. A special focus on the major female sex hormone estrogen will be emphasized particularly its impact on the inflammatory and immune state within the female CF airway. Finally, directions for future basic science and clinical research in the area will be outlined.

2. Past observations

The female gender disadvantage has been observed in CF morbidity and mortality and is reported throughout the early literature. Differences encompass survival, lung function, frequency of infections and microbiological variation however despite investigation explanations have remained elusive. With the lack of adequate explanation persisting over the last decade, controversy has emerged as to whether such disparities in fact ever existed and if such variation could be explained by therapeutic factors or treatment differences alone that exist between countries and care centers worldwide.

The gender dichotomy outlined within early work in CF states that CF females have poorer survival, worse lung function and earlier colonization with *P. aeruginosa*. Early work by Corey *et al* (Corey & Farewell, 1996) assessing almost four thousand individuals with the disease from the Canadian registry illustrated that although regional differences in survival were identified that females had diminished survival of greater than five years when compared to males utilizing cohorts from both the 70's and 80's. The poorer survival in females was associated with poorer weight however the close inter-relation between declining pulmonary function, weight maintainence, gender and mortality was recognized and put forward for further investigation (Corey & Farewell, 1996). Similar results to these were uncovered from an Italian registry and then further confirmed in an independent United Kingdom assessment of mortality and survival in CF extending from 1947-2003 (Bossi et al., 1999; Dodge et al., 2007). In the early 90's, an important demographic shift in CF survival was noted. CF patients who previously were not surviving past childhood were now progressing to young adults. The proportion of adults with CF increased fourfold between the 70's and 90's together with a doubling of median survival from 14 to 28 years of age. Such changes in the age distribution of CF survival at this time provided clinicians further insight into the natural history of the disease that was previously unknown. Despite these improvements to CF survival, female patients continued to show a lower median survival age compared to males (25 versus 30 years of age in 1990) (FitzSimmons, 1993). Subsequent study involving >20,000 patients with CF and utilizing Cox proportional hazards regression analysis to compare age-specific mortality rates between genders again confirmed gender differences in median CF survival (25.3 versus 28.4 years for females versus males respectively) (Rosenfeld et al., 1997). Additionally, this work aimed to identify particular risk factors that may serve as potential explanatory variables for the observed gender related survival differences (Rosenfeld et al., 1997). Despite analysis using a variety of risk factors for death in CF including poor nutritional status, lung function, airway microbiology, pancreatic insufficiency, age at diagnosis, mode of presentation and race, none could account for the gender disparity identified further confirming the existence of a genuine 'gender gap' (Rosenfeld et al., 1997). Consequential to this and other works, it was unsurprising to note that gender was included as a major parameter in a predictive 5-year CF survivorship model developed to help both researchers and clinicians evaluate therapies, improve prospective study design, monitor practice patterns, counsel individual patients and aid determination of suitable candidates for lung transplantation (Liou et al., 2001).

A lack of explanation for such gender differences in CF disease together with a narrowing of this gap recently has ignited controversy with regard to whether the CF 'gender gap' ever existed. Some arguments have been put forward against the phenomena of the female disadvantage in CF which attempt to explain the gender differences based on therapeutic advances occurring over the last decade in the management of the disease. For instance, retrospective cross sectional analysis of annual assessment data from a single center has shown that during childhood and adolescence, the lung function and nutrition of CF patients should be equal between the genders and that individual clinic practice should be reviewed if a gender gap persists. The authors argue that prior studies that have shown poorer prognosis in CF females have generally combined data from several centers and that their aim was to determine whether with modern aggressive treatment of CF this gender difference remains when care is standardized within a single center (Verma et al., 2005). Whilst some of the arguments put forward by this work may be plausible, an important point to consider remains that the gender differences observed in CF were most clearly observed post-puberty and during adulthood and not during the adolescent years, the group assessed by this work. To lend further argument to this, recent data from an Italian registry confirmed the absence of a gender gap in CF survival however this assessment only included patients up to 16 years of age, too early to identify the previously described gender dichotomy (Viviani et al., 2011). As a result, one of the conclusions drawn from this dataset was that the emergence of mortality differences between the genders could not be excluded if this cohort was to be followed into adulthood, the timeframe of interest in older studies (Viviani et al., 2011). Additionally, although Olsen *et al* did acknowledge that females with CF are at higher risks of *P. aeruginosa* and *Burkholderia* colonization, require more intensified treatments with antibiotics and have greater rates of hospitalizations compared to males, they found no gender effect upon survival. It was again reiterated in the conclusions to this work that gender survival differences may in fact follow adolescence, the age group studied (Olesen et al., 2010).

To overcome some of the weaknesses in comparing CF survival data between institutions, a case mix adjustment method may be employed (O'Connor et al., 2002). Such a method accounts for baseline differences in both patient and disease characteristics and although no consensus with regards its use in CF currently exists, the characteristics utilized for such an adjustment should include those that differ across institutions and are associated with patient survival. By accounting for characteristics of disease severity that may be a consequence of treatment effectiveness, this analysis can abolish the argument put forward that improvements to treatment account for gender discrepancies observed in CF disease. Using such case mix adjustment methodologies, O'Connor *et al* have shown that female gender in CF remains associated with an increased risk of death (O'Connor et al., 2002). This conclusion is reached using a model encompassing patient and disease characteristics that are present at the time of diagnosis and not influenced by subsequent treatment strengthening the argument for the existence of a true 'gender gap'.

An alternative argument put forward to refute a true 'gender gap' is greater compliance to therapy among female patients with CF. Masterson *et al* studied adherence to infection control guidelines and medical therapy in a CF cohort and found that although age-related differences exist, gender was importantly not a significant factor for treatment adherence (Masterson et al., 2010).

In view of disagreement about the existence for gender variation in CF, a re-assessment for these differences was performed in early 2000, a time where survival rates were noted to have exponentially improved since the mid 80's. Although survival of both genders was discovered to have benefitted from this trend, females had consistently poorer survival rates compared to male patients re-iterating the existence of genuine gender differences (Kulich et al., 2003). This has been more recently confirmed by data published from our own Irish registry (Jackson et al., 2011). As a consequence, it is clear that female gender is a negative prognostic factor in CF – a finding illustrated across several countries, registries and CF care centers.

In addition to survival variances, differences in the acquisition and conversion of the major pathogen and colonizer *P. aeruginosa* have been described in CF. Females with CF acquire *P. aeruginosa* in advance of males and furthermore convert to their mucoid phenotype earlier conferring worse clinical outcomes (Demko et al., 1995). Longitudinal assessment of this organism in CF has shown a relatively short transition from no *P. aeruginosa* to non-mucoid *P. aeruginosa* however a much more prolonged period, sometimes over a decade preceding mucoid conversion. Transition to mucoid correlated with a deterioration in cough and chest radiography scores along with pulmonary function (Li et al., 2005).

Interestingly, an assessment specifically designed to evaluate whether earlier acquisition of *P. aeruginosa* by females in CF, the greater impact of the organism on lung function or a combination of both factors contributed to the poorer survival in females found that although acquisition of mucoid organism was associated with an increased rate of decline of pulmonary function in both genders males had consistently better FEV_1 (% predicted) and survival rates compared to females. This suggests that alternative factors and not *P. aeruginosa* alone contribute to the gender differences observed in female CF patients (Demko et al., 1995). Separate and independent analysis of the risk factors for initial acquisition of *P. aeruginosa* in children with CF identified by newborn screening found that female gender amongst others represents an important risk for early detection (Maselli et al., 2003). Further study has additionally shown that whilst chronic mucoid *P. aeruginosa* can have prognostic implications in disease outcomes, that female gender again remains an important risk factor for its early detection (Levy et al., 2008).

Whilst these past observations illustrate that gender differences are an important consideration in CF disease, they importantly do not explain why they exist. One important difference between genders and a potential avenue for exploration is the circulating female hormone estrogen. Estrogens are the primary female sex hormone and have fundamental roles during the menstrual cycle. They circulate in three forms: estrone (E_1), estradiol (E_2) and estriol (E_3), with E_2 being the predominant and most active form in the non-pregnant state. Both E_2 and progesterone fluctuations throughout the menstrual cycle have been implicated to impact upon pulmonary function however explanations to address such differences in CF remain lacking (Tam et al., 2011). Our group and others have conducted studies examining E_2 and its effects on infectious, inflammatory and immune consequences in the CF airway. Although such work remains ongoing, its results may provide insight for the first time into reasons for these fundamental gender differences that so far have not been adequately explained.

2.1 Pulmonary innate immunity

The lung constitutes a large surface of the body in contact with the outside environment. It is continuously exposed to a large number of airborne microbes or microbial molecules, and can also be confronted with pathogens approaching via the blood stream. A number of factors including lung structure and physiology and components of the pulmonary innate immune system interact to contribute to effective pulmonary defenses. Individual key factors of pulmonary innate immunity will be outlined following which the effects that E_2 may have on each component will be discussed. These include, but are not limited to the following:

2.1.1 Airway surface liquid (ASL)

The ASL is a protective layer of fluid that covers the airway epithelium. It contains electrolytes, soluble proteins and importantly provides an interface within which cilia can beat and move mucus up through the respiratory tract. The mucociliary escalator together with pulmonary surfactant provides a barrier material at the air-liquid interface of the lungs. Surfactant contains the surfactant proteins A (SP-A), SP-B, SP-C and SP-D which help to lower the surface tension and participate in innate immune defence.

2.1.2 Pattern recognition receptors (PRRs)

Toll-like receptors (TLRs) comprise a major family of PRRs that fulfil key roles in recognising, discriminating and responding to microbial infection (Greene & McElvaney, 2005). They are associated principally with macrophages and dendritic cells, however their expression is widespread and includes, but is not limited to cells of myeloid and lymphoid origin. TLRs are also expressed by pulmonary epithelial cells (Greene et al., 2005). Activation of TLRs by their cognate ligands can lead to induction of proinflammatory cytokine and antimicrobial peptide expression or up regulation of type 1 interferons. TLRs can also communicate with the adaptive immune response via modulation of cell adhesion and co-stimulatory molecules to induce longer term immunity and a range of non-microbial endogenous factors can also activate certain TLRs.

2.1.3 Antimicrobial proteins

A selection of antimicrobial peptides including the human beta-defensins (HBDs), cathelicidin/hCAP-18/LL-37, lactoferrin and lysozyme can be found in the respiratory tract. In addition to their direct bacterial killing activity some of these proteins also have anti-biofilm, anti-inflammatory and anti-viral properties (Rogan et al., 2006).

2.1.4 Proteases

In the healthy lung proteases fulfil basic homeostatic roles and regulate processes such as regeneration and repair. The principal classes of protease present in the lung are the serine, cysteinyl, aspartyl and metalloproteases. These can function to regulate processes as diverse as tissue remodelling, mucin expression, neutrophil chemotaxis and bacterial killing. Members of these protease classes orchestrate a diverse range of changes with respect to infection and inflammation in the lung (Greene & McElvaney, 2009).

2.1.5 Antiprotease protection in the lung

The activity of pulmonary proteases is regulated by antiproteases. There are three major serine antiproteases in the lung – alpha-1 antitrypsin, secretory leucoprotease inhibitor

(SLPI) and elafin. In addition to their anti-protease activities they also possess other intrinsic immunomodulatory, anti-inflammatory and antimicrobial properties (Greene & McElvaney, 2009).

2.2 Dysfunctional pulmonary innate immunity in cystic fibrosis

Pulmonary infection and inflammation in the CF lung are multifaceted processes. Defective chloride ion conductance due to mutant CFTR causes a decrease in the height of the ASL and an increase in both the volume and viscosity of mucus. The most important airway mucins are the secreted mucins, Muc5AC and Muc5B which are produced by goblet cells of the superficial airway epithelium. Their expression is increased in the CF lung and the overall composition of CF mucus is altered due to an increased content of macromolecules such as DNA, filamentous actin, lipids, and proteoglycans. Together these contribute to mucus plugging within the CF lung (Rose & Voynow, 2006; Voynow & Rubin, 2009). This also facilitates microbial colonisation with *P. aeruginosa, Staphylococcus aureus, Burkholderia cepacia, Prevotella* spp, *Candida* spp, and *Aspergillus* spp. One remarkable consequence of these events is an exaggerated influx of activated neutrophils into the lung. Due to the large numbers of infiltrating neutrophils higher than normal levels of neutrophil-derived reactive oxidant species and proteases are reached. The consequences of these events include (i) an imbalance in the lung's redox balance which can be further exaggerated due to reduced glutathione levels (Roum et al., 1993) that together lead to oxidative damage, and (ii) an imbalance in the normal protease-antiprotease balance due to the combined effects of oxidative inactivation of the normal anti-protease defences and the presence not only of excess neutrophil-derived but also bacterial-derived proteases (Greene & McElvaney, 2009).

Neutrophil elastase (NE) is the major protease released by neutrophils in the CF lung. It has significant effects (Kelly et al., 2008). Not only does it up regulate the expression of other proteases including metalloproteases and cysteinyl cathepsins (Geraghty et al., 2007), it can also inactivate certain serine antiproteases (elafin and SLPI) and abrogate their anti-inflammatory and immunomodulatory properties (Kelly et al., 2008; Weldon et al., 2009). In concert with proteinase-3, macrophage-derived metalloelastases and elastolytic proteases expressed by *P. aeruginosa*, NE can promote secretion of mucus and degrade surfactant proteins and antimicrobials. NE can also directly injure epithelial cells and reduce ciliary beat frequency, cleave haemoglobin, complement components and immunoglobulins and interfere with effective neutrophil killing of microbes (Kelly et al., 2008). NE also contributes not only to the intracellular killing of gram-negative bacteria by neutrophils but also, once released extracellularly, can play a role in bacterial killing by comprising a key component of neutrophil extracellular traps (NETs). NETs are involved in host defense (Brinkmann et al., 2004). They bind gram-positive and gram-negative bacteria and allow neutrophils to directly deliver high concentrations of serine proteases that degrade virulence factors and kill bacteria.

The high protease milieu of the CF lung can also impact deleteriously on antimicrobial protein activity. Defensins, lactoferrin, LL-37 and SLPI are all susceptible to proteolytic degradation particularly by cysteinyl cathepsins (Bergsson et al., 2009).

Pulmonary inflammation in CF is also mediated by proinflammatory molecules such as C5a, LTB4, ceramide, and the chemotactic tripeptide Proline-Glycine-Proline (Greene, 2010), which together contribute to the highly proinflammatory milieu in the CF lung. Furthermore the CF lung is a TLR agonist-rich milieu, represented by microbial-derived factors (bacterial, viral and fungal) and neutrophil elastase (NE), respectively (Greene et al., 2008). The chronic inflammatory phenotype evident in CF airway epithelial cells is likely due in large part to activation of TLRs (Greene et al., 2008). In the CF lung NE–induced activation of TLR signalling is mediated via EGFR ligand generation and EGFR activation (Bergin et al., 2008).

Overall the CF lung is highly prone to exaggerated inflammation. Although it is a neutrophil-rich environment, neutrophil degranulation and killing activity are dysfunctional. With inadequate anti-inflammatory mechanisms due to oxidation and proteolytic inactivation, incomplete resolution of infection occurs, bacterial biofilms remain established and infective exacerbations induce more severe symptoms. In females with CF these events may be further complicated due to gender-specific effects mediated in part by the female sex hormone estrogen which will now be discussed.

3. Present understanding

Estrogen, the predominant female hormone is released from the ovaries and subsequently circulates bound to sex hormone binding globulin (SHBG). Free E_2 interacts with its specific estrogen receptors (ERs) to affect human physiological responses. ERs are predominantly based in the cell cytoplasm however more recently, an association with the cell plasma membrane has been described (Levin, 2009). The major ERs are ERα and ERβ, which share structural similarities however can effect opposing responses based on tissue type and location (Weihua et al., 2003).

Traditional effector mechanisms associated with ERs are genomic where the hormone following binding to its receptor within the cell cytoplasm shuttles as a complex into the cell nucleus to induce gene transcription of estrogen-responsive genes (Metivier et al., 2006). Membrane associated ERs however act through non-genomic pathways that are more rapid affecting protein kinases and mobilizing intracellular calcium stores (Morley et al., 1992; Pedram et al., 2006; Pietras & Szego, 1975; Pietras et al., 2005; Razandi et al., 2000, 2004). Genomic and non-genomic pathways may interact with one another resulting in modification of gene transcription as the end-event.

ERs are distributed throughout the human body however proportions vary by organ system. In some settings, both receptors are expressed whereas in others one subtype predominates. For example, ERα is related to reproductive tissues, bone, liver and the kidney whilst ERβ is more abundant in the colon, bladder and lung. Its role in the lung, particularly one that is chronically inflamed is a subject of continuing research in the context of CF (Chotirmall et al., 2010). Emerging inflammatory, immune and microbiological data suggests a potential role for E_2 in the cause and course of chronic inflammatory lung diseases such as CF.

Over a monthly menstrual cycle, *in vivo* E_2 concentrations fluctuate with highest levels preceding ovulation with the lowest around menstruation. In view of its physiological role, ability to fluctuate in concentration, coupled to its capability to modulate cellular functions, responses and gene expression in those containing estrogen response elements (EREs), E_2

represents an attractive avenue for investigation in terms of the gender differences observed in CF disease.

Our current understanding of the role that E_2 plays within the female CF lung is driven by investigations focused on its effects upon the dysfunctional pulmonary innate immune system and specifically some of its key components as described above. One such component is the ASL which is already known to be compromised in the setting of CFTR dysfunction. Coakley *et al* (Coakley et al., 2008) have recently shown that in the setting of E_2 exposure ASL is further compromised by dehydration and an increased risk of infection and subsequent exacerbation during high circulating E_2 states. Therefore the two-week period of a single menstrual cycle where E_2 concentrations are highest represents a high risk time-frame of acquiring infection and promoting exacerbation (Coakley et al., 2008). To date however, this proposed relationship between E_2 concentration, menstrual cycle phase and infective exacerbations is yet to be illustrated by *in vivo* study and represents a future direction for clinical research.

We have added to the understanding of E_2's role within the innate immune system in CF by demonstrating that high circulating E_2 states confer a TLR hyporesponsiveness to a range of bacterial agonists manifested by an inhibition of IL-8 release. We found that the mechanism by which this phenomenon occurs is through ERβ-mediated upregulation of SLPI, an important anti-protease/anti-inflammatory described above that is widely expressed within the respiratory tract (Chotirmall et al., 2010). SLPI, in separate work has been shown to competitively inhibit NF-κB p-65 subunit binding to DNA inhibiting the transcription of NF-κB regulated genes such as IL-8 (Taggart et al., 2005). It is also important to note that in the non-CF context NF-κB has long been described to affect E_2 signaling pathways, for example within circulating monocytes or tissue macrophages E_2 can block LPS-induced NF-κB activity (Ghisletti et al., 2005). As we have demonstrated E_2 to have an anti-inflammatory role in the context of the female CF lung, we hypothesized that although an environment of chronic uncontrolled inflammation may be damaging over the course of lifelong disease, acute surges in inflammation particularly in the setting of an acute infection may in fact provide protection and play a crucial role in facilitating bacterial clearance. Our published data would suggest however that in CF females this acute inflammatory response to an infective exacerbation is blunted by the presence of circulating E_2 and when taken together with the compromised ASL, high circulating E_2 states create an environment prone to both acquisition of infection and a subsequently compromised response to it (Chotirmall et al., 2010). It is becoming clearer with studies such as those described that E_2 plays an important role in some of the observed gender differences in CF disease probably in tandem with other factors influencing clinical outcomes. One important offshoot from our work illustrating the hyporesponsive state induced by E_2 exposure is in potentially elucidating why anti-inflammatory agents such as the leukotriene B4 antagonist have been unsuccessful in clinical trial, in fact causing premature trial termination (trial registration: NCT00060801) owing to increased infection within the treatment arm (Schmitt-Grohe & Zielen, 2005). Despite this, it remains important to highlight that clinical benefit has been shown following use of high-dose Ibuprofen however mechanisms to explain these outcomes are still sought (Konstan et al., 1995). Notably, we detected ERβ to be the predominant ER within the CF airway by use of bronchial brushings obtained via bronchoscopy (Chotirmall et al., 2010). An increased ERβ expression is associated with oxidative stress and hypoxic conditions explaining why it probably predominates in the CF context (Chotirmall et al., 2010; Schneider et al., 2000).

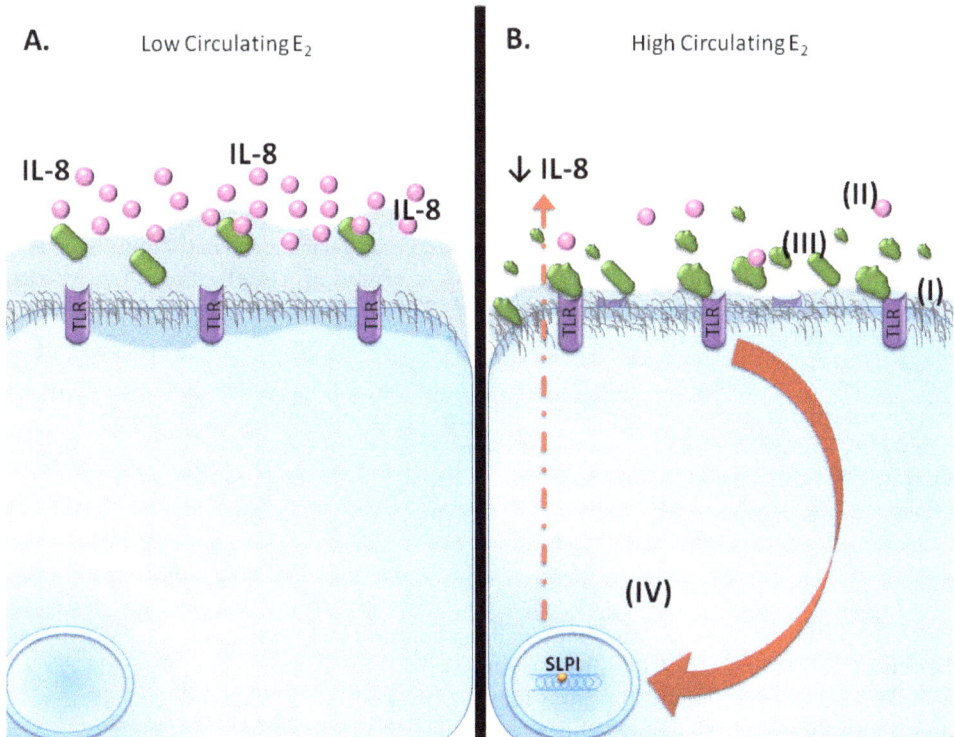

Fig. 1. The effect of 17β-estradiol (E_2) within the female CF airway. (A) In states of low circulating E_2 (luteal phase), a dehydrated airway surface liquid (ASL) overlies the CF female airway epithelium. Within the lumen, antimicrobials (pink) such as lactoferrin and neutrophil chemokines e.g. interleukin-8 (IL-8) are detected along-with potential *Pseudomonas aeruginosa* colonization. (B) During high circulating E_2 states (follicular phase), (I) a further disadvantaged and diminished ASL (Coakley et al; 2008) coupled with (II) an inhibitory effect and consequent dearth of anti-microbial peptides (Wang et al; 2010) combine to create an ideal environment primed for infection and exacerbation (III). (IV) Following infection, a blunted response to microbial agonists occur resulting in diminished luminal IL-8 and a hypo-responsive immune state (Chotirmall et al; 2010). These factors (I-IV) combine to confer an elevated risk of infection and subsequent exacerbation in the E_2 exposed CF airway.

More recent work additionally highlights a role for E_2 in *P. aeruginosa* infection. Proposed mechanisms include an enhanced Th17 regulated inflammatory response and suppression of innate antibacterial defences including the anti-microbial peptide lactoferrin (Wang et al., 2010). When assessed in unison, our work and others may provide an important mechanistic basis for some of the gender differences observed in CF disease. For instance, in CF, a dehydrated ASL overlies the female airway epithelium whilst within the lumen, antimicrobials and the neutrophil chemokines (e.g. IL-8, LTB4, C5a and Proline-Glycine-Proline) may be detected along with *P. aeruginosa* colonization. During high circulating E_2 states (follicular phase of the menstrual cycle), a further disadvantaged and diminished ASL (Coakley et al., 2008) coupled with impaired antimicrobial defences (Wang et al., 2010) combine to create an ideal environment primed for infection and exacerbation. Following infection, a blunted response to microbial agonists occurs resulting in diminished luminal IL-8 and a hypo-responsive immune state due to up-regulation of SLPI (Chotirmall et al., 2010). In tandem, these factors combine to confer an elevated risk of infection and subsequent exacerbation in the E_2 exposed CF airway (Figure 1). The effect of E_2 however on other antimicrobial peptides, proteases and anti-proteases within the pulmonary environment is yet to be fully established.

An alternate but critical avenue to further address gender differences in CF is by investigating the relationship between E_2 and microorganisms within the CF airway. The CF microbiome is complex and encompasses interplay between various bacteria, viruses and fungi that co-exist some to detrimental effect. Whether circulating hormones such as E_2 may influence this organism-rich milieu is an area of ongoing investigation. Microbial endocrinology, an emerging field has begun to address some of these important questions. This particular area of research focuses upon examining the effect of hormones on microorganisms such as *P. aeruginosa*. Thus far, published work in the field has described the effects of hormones such as noradrenaline and norepinephrine upon microorganisms that impact upon their adhesion proteins among other virulence factors (Freestone et al., 1999, 2008). Despite the crucial functions that E_2 carries out in its eukaryotic host, its impact upon prokaryotes are less clearly understood. Whilst E_2 mediates its effects in eukaryotes through its major receptors –α and –β, comparable structures have been sought within prokaryotes. Estrogen binding proteins have been identified in *P. aeruginosa* whilst *Escherichia coli* possesses enzymes with analogous homology to human ERs (Baker, 1989; Rowland et al., 1992; Sugarman et al., 1990). Additionally, it is known that *P. aeruginosa* actively breaks down E_2 to its major metabolite estriol (E_3) and whether such metabolites can impact upon microorganisms particularly in the CF context remains to be determined (Fishman et al., 1960). Importantly, certain fungi are capable of producing estrogenic-like substances termed myco-estrogens however, whether these have any relevance for pulmonary environment in CF remain undetermined.

4. Future directions

Our understanding of the role that E_2 may potentially play within the female CF airway has exponentially grown. Studies performed to date have implicated the hormone as a potential explanation for the long-observed gender differences in CF disease. With such advances to our understanding come further avenues for future exploration.

One such avenue is the role of modifying the endogenous concentration of E_2 to alleviate its detrimental effects. Use of the anti-estrogen agent Tamoxifen or the oral contraceptive pill (OCP) can achieve this albeit by differing mechanisms. Tamoxifen *in vitro* is able to re-instate the ASL to its pre-E_2 state confirming the importance of E_2 in mediating its negative effect (Coakley et al., 2008). Use of the OCP to modulate endogenous E_2 concentrations would be a preferred and safer option although no studies to date have examined use of the OCP in CF in terms of effects on ASL or infection frequency. Such studies will undoubtedly emerge in due course and may provide a valuable potential future therapeutic option for CF females.

Although E_2 in its most active form is the chosen compound for most studies to date, it must be considered that through its natural metabolic process that E_2 is broken down into metabolites such as E_3. Whether such metabolites have effects within the CF airway on immune, inflammatory or infectious consequences is another area for future focus. In terms of innate immunity, prior publications in the non-respiratory setting have shown that E_2 has a major influence on antimicrobial peptides such as lactoferrin, elafin and SLPI (Fahey et al., 2008).

Whilst we have shown in our work that E_2 up-regulates SLPI in CF bronchial epithelium, the effects of E_2 on other anti-microbials have yet to be fully established (Chotirmall et al., 2010). Furthermore, the functional consequence of E_2 exposure on the various anti-microbial peptides has not been addressed.

The complex effects of E_2 on inflammation continue to be deciphered and consequently ERβ agonists have emerged as anti-inflammatory candidates. The development of such a compound however remains a pharmacological challenge that the forthcoming decade should address. Other important estrogen-based chemical compounds include the estrogen dendrimer conjugate (EDC) that binds ERs but excludes them from accessing the cell nucleus and exerting genomic effects (Harrington et al., 2006). Future research utilizing compounds such as the EDC will evaluate the precise contributions of genomic versus non-genomic mechanisms in a variety of *in vitro* and *vivo* settings that will provide further insight into the mechanistic explanations for the gender disparities acknowledged.

Finally, an exciting new development in CF therapeutics is targeting of the basic genetic defect by the use of channel potentiators such as VX-770 (Accurso et al., 2010). Whether E_2 or gender appears to impact upon these emerging agents and their effects represents another exciting direction for both CF basic science and clinical research leading us into the next decade of CF care.

5. Acknowledgments

Funding for our cystic fibrosis research is gratefully acknowledged from the Higher Education Authority (HEA)-PRTLI Cycle 4, through a Molecular Medicine Ireland (MMI) Clinician-Scientist Fellowship Programme (CSFP) grant 2008-2011, the Irish CF Research Trust, the Medical Research Charities Group and the Health Research Board of Ireland, the Children's Medical and Research Centre, Crumlin Hospital and Science Foundation Ireland.

6. References

Accurso FJ, Rowe SM, Clancy JP, Boyle MP, Dunitz JM, Durie PR, Sagel SD, Hornick DB, Konstan MW, Donaldson SH, Moss RB, Pilewski JM, Rubenstein RC, Uluer AZ, Aitken ML, Freedman SD, Rose LM, Mayer-Hamblett N, Dong Q,Zha J, Stone AJ, Olson ER, Ordonez CL, Campbell PW, Ashlock MA & Ramsey BW. 2010. Effect of VX-770 in persons with cystic fibrosis and the G551D-CFTR mutation. *N Engl J Med.* Vol. 363, No. 21, pp1991-2003.

Baker ME. 1989. Similarity between tyrosyl-tRNA synthetase and the estrogen receptor. *FASEB J.* Vol. 3, No. 9, pp2086-8.

Bergin DA, Greene CM, Sterchi EE, Kenna C, Geraghty P, Belaaouaj A, Taggart CC, O'Neill SJ & McElvaney NG. 2008. Activation of the epidermal growth factor receptor (EGFR) by a novel metalloprotease pathway. *J Biol Chem.* Vol. 283, No. 46, pp31736-44.

Bergsson G, Reeves EP, McNally P, Chotirmall SH, Greene CM, Greally P, Murphy P, O'Neill SJ & McElvaney NG. 2009. LL-37 complexation with glycosaminoglycans in cystic fibrosis lungs inhibits antimicrobial activity, which can be restored by hypertonic saline. *J Immunol.* Vol. 183, No.1, pp543-51.

Bossi A, Battistini F, Braggion C, Magno EC, Cosimi A, de Candussio G, Gagliardini R, Giglio L, Giunta A, Grzincich GL, La Rosa M, Lombardo M, Lucidi V, Manca A, Mastella G, Moretti P, Padoan R, Pardo F, Quattrucci S, Raia V, Romano L, Salvatore D, Taccetti G & Zanda, M. 1992. [Italian Cystic Fibrosis Registry: 10 years of activity]. *Epidemiol Prev.* Vol. 23, No.1, pp5-16.

Brinkmann V, Reichard U, Goosmann C, Fauler B, Uhlemann Y, Weiss DS, Weinrauch Y & Zychlinsky A. 2004. Neutrophil extracellular traps kill bacteria. *Science.* 2004. Vol 5, No. 303(5663), pp1532-5.

Chotirmall SH, Greene CM, Oglesby IK, Thomas W, O'Neill SJ, Harvey BJ & McElvaney NG. 2010. 17Beta-estradiol inhibits IL-8 in cystic fibrosis by up-regulating secretory leucoprotease inhibitor. *Am J Respir Crit Care Med.* Vol. 182, No. 1, pp62-72.

Coakley RD, Sun H, Clunes LA, Rasmussen JE, Stackhouse JR, Okada SF, Fricks I, Young SL & Tarran R. 2008. 17beta-Estradiol inhibits Ca2+-dependent homeostasis of airway surface liquid volume in human cystic fibrosis airway epithelia. *J Clin Invest.* Vol. 118, No. 12, pp4025-35.

Corey M & Farewell V. 1996. Determinants of mortality from cystic fibrosis in Canada, 1970-1989. *Am J Epidemiol.* Vol. 143, No. 10, pp1007-17.

Davis PB, Drumm ML & Konstan MW.1996. State of the art: Cystic fibrosis. *Am J Respir Crit Care Med.* Vol. 154, No. 5, pp1229-56.

Demko CA, Byard PJ & Davis PB. 1995. Gender differences in cystic fibrosis: Pseudomonas aeruginosa infection. *J Clin Epidemiol.* Vol. 48, No. 8, pp1041-9.

Dodge JA, Lewis PA, Stanton M & Wilsher J. 2007. Cystic fibrosis mortality and survival in the UK: 1947-2003. *Eur Respir J.* Vol. 29, No. 3, pp522-6.

Fahey JV, Wright JA, Shen L, Smith JM, Ghosh M, Rossoll RM & Wira CR. 2008. Estradiol selectively regulates innate immune function by polarized human uterine epithelial cells in culture. *Mucosal Immunol.* Vol. 1, No.4, pp317-25.

Farrell PM. 2008. The prevalence of cystic fibrosis in the European Union. *J Cyst Fibros.* Vol. 7, No. 5, pp450-3.

Fishman J, Bradlow HL & Gallagher TF. 1960. Oxidative metabolism of estradiol. *J Biol Chem.* Vol. 235, pp3104-7.

FitzSimmons SC. 1993. The changing epidemiology of cystic fibrosis. *J Pediatr.* Vol. 122, No. 1, pp1-9.

Freestone PP, Haigh RD, Williams PH & Lyte M. 1999. Stimulation of bacterial growth by heat-stable, norepinephrine-induced autoinducers. *FEMS Microbiol Lett.* Vol. 172, No. 1, pp53-60.

Freestone PP, Sandrini SM, Haigh RD & Lyte M. 2008. Microbial endocrinology: how stress influences susceptibility to infection. *Trends Microbiol.* Vol. 16, No.2, pp55-64.

Geraghty P, Rogan MP, Greene CM, Boxio RM, Poiriert T, O'Mahony M, Belaaouaj A, O'Neill SJ, Taggart CC & McElvaney NG. 2007. Neutrophil elastase up-regulates cathepsin B and matrix metalloprotease-2 expression. *J Immunol.* Vol. 178, No. 9, pp5871-8.

Ghisletti S, Meda C, Maggi A & Vegeto E. 2005. 17beta-estradiol inhibits inflammatory gene expression by controlling NF-kappaB intracellular localization. *Mol Cell Biol.* Vol. 25, No. 8, pp2957-68.

Greene CM, Carroll TP, Smith SG, Taggart CC, Devaney J, Griffin S, O'Neill SJ & McElvaney NG. 2005. TLR-induced inflammation in cystic fibrosis and non-cystic fibrosis airway epithelial cells. *J Immunol.* Vol. 174, No. 3, pp1638-46.

Greene CM & McElvaney NG. 2005. Toll-like receptor expression and function in airway epithelial cells. *Arch Immunol Ther Exp (Warsz).* Vol. 53, No. 5, pp418-27.

Greene CM, Branagan P & McElvaney NG. 2008. Toll-like receptors as therapeutic targets in cystic fibrosis. *Expert Opin Ther Targets.* Vol. 12, No. 12, pp1481-95.

Greene CM & McElvaney NG. 2009. Proteases and antiproteases in chronic neutrophilic lung disease - relevance to drug discovery. *Br J Pharmacol.* Vol. 158, No. 4, pp1048-58.

Greene CM. 2010. How can we target pulmonary inflammation in cystic fibrosis? *Open Respir Med J.* Vol.4, pp18-9.

Harrington WR, Kim SH, Funk CC, Madak-Erdogan Z, Schiff R, Katzenellenbogen JA & Katzenellenbogen BS. 2006. Estrogen dendrimer conjugates that preferentially activate extranuclear, nongenomic versus genomic pathways of estrogen action. *Mol Endocrinol.* Vol. 20, No. 3, pp491-502.

Jackson AD, Daly L, Jackson AL, Kelleher C, Marshall BC, Quinton HB, Fletcher G, Harrington M, Zhou S, McKone EF, Gallagher C, Foley L & Fitzpatrick P. 2011. Validation and use of a parametric model for projecting cystic fibrosis survivorship beyond observed data: a birth cohort analysis. *Thorax.*Vol. 66, No. 8, pp674-9.

Kelly E, Greene CM & McElvaney NG. 2008. Targeting neutrophil elastase in cystic fibrosis. *Expert Opin Ther Targets.* Vol. 12, No. 2, pp145-57.

Konstan MW, Byard PJ, Hoppel CL & Davis PB. 1995. Effect of high-dose ibuprofen in patients with cystic fibrosis. *N Engl J Med.* Vol. 332, No. 13, pp848-54.

Kulich M, Rosenfeld M, Goss CH & Wilmott R. 2003. Improved survival among young patients with cystic fibrosis. *J Pediatr.* Vol. 142, No. 6, pp631-6.

Levin ER. 2009. Plasma membrane estrogen receptors. *Trends Endocrinol Metab.* Vol. 20, No. 10, pp477-82.

Levy H, Kalish LA, Cannon CL, Garcia KC, Gerard C, Goldmann D, Pier GB, Weiss ST & Colin AA. 2008. Predictors of mucoid Pseudomonas colonization in cystic fibrosis patients. *Pediatr Pulmonol.* Vol. 43, No.5, pp463-71.

Li Z, Kosorok MR, Farrell PM, Laxova A, West SE, Green CG, Collins J, Rock MJ & Splaingard ML. 2005. Longitudinal development of mucoid Pseudomonas aeruginosa infection and lung disease progression in children with cystic fibrosis. *JAMA.* Vol. 293, No. 5, pp581-8.

Liou TG, Adler FR, Fitzsimmons SC, Cahill BC, Hibbs JR & Marshall BC. 2001. Predictive 5-year survivorship model of cystic fibrosis. *Am J Epidemiol.* Vol. 153, No. 4, pp345-52.

Maselli JH, Sontag MK, Norris JM, MacKenzie T, Wagener JS & Accurso FJ. 2003. Risk factors for initial acquisition of Pseudomonas aeruginosa in children with cystic fibrosis identified by newborn screening. *Pediatr Pulmonol.* Vol. 35, No. 4, pp257-62.

Masterson TL, Wildman BG, Newberry BH & Omlor GJ. 2010. Impact of age and gender on adherence to infection control guidelines and medical regimens in cystic fibrosis. *Pediatr Pulmonol.* [Epub ahead of print].

Metivier R, Reid G & Gannon F. 2006. Transcription in four dimensions: nuclear receptor-directed initiation of gene expression. *EMBO Rep.* Vol. 7, No. 2, pp161-7.

Morley P, Whitfield JF, Vanderhyden BC, Tsang BK & Schwartz JL. 1992. A new, nongenomic estrogen action: the rapid release of intracellular calcium. *Endocrinology.* Vol. 131, No. 3, pp1305-12.

O'Connor GT, Quinton HB, Kahn R, Robichaud P, Maddock J, Lever T, Detzer M & Brooks JG. 2002. Case-mix adjustment for evaluation of mortality in cystic fibrosis. *Pediatr Pulmonol.* Vol. 33, No. 2, pp99-105.

Olesen HV, Pressler T, Hjelte L, Mared L, Lindblad A, Knudsen PK, Laerum BN & Johannesson M; Scandinavian Cystic Fibrosis Study Consortium. 2010. Gender differences in the Scandinavian cystic fibrosis population. *Pediatr Pulmonol.* Vol. 45, No. 10, pp959-65.

Pedram A, Razandi M & Levin ER. Nature of functional estrogen receptors at the plasma membrane. 2006. *Mol Endocrinol.* Vol. 20, No. 9, pp1996-2009.

Pietras RJ & Szego CM. Endometrial cell calcium and oestrogen action. 1975. *Nature.* Vol. 253(5490), pp357-9.

Pietras RJ, Levin ER & Szego CM. 2005. Estrogen receptors and cell signaling. *Science.* Vol. 7, No. 310(5745), pp51-3.

Razandi M, Pedram A & Levin ER. 2000. Plasma membrane estrogen receptors signal to antiapoptosis in breast cancer. *Mol Endocrinol.* Vol. 14, No. 9, pp1434-47.

Razandi M, Pedram A, Merchenthaler I, Greene GL & Levin ER. 2004. Plasma membrane estrogen receptors exist and functions as dimers. *Mol Endocrinol.* Vol. 18, No. 12, pp2854-65.

Rogan MP, Geraghty P, Greene CM, O'Neill SJ, Taggart CC & McElvaney NG. 2006. Antimicrobial proteins and polypeptides in pulmonary innate defence. *Respir Res.* Vol. 7, pp29.

Rose MC & Voynow JA. 2006. Respiratory tract mucin genes and mucin glycoproteins in health and disease. *Physiol Rev.* Vol. 86, No.1, pp245-78.

Rosenfeld M, Davis R, FitzSimmons S, Pepe M & Ramsey B. 1997. Gender gap in cystic fibrosis mortality. *Am J Epidemiol.* Vol. 145, No. 9, pp794-803.

Roum JH, Buhl R, McElvaney NG, Borok Z & Crystal RG. 1993. Systemic deficiency of glutathione in cystic fibrosis. *J Appl Physiol.* Vol. 75, No.6, pp2419-24.

Rowe SM, Miller S & Sorscher EJ. 2005. Cystic fibrosis. *N Engl J Med.* Vol. 352, No.19, pp1992-2001.

Rowland SS, Falkler WA Jr & Bashirelahi N. 1992. Identification of an estrogen-binding protein in Pseudomonas aeruginosa. *J Steroid Biochem Mol Biol.* Vol. 42, No. 7, pp721-7.

Schmitt-Grohe S & Zielen S. 2005.Leukotriene receptor antagonists in children with cystic fibrosis lung disease : anti-inflammatory and clinical effects. *Paediatr Drugs.* Vol. 7, No. 6, pp353-63.

Schneider CP, Nickel EA, Samy TS, Schwacha MG, Cioffi WG, Bland KI & Chaudry IH. 2000. The aromatase inhibitor, 4-hydroxyandrostenedione, restores immune responses following trauma-hemorrhage in males and decreases mortality from subsequent sepsis. *Shock.* Vol. 14, No. 3, pp347-53.

Sugarman B & Mummaw N. 1990. Oestrogen binding by and effect of oestrogen on trichomonads and bacteria. *J Med Microbiol.* Vol. 32, No. 4, pp227-32.

Taggart CC, Cryan SA, Weldon S, Gibbons A, Greene CM, Kelly E, Low TB, O'Neill SJ & McElvaney NG. 2005. Secretory leucoprotease inhibitor binds to NF-kappaB binding sites in monocytes and inhibits p65 binding. *J Exp Med.* Vol. 202, No.12, pp1659-68.

Tam A, Morrish D, Wadsworth S, Dorscheid D, Man SF & Sin DD. 2011. The role of female hormones on lung function in chronic lung diseases. *BMC Womens Health.* Vol. 11, No.24.

Verma N, Bush A & Buchdahl R. 2005. Is there still a gender gap in cystic fibrosis? *Chest.* Vol. 128, No.4, pp2824-34.

Viviani L, Bossi A & Assael BM; On behalf of the Italian Registry for Cystic Fibrosis Collaborative Group. 2011. Absence of a gender gap in survival. An analysis of the Italian registry for cystic fibrosis in the paediatric age. *J Cyst Fibros.* Vol. 10, No.5, pp313-7.

Voynow JA & Rubin BK. 2009. Mucins, mucus, and sputum. *Chest.* Vol. 135, No. 2, pp505-12.

Wang Y, Cela E, Gagnon S & Sweezey NB. 2010. Estrogen aggravates inflammation in Pseudomonas aeruginosa pneumonia in cystic fibrosis mice. *Respir Res.* Vol. 11, pp166.

Weldon S, McNally P, McElvaney NG, Elborn JS, McAuley DF, Wartelle J, Belaaouaj A, Levine RL & Taggart CC. 2009. Decreased levels of secretory leucoprotease inhibitor in the pseudomonas-infected cystic fibrosis lung are due to neutrophil elastase degradation. *J Immunol.* Vol. 183, No. 12, pp8148-56.

Weihua Z, Andersson S, Cheng G, Simpson ER, Warner M & Gustafsson JA. 2003. Update on estrogen signaling. *FEBS Lett.* Vol. 546, No. 1, pp17-24.

Part 2

CFTR – Genetics and Biochemistry

5

The Genetics of CFTR: Genotype – Phenotype Relationship, Diagnostic Challenge and Therapeutic Implications

Marco Lucarelli, Silvia Pierandrei, Sabina Maria Bruno and Roberto Strom
Dept. of Cellular Biotechnologies and Haematology - Sapienza University of Rome
Italy

1. Introduction

Cystic fibrosis (CF; OMIM 602421, see OMIM link in the website section) is the most common lethal genetic disease of the Caucasian population, with a very variable prevalence, from 1/25000 to 1/900, depending on the geographical region (O'Sullivan & Freedman, 2009; Riordan, 2008). CF is caused by mutations of the cystic fibrosis transmembrane conductance regulator (CFTR) gene (Kerem et al., 1989; Rommens et al., 1989; Zielenski et al., 1991) (see Ensembl link in the website section), which encodes for a transmembrane multifunctional protein expressed mainly in epithelia (Trezise et al., 1993a; Yoshimura et al., 1991b) but also in several cell types of nonepithelial origin (Yoshimura et al., 1991a). It is an ATP- and cAMP-dependent Cl⁻ channel with the main function performed at the apical membrane of epithelial cells. This function is the Cl⁻ ion secretion in the colon and airways, or its reabsorption in sweat glands (Riordan, 2008; Vankeerberghen et al., 2002). In the lung, the main targeted organ of CF, an additional crucial function performed by CFTR is the regulation of the epithelial Na⁺ channel (ENaC) activity. The exact mechanism of CFTR – ENaC interaction is not completely understood and contrasting evidences exist about the role of ENaC in CF. The most reliable vision of the basic defect is that, in the airway epithelia of CF patients, a CFTR deficiency causes an anomalous dual ion transport associated to an altered water absorption (Mall et al., 1998; Stutts et al., 1995; Berdiev et al., 2009) that, in turn, leads to sticky mucus and impaired mucociliary clearance (Donaldson et al., 2002; Matsui et al., 1998). The immune response greatly contributes to increased mucus viscosity through bacterial lysis and DNA release, as well as through immune cell death in the airways. Bacterial infections and inflammation produce bronchial obstruction, bronchiectasis, atrophy and, eventually, lung insufficiency. A probably non-exhaustive list of other CFTR functions includes: the bicarbonate secretion (Kim & Steward, 2009); the regulation of several other ionic channels and of the ion composition of intracellular compartments, as well the control of intracellular vesicle transport (Vankeerberghen et al., 2002); antibacterial activity exerted by epithelial cells (Pier et al., 1997; Schroeder et al., 2002) and macrophages (Del Porto et al., 2011; Di et al., 2006); maintenance of a correct level of hydration, essential for a physiologic development of male reproductive apparatus (Dube et al., 2008; Patrizio & Salameh, 1998; Trezise et al., 1993a), testis, pancreas, liver and intestine (O'Sullivan & Freedman, 2009; Ratjen & Doring, 2003); critical role in spermatogenesis (Trezise et al., 1993a; Trezise et al., 1993b; Xu et al., 2011b), sperm fertilizing capacity (Xu et al., 2007) and inflammatory response (Belcher & Vij, 2010; Buchanan et al., 2009; Campodonico et al., 2008; Mattoscio et al., 2010). The phenotypic severity of CF is essentially referable to CFTR residual function (Estivill, 1996; Zhang et al., 2009) that in turn depends on a combination of variables acting on the CFTR gene, transcript and/or protein, as well as to the action of variables external to CFTR. Random variability and the effect of the environment also influence the final phenotype (Figure 1). Depending on this complex situation, clinical manifestations of CF are highly variable. Some mono- or oligo-symptomatic phenotypes, namely the CFTR-related disorders (CFTR-RD), should have to be distinguished from poly-symptomatic classic CF (Dequeker et al., 2009). Nearly all male CF patients and several CFTR-RD male subjects show obstructive azoospermia due to congenital bilateral absence of the vas deferens (CBAVD); over 80% of CF patients show pancreatic insufficiency. The clinical history of CF patients is characterized by progressive, age-dependent, multiresistant bacterial infections of the lung, where the main pathogens are *Pseudomonas aeruginosa*, *Staphylococcus aureus*, *Haemophilus influenzae*, and the *Burkholderia cepacia* complex. Lung colonization causes the clinical decline, characterized by respiratory impairment, that is the main cause of morbidity and mortality. Despite advances in the treatment of CF, there is no definitive cure, the survival median of CF patients being at present limited to approximately 40 years .

2. The genetics of cystic fibrosis

The CFTR gene is located on the long arm of chromosome 7 (7q31.2), spans about 250 kb and contains 27 exons (Zielenski et al., 1991). The most common transcript is 6128 bases long and it is translated to a protein of 1480 aminoacids. The CFTR is under control of an housekeeping-type promoter with a time- and tissue-specific regulated expression established by alternative transcription start sites and/or alternative splicing (Vankeerberghen et al., 2002). CF is a monogenic autosomal recessive disease. Affected subjects have both the alleles mutated. When the same mutation is present on both alleles they are called homozygotes, whereas when different mutations are present on the 2 alleles they are called compound heterozygotes. A carrier of only 1 mutation on 1 allele has no clinical symptoms but has a genetic risk. Two carriers have a high risk of 1/4 (25%) of having an affected child and a risk of 1/2 (50%) of having a healthy carrier child, with a residual probability of 1/4 (25%) of having a healthy non-carrier child. In a given population, the frequency of couples at high risk depends on the frequency of carrier individuals. The prevalence of CFTR mutations and carrier frequency, as well as the incidence of CF, are highly variable depending on geographical region and ethnic group. The disease is very common among Europeans and white Americans with an incidence of about 1/3000 (about 1/27 carriers), whereas the incidence is lower in African Americans (1/17000) and Asian Americans (1/30000). It is uncommon in Africa and Asia with, for example, an incidence as low as 1/350000 in Japan. A comprehensive analysis of worldwide CF incidence and ethnic variations is available (Bobadilla et al., 2002; O'Sullivan & Freedman, 2009).

The basic view of the CF genetics explained above is complicated by biological variability, gene network and technical limitations in the mutational search. A more complex view is reported below.

2.1 Maturation, protein domains and mutational classes

The CFTR gene codes for a symmetric transmembrane protein of 1480 aminoacids that belongs to the family of ATP-binding cassette transporters (ABC transporters). The CFTR protein undergoes a complex transport and maturation process within the cell (Rogan et al., 2011; Vankeerberghen et al., 2002). Through an initial co-translational transport, the polypeptide is included in the membranes of the endoplasmic reticulum (130 kDa form) and is N-glycosylated (150 kDa form). By interacting with chaperones the polypeptide assumes the correct folding with a relatively low efficiency of about 25%, the remainder being degraded by the proteasome. Then it is transported to Golgi apparatus where, after further glycosylation, it becomes the mature CFTR (170 kDa form). It is then transported to the cell membrane where it performs its multiple functions, with a half-life of about 12 to 24 h. The CFTR protein exists in a cAMP-regulated dynamic condition of endocytosis and recycling in clathrin-coated vesicles. Finally it is degraded within lysosomes. After this complex pathway to intracellular and plasma membranes and owing to its multiple functions, the CFTR protein contains a number of different domains, each functionally specialized (Rogan et al., 2011; Vankeerberghen et al., 2002). Its NH_2-end interacts with the SNARE-proteins Syntaxin 1A (STX1A) and synaptosome-associated protein of 23 kDa (SNAP23) (Peters et al., 2001; Tang et al., 2011). The first (TMD1) and the second (TMD2) transmembrane domains, both consisting of six transmembrane helices, form the physical pore through the membrane. The nucleotide binding domains 1 (NBD1) and 2 (NBD2), functionally interacting, contain the sites for ATP binding and hydrolysis. The ATP binding to NBD1 site initiates channel activity, whereas the ATP binding to NBD2 site allows the formation of the intramolecular NBD1 – NBD2 tight heterodimer that turns the channel in a stable open state; the hydrolysis of the ATP bound at NBD2 starts the disruption of the heterodimer interface and finally leads to channel closure (Gadsby et al., 2006). The regulatory domain (R) contains most of the PKA, PKC and PKG phosphorylation sites and has a regulatory role in channel opening/closing. The ATP binding is allowed only after channel activation by PKA-dependent phosphorylation of the R domain. It also interacts with the SNARE protein Syntaxin 8 (STX8) (Bilan et al., 2004). The COOH-end interacts with PDZ domains of the CFTR-associated protein 70 (CAP70) (Wang et al., 2000a), of the Na^+/H^+ exchanger regulatory factor (NHERF, which in turn interacts with ezrin) (Seidler et al., 2009) and of the CFTR associated ligand (CAL) (Cheng et al., 2002). It also interacts with the α1 AMP-activated protein kinase (AMPK) (Hallows et al., 2000) and contains an internalization signal (Prince et al., 1999) and a binding site for the AP-2 adaptor complex (Weixel & Bradbury, 2000), needed for correct endocytosis.

CFTR mutations are at the present grouped into 6 classes (Table 1), according to their effects on transcription, cellular processing, final localization and quantitative level of functional protein (Amaral & Kunzelmann, 2007; O'Sullivan & Freedman, 2009; Rogan et al., 2011; Vankeerberghen et al., 2002). Class I identifies mutations with a complete lack of protein production. Usually they are nonsense mutations, severe splicing mutations (which produce only aberrant mRNA), small or large deletions or insertions. They act by generating in-frame or frameshift premature stop codons. The unstable transcripts and/or proteins formed are rapidly degraded or retain no functionality. In the class II are grouped protein trafficking defects based on ubiquitination and increased degradation, within the endoplasmic reticulum, of the misfolded protein. These are processing/maturation defects that severely decrease the protein quantity in the apical membrane, although often in a tissue-specific manner. In class III are included mutations leading to defective regulation that impair channel opening. Although the CFTR protein is able to reach the apical membrane, it is not properly activated by ATP or cAMP. The effect is a decrease or absence of functional CFTR protein. In class IV are grouped the defects of reduced Cl⁻ transport through CFTR. In this case the CFTR is present at the apical membrane but it is unable to properly sustain the Cl⁻ flux. Most of mutations included in classes II, III or IV are missense ones, that produce different degrees of CFTR impairment in reaching the cell apical membrane or in functioning although correctly localized. In some cases, however, also small deletions or insertions can be found. Class V mutations are splicing defects that cause a reduction of wild-type CFTR mRNA. At variance from the splicing mutations belonging to class I, the splicing mutations grouped in this class V do not completely abolish the correctly spliced form. Mutations of class VI decrease the stability of CFTR or affect the regulation of other channels. They can be missense mutations but also nonsense mutations possibly generating overdue stop codons, that allow the production of a protein that retains a partial Cl⁻ transport ability but is unable to correctly regulate other proteins.

2.2 The significance of genetics for personalized therapies

The increased knowledge about CFTR derived from over 20 years of basic and applied researches. This allowed both the development of symptom-based treatments, already in use, that greatly enhanced the life quality and lifespan of patients and the actual possibility of more effective personalized therapies. As well, a promise of primary defect correction also arose. As the most severe clinical aspect is respiratory impairment, the target tissue of these therapies is the pseudostratified epithelia of airways. A normalization of ion and water transport in respiratory epithelium can be achieved with the correction of less than 25% of the airway epithelial cells (Farmen et al., 2005; Johnson et al., 1992; Zhang et al., 2009). To classify a CFTR mutation in a functional class has recently become meaningful for a restoring strategy based on drugs acting on specific functional impairment (the so-called mutation-specific therapy) (Amaral & Kunzelmann, 2007; Becq et al., 2011; Kerem, 2005; Rogan et al., 2011) (Table 1). Particularly studied are the in-frame premature termination codons (class I). In general, many kind of tumours and more than a third of genetic diseases are originated by premature termination codons (Frischmeyer & Dietz, 1999). Also in CF, about 20% of affected subjects have at least 1 mutation that is an in-frame premature termination codon. Aminoglycoside antibiotics have shown to be useful to suppress in-frame premature termination codons by read-through and production of full-length CFTR protein (although a wrong aminoacid is inserted in each individual protein) allowing the targeting of class I mutations. The rationale of this approach is that a population of CFTR proteins each with a different wrong aminoacid will show an overall functionality greater than a population of identically truncated CFTR proteins. In this regard, recent findings, although not specifically obtained for CF, highlighted a surprisingly therapeutic potentiality for ribonucleoproteins. The authors (Karijolich & Yu, 2011) demonstrated the possibility, in vitro and in yeast, of the conversion of uridine into pseudouridine, a chemical transformation known as pseudouridylation. As all three translation termination codons contain a uridine residue at first position and the pseudouridylated nonsense codons code for serine, threonine tyrosine or phenylalanine, this may be a tool for converting nonsense into sense codons. Also in this case a wrong aminoacid will be inserted, although within a reduced choice of 4 aminoacids. Notably, the ribonucleoprotein complex used by the authors contain a RNA guide able to target the complex to a specific nonsense mutation. Chemical, molecular or pharmacological chaperones, usually called correctors (of trafficking), have been reported to be useful, by promoting protein folding and stabilizing CFTR structure, in the targeting of class II mutations. By increasing the activation of mutated CFTR correctly localized at the apical membrane and/or by extending its half-life, some drugs act as potentiators (of function) and are suitable for the targeting of class III, IV and V mutations. Class VI mutations may be targeted by either potentiators or suppressors of in-frame termination codons. Extensive lists of promising compound are available (Amaral & Kunzelmann, 2007; Becq et al., 2011; Rogan et al., 2011). For an up-to-date description of CF clinical trials see, in the website section, the links to the U.S. National Institutes of Health Clinical trials registry and database, and to the U.S. CF Foundation drug development pipeline.

The topic of mutational classes and personalized therapy is not devoid of problems. Some mutations produce multiple effects and should be classified in multiple classes. An emblematic example is the CFTR worldwide most common mutation, the F508del, a deletion of phenylalanine at position 508 of the CFTR protein. It is a class II mutation, because most of the protein is degraded within the endoplasmic reticulum; a small proportion of it reaches however the apical membrane where it behaves as a class III mutation, with only a limited capacity to bind ATP. In addition, the F508del protein has shown a decreased stability and an enhanced degradation also in post-endoplasmic reticulum compartments (Sharma et al., 2001), a behaviour that would point to the mutational class VI. It is in general quite difficult to classify a mutation without specific experimental studies aimed to its functional characterization. Due to the complexity of such studies, they have been performed only for a very limited number of the over 1800 sequence variations found in the CFTR gene. On the other hand, only in a limited number of cases it is possible to infer, by a theoretical approach, a relationship between the functional impairment and the protein domain where the mutation is located, as well a relationship between a specific DNA sequence variation and the class it should belong to. For example, although most of class III mutations localize in the R, NBD1 or NDB2 domains and most of class IV mutations localize in TMD1 or TMD2, if a missense mutation in these domains has been found, it cannot be assumed that the effect will effectively correspond to class III or IV, since that mutation might have a prevalent effect on protein trafficking and should therefore be classified as class II. Likewise, only for nonsense and frameshift mutations it is possible to reasonably assume a direct classification in class I, while for all other kinds of mutations it is very difficult to recognize the mutational class just from DNA sequence variation. For example, for splicing mutations it can be hazardous to deduce the possible amount of anomalous splicing only by software analysis, since just a limited amount of wild type mRNA would cause the shift of that mutation from class I to class V. Taking into account these considerations, although the class-specific personalized therapeutic approach can be at the moment applied only to a limited amount of CFTR mutations, its enhancement is foreseeable when the gap between the knowledge of the structure and the effect of a mutation will be filled by increasing numbers of mutation-specific functional studies.

Gene therapy would be the resolutive therapeutic intervention. Although, since the discovery of CFTR gene in 1989 more than 30 clinical trials of gene therapy have been undertaken, no gene therapy has been so far approved for clinical use (Conese et al., 2011; Davies & Alton, 2011; Griesenbach & Alton, 2011). The problems arose from the repeated administration of adenovirus- and adeno-associated virus-based vectors shifted the approaches to lentiviral vectors and non-viral strategies, as well as cell therapy. The evidence that a lot of work is still to be done in laboratory to optimize gene therapy tools arose. Two opposite approaches can be distinguished in gene therapy: the gene augmentation and the gene targeting. By the former approach, the entire wild-type CFTR gene, producing a normal gene function, is introduced into the cell without the need to know the specific CFTR mutation. On the contrary, the latter approach is a mutation-specific gene therapy strategy, as only the zone of mutation is targeted in situ, allowing the correction of the mutated zone of the gene. A recent study (Auriche et al., 2010) of gene augmentation in CF used the entire CFTR locus, including regulatory regions, cloned and delivered by a bacterial artificial chromosome (BAC), a non-viral vector. The possibility to obtain a physiologically regulated CFTR expression and activity, also of Pseudomonas internalization, in an in vitro cellular system has been demonstrated. The control of CFTR activity by naturally occurring regulatory elements appeared a critical aspect to obtain a physiologic CFTR expression pattern, to be taken under consideration in the planning of gene augmentation strategies. By the gene targeting, the corrected gene remains regulated by its endogenous regulatory machinery maintaining its physiologic expression pattern. Recent researches (Gruenert et al., 2003; Sangiuolo et al., 2008; Sangiuolo et al., 2002) applied to CF an intriguing gene targeting strategy, the Small Fragment Homologous Replacement (SFHR), that exchange a wild-type corrector DNA fragment with the endogenous mutated sequence, through a still undefined mechanism probably based on homologous recombination. Both approaches have to be enhanced before clinical application. The main difficulties encountered in the BAC approach are efficient manipulation and delivering to the proper cell population. The main hitches with SFHR are the low reproducibility and recombination efficiency, ranging from 0.01% to 5% (Gruenert et al., 2003). In both cases additional studies are needed to clarify the respective driving molecular mechanisms, to ameliorate our applicatory ability.

Mutation class	Functional effect	Kind of mutations	Mutation-specific therapy
I	Complete lack of protein production	Premature stop codons by: - nonsense - severe splicing - small or large deletions or insertions	Suppressors of in-frame premature termination codons
II	Processing and/or maturation protein defects	- missense - small deletions or insertions	Correctors (chemical, molecular or pharmacological chaperones)
III	Defective regulation of channel opening	- missense - small deletions or insertions	Potentiators
IV	Reduced Cl- transport	- missense - small deletions or insertions	Potentiators
V	Reduction of wild-type mRNA	- partial splicing	Potentiators
VI	Protein decreased stability or impaired ability of other channel regulation	- missense - nonsense (overdue stop codons)	Potentiators or suppressors of in-frame overdue termination codons

Table 1. Classes of CFTR mutations and possible personalized therapeutic interventions.

2.3 The complexity and sources of variability in the genotype – Phenotype relationship of the CF and CFTR-RD

Separation of classic CF from CFTR-RD only represents a starting attempt to organize the great clinical variability of CF (Bombieri et al., 2011; Dequeker et al., 2009; Estivill, 1996; Noone & Knowles, 2001). In fact, within classic CF are usually grouped both poly-symptomatic and oligo-symptomatic forms greatly differing in the involvement of lung, pancreas, liver, sweat gland and reproductive apparatus (to consider only the main CF targets). Not easier is the task of categorizing the even more heterogeneous oligo- and mono-symptomatic CFTR-RD. In this regard CFTR mutations have been linked to a wide series of pathologies: obstructive azoospermia for CBAVD (Claustres, 2005; Cuppens & Cassiman, 2004; Stuhrmann & Dork, 2000); non-obstructive azoospermia, reduced sperm quality and spermatogenesis defects (Boucher et al., 1999; Dohle et al., 2002; Jakubiczka et al., 1999; Jarvi et al., 1998; Mak et al., 2000; Pallares-Ruiz et al., 1999; van der Ven et al., 1996); male hypofertility due to idiopathic seminal hyperviscosity (Elia et al., 2009; Rossi et al., 2004); female hypofertility due to thick cervical mucus (Gervais et al., 1996; Hayslip et al., 1997); neonatal hypertrypsinaemia with normal sweat test (Castellani et al., 2001a; Gomez Lira et al., 2000; Narzi et al., 2007; Padoan et al., 2002); idiopathic pancreatitis (Castellani et al., 2001b; Gomez Lira et al., 2000; Maire et al., 2003; Pallares-Ruiz et al., 2000); pulmonary diseases (Bombieri et al., 1998; Bombieri et al., 2000); disseminated bronchiectasis (Girodon et al., 1997; Pignatti et al., 1995); chronic rhinosinusitis (Raman et al., 2002; Southern, 2007; Wang et al., 2000b); nasal polyposis (Kerem, 2006; Pawankar, 2003); metabolic alkalosis, hypochloremia, hyponatriemia, hypokalemia and dehydration (Augusto et al., 2008; Kerem, 2006; Leoni et al., 1995; Priou-Guesdon et al., 2010; Salvatore et al., 2004); primary sclerosing cholangitis, biliary cirrhosis and portal hypertension (Collardeau-Frachon et al., 2007; Gallegos-Orozco et al., 2005; Girodon et al., 2002; Kerem, 2006; Sheth et al., 2003). Several CFTR-RD are still debated, as the involvement of CFTR mutations is often inferred from small case series or even isolated case reports, as well for controversial results (as for example for non-CBAVD male reproductive defects). In addition, in several cases only one mutated allele could be found by quite non homogeneous methodological approaches of mutational search. This raises the troublesome question whether it should be assumed that 2 mutated alleles are indeed present, but the mutational search protocol applied was unable to identify both of them, or if the possibility of CFTR-RD arising in heterozygotes might also be taken into consideration. Rather than an approach for categories, a vision of a mosaic of different clinical manifestations combined in a peculiar way in each patient, overall constituting a continuous gradient of disease clinical severity, seems to better reflect the reality.

Only a rough correspondence between mutational classes and clinical outcome can be found with, for example, more severe phenotypes generated by the combination of class I and class III mutations and milder phenotypes originated by class IV and V. The variability is however so high that clinicians usually do not use genotypes for prognosis. The problem of the relationship between genotype and phenotype in CF can be partitioned in, at least, 2 steps (Figure 1). The first step concerns the production of a CFTR protein with reduced functionality starting from a mutated CFTR genotype. The second step concerns the clinical manifestations that originate owing to the protein malfunction. It is generally accepted that the clinical severity of CF and CFTR-RD is correlated with the residual function of CFTR

(Estivill, 1996; Zhang et al., 2009). It is easy to collocate high (almost physiological) levels of CFTR protein at the same end of the spectrum of the strictly mono-symptomatic patients and very low (almost absent) levels to the other end, where the poly-symptomatic patients with severe clinical manifestations are ideally collocated. Within these extreme conditions, it is however very difficult to link the values of CFTR residual activity to the severity of clinical manifestations. This not only because of the lack of systematic studies, but also for the difficulty of measuring in a real quantitative manner both the CFTR residual function and the clinical severity. Although CFTR mutated genotypes responsible for intermediate levels of residual activity often consist of a classic mutation on one allele and a mild mutation, retaining some CFTR activity, on the other allele, also the link between a specific mutated genotype and its effect on the protein functionality is elusive. Again, also in this case, the lack of systematic functional studies, addressing in vitro the effect of the mutated genotype on the protein cellular fate, have greatly hampered the knowledge at this level.

Several sources of variability influence both steps and make the overall picture unclear (Figure 1).

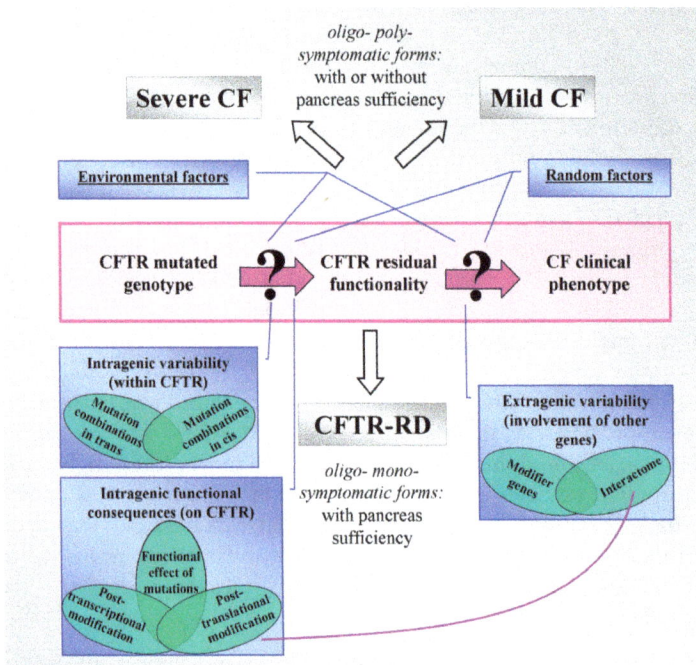

Fig. 1. The variability determinants of the genotype – phenotype relationship in CF and CFTR-RD.

The first step (from mutated genotype to residual function) is mainly influenced by structural and functional intragenic (CFTR-depending) variability. The structural intragenic variability is due to the large number of mutations and to the even larger number of their combinations both in trans, to originate homozygous and compound heterozygous genotypes, and in cis, with more than one mutation on the same allele to form the complex alleles. Trans and cis variability may also combine leading, for instance, to genotypes with 2 complex alleles and 4 different mutations each belonging to a different mutational class. The functional intragenic variability is due on one side to the variable impairment effect of mutations and, on the other side, to the influence of both post-transcriptional and post-translational modifications, possibly with overlapping effects and interacting mechanisms. The second step (from residual function to clinical phenotype) is more likely to be influenced by extragenic variability due to genes different from CFTR. Modifier genes can indeed modulate the original effect of CFTR mutations (Collaco & Cutting, 2008; Cutting, 2010; Merlo & Boyle, 2003; Salvatore et al., 2002; Slieker et al., 2005), as evidenced by the high phenotypic variability found in some subjects with identical CFTR mutated genotypes. Reciprocal influence between modifier genes and interactome (Wang et al., 2006), as well as an effect of interactome on intragenic functional variability, might also influence this step. Furthermore, it should be taken under consideration that the CFTR levels physiologically required can be tissue-specific, with only some organs affected despite the same CFTR residual function (Estivill, 1996). For example, the male reproductive apparatus appears as the most sensitive district to CFTR impairment, as nearly all men with CF (lower levels of functional CFTR) exhibit also CBAVD while, on the contrary, men with only CBAVD (higher level of functional CFTR) do not have other organs targeted. Superimposed to these genetic sources of variability the powerful role of environmental and random factors on both steps should not be undervalued. Due to these sources of variability, the genotype - phenotype relationship in CF is still poorly understood (Salvatore et al., 2011) with, therefore, our diagnostic, prognostic and therapeutic abilities severely limited.

3. Complex alleles and modifier genes

3.1 The relevance of complex alleles

The least addressed aspect of CFTR intragenic structural variability probably is the involvement of complex alleles, with two (or more) mutations in cis (on the same allele). Unfortunately, the most widely used protocols for a mutational search within the CFTR gene are designed only with the aim of finding the first two mutations on different alleles; additional mutations, possibly in cis with the already found mutations, may escape detection. The result is that the mutated genotypes of CF subjects with varying clinical presentations may appear identical, despite the presence of unfound complex alleles that might explain the divergent phenotypes. Undetected complex alleles may have important consequences. For example, if 2 already known disease-causing mutations have been found on both alleles (also on the allele with an in cis undetected additional mutation), the consequences will be an unclear genotype – phenotype relationship with prognostic failure. If at least 1 sequence variation with unclear functional significance in cis with an undetected additional disease-causing mutation has been found, a diagnostic error and/or misclassification of the sequence variation will arise. A systematic experimental search for complex alleles has not yet been undertaken. Probably for this reason only few complex alleles have been found so far and their prevalence is unknown. A probably non exhaustive list of CFTR complex alleles at the moment known is reported in Table 2. They have been more frequently found in patients with CF than CFTR-RD. Only in some cases an in vitro functional characterization has been performed, with the consequence that only in a limited number of these alleles it is possible to distinguish the relative functional contribution of

Complex allele	Bibliographic source
[R75Q;S549N]	Consortium for CF genetic analysis database
[(TG)$_m$T$_5$;2184insA]	Consortium for CF genetic analysis database
[129G>C;R117H]	Consortium for CF genetic analysis database
[F508del;R553Q]	(Dork et al., 1991);(Teem et al., 1993)
[3732delA;K1200E]	Consortium for CF genetic analysis database
[F508C;S1251N]	(Kalin et al., 1992)
[F508del;R553M]	(Teem et al., 1993)
[R117H;(TG)$_m$T$_n$]	(Kiesewetter et al., 1993; Massie et al., 2001; Peckham et al., 2006)
[125G>C;R75X]	Consortium for CF genetic analysis database
[R297Q;(TG)$_m$T$_n$]	Consortium for CF genetic analysis database
[R668C;3849+10kbC>T]	Consortium for CF genetic analysis database
[deleD7S8 (CFTR 3' 500 kb); F508del]	(Wagner et al., 1994)
[1716G>A;L619S]	Consortium for CF genetic analysis database
[405+1G>A;3030G>A]	Consortium for CF genetic analysis database
[G576A;R668C]	(McGinniss et al., 2005; Pignatti et al., 1995)
[(TG)$_m$T$_5$;A800G]	(Chillon et al., 1995)
[L88X;G1069R]	(Savov et al., 1995)
[S912L;G1244V]	(Clain et al., 2005; Savov et al., 1995)
[R334W;R1158X]	(Duarte et al., 1996)
[R347H;D979A]	(Clain et al., 2001; Hojo et al., 1998)
[-102T;S549R(T>G)]	(Romey et al., 1999)
[R74W;D1270N]	(Fanen et al., 1999)
[G628R;S1235R]	(Mercier et al., 1995; Wei et al., 2000)
[R117C;(TG)$_m$T$_n$]	(Massie et al., 2001)
[M470V;S1235R]	(Wei et al., 2000)
[I148T;3199del6]	(Rohlfs et al., 2002)
[S1235R;(TG)$_m$T$_5$]	(Feldmann et al., 2003)
[L24F;296+2T>G]	Consortium for CF genetic analysis database
[W356_A357del;V358I]	(McGinniss et al., 2005)
[V562I;A1006E]	(McGinniss et al., 2005)
[R352W;P750L]	(McGinniss et al., 2005)
[1198_1203delTGGGCT;1204G>A]	(McGinniss et al., 2005)
[V754M;CFTRdele3_10,14b_16]	(Niel et al., 2006)
[F508del;I1027T]	(Fichou et al., 2008)
[R74W;R1070W;D1270N]	(de Prada et al., 2010)
[(TG)$_{11}$T$_5$;A1006E]	(Tomaiuolo et al., 2010)
[R117L;L997F]	(Lucarelli et al., 2010)

Nucleotide notation: A = adenine, C = cytosine, G = guanine, T = thymine.
Aminoacid notation: A = alanine, C = cysteine, D = aspartic acid, E = glutamic acid, I = isoleucine, K = lysine, E = glutamic acid, , F = phenylalanine, G = glycine, L = leucine, M = methionine, N = asparagine, H = histidine, P = proline, Q = glutamine, R = arginine, S = serine, T = threonine, V = valine, W = tryptophan, X = stop codon (nonsense).
The link to the Consortium for CF genetic analysis database is reported in the website section.

Table 2. Complex alleles of CFTR (in chronological order of discovery).

each mutation. They often result in a combination of two mild mutations that, if isolated, cause CFTR-RD but if combined in cis originate CF. In some cases there is one main mutation whose phenotypic effect is worsened by a second sequence variation that may even be a neutral variant if isolated, such as F508C , R74W , S912L or M470V. Also variants that have a suppressive effect when in cis but originate a hyperactive CFTR when combined in trans, as for example the M470 and R1235, have been described. On the other hand, the finding of complex alleles also in CFTR-RD suggests the possibility that an additional mutation in cis may even lead to a lessening of the phenotypic severity (Mercier et al., 1995). This effect has been demonstrated for -102T, R553Q, R553M and R334W. The situation is further complicated by the fact that some CFTR polymorphisms, combined in specific haplotypes, may have at least CFTR-RD as phenotypic consequences (Steiner et al., 2004; Steiner et al., 2011).

3.2 The relevance of modifier genes

A small fraction of CF patients and a higher amount of CFTR-RD subjects remain with no CFTR mutations, also when high sensitivity methods of mutational search are used. In addition, CF and CFTR-RD patients with the same mutated CFTR genotypes often show divergent phenotypes. Also some intriguing cases have been reported: an unaffected sister who inherited the same CFTR alleles, without mutations, of her CF brother (Mekus et al., 1998) and two CF sibs, with no CFTR mutation found, who had inherited different parental CFTR allele (Groman et al., 2002). This suggested that genes different from CFTR may cause CF or CFTR-RD. The involvement of other genes in the definition of these phenotypes is relevant for the comprehension of both the molecular pathogenesis and the genotype – phenotype relationship. However, the widest action of the modifier genes probably is to modulate the CF final clinical phenotype in patients with both CFTR mutations found. Even more important, the modifier genes can represent excellent therapeutic targets, as they are able, by definition, to modify the clinical outcome of the disease but they are not mutated (on the contrary to the CFTR). A so-called bypassing approach has been proposed to correct the CF ionic imbalance by stimulating alternative ionic pathways that might compensate the impaired CFTR (Amaral & Kunzelmann, 2007). At present a comprehensive list of these genes does not exist and little is known about their effects and molecular mechanisms of action, as well as about their exact kind of interaction, if any, with the CFTR. Several putative modifier genes have been reported (Collaco & Cutting, 2008; Cutting, 2010; Merlo & Boyle, 2003; Slieker et al., 2005) to influence the second step, from CFTR residual functionality to clinical outcome. On the other hand, microRNA, known to exert a post-transcriptional regulation, have recently been shown to potentially influence the CFTR protein levels (Gillen et al., 2011; Xu et al., 2011a). Together with complex alleles, it is these genes that most probably represent the greatest source of variability in CF. Furthermore, modifier genes show tissue-specific levels of activity, that combine with equally tissue-specific CFTR levels, thus amplifying the complexity of the network. They may also influence the different CFTR functions, even in a tissue-specific manner. One of the most interesting gene complex proposed as CF modifier is the epithelial Na^+ channel (ENaC).

3.2.1 The ENaC genes

The human functional ENaC is composed of 3 subunits coded by 3 genes with sequence similarities: α (SCNN1A gene) (Voilley et al., 1994), β (SCNN1B gene) and γ (SCNN1G gene)

(Voilley et al., 1995). The ENaC protein has the functional properties of a Na^+ channel with high Na^+ selectivity, low conductance and amiloride sensitivity. It is expressed in human epithelial cells that line the distal renal tubule, distal colon and several exocrine glands; an ENaC-mediated amiloride-sensitive electrogenic Na^+ reabsorbtion has been documented in the upper and lower airways (Hummler et al., 1996). Genetic diseases are caused by either loss- or gain-of-function mutations in the ENaC genes: loss-of-function mutations in one of the three subunits cause pseudohypoaldosteronism type I (PHA-I) (Chang et al., 1996) characterized by severe renal dysfunction, arterial hypotension and reduced reabsorbtive capacity of both kidney and lung; gain-of-function mutations in either SCNN1B or SCNN1G are responsible for Liddle's syndrome, a severe form of hypertension (Shimkets et al., 1994). Interestingly, some PHA-I patients, without CFTR mutations, also exhibit CF-like lung symptoms, such as recurrent bacterial infection of the airways (Hanukoglu et al., 1994).

Because of the involvement of both CFTR and ENaC in the physiologic dual ion transport, it was supposed that also ENaC deregulation and/or molecular lesions might sustain CF or CFTR-RD. There are indeed experimental evidences validating this hypothesis. The over-expressing β-ENaC mouse model has CF-like pulmonary symptoms, with morbidity and mortality partially reduced by preventive treatment with amiloride, an inhibitor of the ENaC channel (Zhou et al., 2008). Wild type CFTR has been shown, in a heterologous cellular system and in polarized primary human bronchial epithelial cultures, to prevent the proteolitic stimulation of ENaC, thus downregulating Na^+ absorption (Gentzsch et al., 2010). Enhanced expression of all the 3 ENaC genes was shown in the nasal epithelium of CF patients (Bangel et al., 2008). In human bronchial epithelial cells, the CFTR regulates the functional surface expression of endogenous ENaC, by influencing its trafficking (Butterworth, 2010; Rubenstein et al., 2011). However, also experimental evidences against a direct involvement of ENaC and/or of CFTR - ENaC interaction in CF pathogenesis have been provided. According to one study (Joo et al., 2006), CF airway submucosal glands do not display ENaC-mediated fluid hyperabsorption, differently from the ciliated cells of the airway surface. Another study (Nagel et al., 2005) evidenced that human CFTR fails to inhibit the human ENaC channel in a heterologous experimental system of Xenopus oocytes. Finally, no increased sodium absorption has been found in newborn CFTR$^{-/-}$ pigs, an animal model with features resembling those of human CF disease (Chen et al., 2010). The differences between CF and CFTR action in humans and pigs, the fact that the study has been conducted only shortly after birth and that CF patients have a mutated CFTR and not a CFTR$^{-/-}$, should however be taken into account. Following the above considerations, mutational search in the ENaC genes have been performed in CF and CFTR-RD patients. Both, loss-of-function (Huber et al., 2010; Sheridan et al., 2005) and gain-of-function (Mutesa et al., 2008; Sheridan et al., 2005) mutations have been found in the SCNN1B gene of CFTR-RD patients. Several variants of SCNN1B and SCNN1G have been also found in bronchiectasis patients, some of them with only one CFTR mutation. A significantly increased prevalence of ENaC rare polymorphisms have been found in CFTR-RD patients (Azad et al., 2009), with some of these variants producing alterations of ENaC activity (Azad et al., 2009; Huber et al., 2010). The bulk of these data allows to ascribe to ENaC some roles in CF and/or CFTR-RD. This is reinforced also by the findings of physical and functional co-regulatory interactions between SNARE proteins (in particular Syntaxin 1A) and both the CFTR and ENaC (Peters et al., 2001). It is likely that wild-type ENaC is deregulated by the mutated CFTR. Moreover, ENaC genes can also act as additional mutated genes either when only one or no copy of CFTR is mutated (the ENaC genes behaving as concomitant pathogenetic factors with respect to CFTR) or when both copies of the CFTR gene are mutated (the ENaC genes as modifiers, modulating the CF phenotype). Little is known about the prevalence and kind of mutations, as well as about the role of other kind of ENaC alterations, such as transcriptional modifications. This last point is quite intriguing considering that a deregulation of ENaC, rather than mutations of it, seems more frequently the main pathogenic mechanism. The topic of the regulation of ENaC activity further increases the complexity of the puzzle, as multiple biochemical and cellular pathways are involved in the lung (Bhalla & Hallows, 2008; Butterworth, 2010; Eaton et al., 2010; Edinger et al., 2006; Gaillard et al., 2010; Gentzsch et al., 2010). However, little is known about the tissue-specific expression of ENaC and the coordinated transcriptional regulation of the 3 SCNN1 genes. The structure of these genes suggested a role for DNA methylation. The SCNN1G gene has 2 CpG islands in its promoter region and exon 1 (Auerbach et al., 2000; Zhang et al., 2004), the SCNN1B gene has 1 CpG island in its promoter and exon 1 (Thomas et al., 2002) and the SCNN1A gene has a high density of CpG sites, that are however not organized in a CpG island (Ludwig et al., 1998). In effect, experimental evidences suggest that DNA methylation can control transcription of the SCNN1G gene (Zhang et al., 2004).

In general, the search for new genes involved in genetic diseases, in addition to the identification and characterization of new pathogenetic mechanisms, allows the identification of new therapeutic targets. The functional interaction between CFTR and ENaC evidenced by the vast majority of experimental data makes ENaC genes attractive therapeutic targets, since it looks easier to attempt the correction of the regulation of wild type ENaC than the correction of the mutated CFTR. The ENaC gene activity repression has been tempted by amiloride, with partially contrasting results obtained in humans (Burrows et al., 2006) and animal models (Zhou et al., 2008). Also RNA interference seems a valuable and specific tool (Caci et al., 2009; Yueksekdag et al., 2010). The experimental evidences that ENaC genes undergo a DNA methylation-dependent transcription, raised new therapeutic opportunity in epigenetics and chromatin remodelling.

4. The genetics, biochemistry and clinics in the diagnosis of CF

Due to the wide range of signs and symptoms, CF and CFTR-RD diagnosis is difficult, particularly in infancy. On the other hand, CF early diagnosis, revealing pancreas insufficiency, preventing malnutrition and allowing a prompt treatment of lung infections, improves both lifespan and quality of life. In addition, it allows the early selection of high risk couples. For these reasons, neonatal screening programs have been activated worldwide (Castellani & Massie, 2010; Lai et al., 2005; Southern et al., 2007). The most used neonatal screening procedure is based on a single or double dosages (at birth and later on, between the third and fifth week of life) of immunoreactive trypsinogen (IRT), possibly combined with a I level mutational analysis (Castellani et al., 2009; Narzi et al., 2002). In addition to CF newborns, it has been demonstrated that also CFTR-RD newborns are selected by the screening programs (Boyne et al., 2000; Castellani et al., 2001a; Massie et al., 2000; Narzi et al., 2007; Padoan et al., 2002). In a part of newborns positive to the neonatal screening, only one or even no CFTR mutation, sometimes linked to borderline sweat test values, are found. This raises diagnostic uncertainty (Parad & Comeau, 2005) and provides evidence that some carriers are selected by neonatal screening (Castellani et al., 2005; Laroche & Travert, 1991;

Scotet et al., 2001). A common effect of the introduction of CF neonatal screening is the progressively increasing number of CF diagnoses performed each year by screening and the decreasing number of diagnoses performed by symptoms. By definition, neonatal screening selects a lot of false positive subjects and, consequently, is not a diagnostic procedure. On the other hand, also several other pathologies different from CF have a positive sweat test, as well as some CF and a lot of CFTR-RD subjects have a borderline or even negative sweat test. In some cases measurements of the nasal potential difference and/or intestinal Cl⁻ flux appear to be quite useful procedures. Taking into account also the highly variable clinical manifestations of CF and CFTR-RD, some of which superimposable to those of other pathologies, it became clear that none of this measurements alone allows a full diagnosis of CF or CFTR-RD. For these reasons, as stated by recent general (Farrell et al., 2008), neonatal screening-oriented (Castellani et al., 2009; Mayell et al., 2009; Sermet-Gaudelus et al., 2010), sweat test-oriented (Green & Kirk, 2007; Legrys et al., 2007) and genetic-oriented (Castellani et al., 2008; Dequeker et al., 2009) guidelines, the diagnosis of CF and CFTR-RD may only be made by a coordinated evaluation of clinical, biochemical and genetic data (Figure 2 upper part). In the last years genetic assessment has been clearly emerging as the most crucial point. In fact if 2 CF or CFTR-RD disease-causing mutations on the different alleles are found, a reliable diagnosis can be defined. Both the finding of the CFTR mutations and their functional interpretation are however very critical points, as described below.

4.1 The technical complexity of the mutational search in the CFTR gene

Over 1500 CFTR mutations and 300 polymorphisms are at moment known (in the website section see the links to the Consortium for CF genetic analysis database and to the human gene mutation database (HGMD)). The F508del is the worldwide most common mutation, accounting, on average, for about 60% of mutated alleles in northern European and North American populations. Few other single mutations account for more than about 5%. In addition the frequencies of CFTR mutations are very different depending on the geographical area (Bobadilla et al., 2002; O'Sullivan & Freedman, 2009). The simplest approach of mutational search would be to define a panel of mutations to be included in a rapid and low-cost test allowing a direct search. However, the high genetic heterogeneity has at least 2 consequences that limit such an approach. First, it is impossible to establish a general mutational panel applicable worldwide; second, the allelic detection rate, also of geographical optimized mutational panels, rarely exceeds the 80% and often is quite lower (Bobadilla et al., 2002; O'Sullivan & Freedman, 2009; Tomaiuolo et al., 2003). The detection rate is the genetic equivalent of the laboratory operative characteristics called diagnostic sensitivity. In this case it represents the proportion of mutated alleles that the specific genetic test is able to evidence. The practical consequence of a limited detection rate is that in case of a negative test, the presence of a mutation not included in the analyzed panel of mutations can not be excluded. A widely accepted approach of mutational search is the multistep one. Usually, methods of I, II and III levels are recognized (Figure 2 lower part). The I level methods are based on the search panels of the most common CFTR mutations by entry-level techniques. They are the most commonly used methods worldwide. However, due to technical and cost limitations, they show a low detection rate as at best they search for the most common CFTR mutations of the specific geographical area. At the moment commercial methods able to search near all CFTR mutations of specific geographic areas are not available. The I level genetic tests are therefore of limited prognostic and diagnostic usefulness, particularly in CFTR-RD subjects with borderline clinical and/or biochemical values. In this case, the use of methods with higher detection rate are fundamental to resolve uncertain diagnoses. The II level methods are scanning procedures usually able to analyze all the exons, adjacent intronic zones and proximal 5'-flanking of the CFTR gene. In last years, several enhanced methods specific for CFTR scanning have been developed as for example denaturing gradient gel electrophoresis (Costes et al., 1993; Fanen et al., 1992), single-strand conformation polymorphism and heteroduplex analysis (Ravnik-Glavac et al., 1994), denaturing high pressure liquid chromatography (D'Apice et al., 2004; Le Marechal et al., 2001; Ravnik-Glavac et al., 2002), and re-sequencing (Lucarelli et al., 2002; Lucarelli et al., 2006). Due to the progressively reducing costs of the re-sequencing and to the need of further characterization by re-sequencing of positive findings of other scanning techniques, the re-sequencing has become the most used II level method. However, no mutational scan technique able to detect all the CFTR mutations exists. Also the re-sequencing, at the moment the method of mutational search with the highest detection rate, is able to select about 97% of CFTR mutations. The remaining 3% of alleles carry mutations not identified. These may be large deletions, completely intronic mutations that may reveal cryptic exons and mutations in the distal 5'-flanking as well as 3'-UTR zones. Although little is known about the geographical variability of the prevalence of this kind of mutations, due to their overall limited amount and to the extended analysis of the CFTR gene, the re-sequencing shows not only a higher, but also a more constant detection rate than mutational panel-based techniques. Automated protocol of re-sequencing, as well as software templates for automated analysis of re-sequencing data (Ferraguti et al., 2011), have also greatly reduced the time and efforts needed for both the experimental and data processing phases. It should be clear that the use of scanning techniques may raise the problem of functional interpretation of sequence variations found. In fact, whereas the mutational panels are usually planned as to include only disease-causing CFTR mutations, by using scanning procedures also sequence variations not previously characterized from functional point of view may be selected. This may complicate the genetic counselling. The III level methods should be aimed to the search for large deletions, full intronic and distal 5'-flanking, as well as 3'-UTR, mutations. In practise, commercially available products only exist either for the search of most common CFTR large deletions or for the CFTR scanning for gene dosage (gain or loss of genetic material). Although full intronic, distal 5'-flanking and 3'-UTR mutations are assessable by re-sequencing, only recently some efforts have been done to value the pathogenetic contribution of these kind of mutations to CF and CFTR-RD. Whatever technique based on PCR and/or hybridization is applied, the possibility that polymorphisms within the primer/probe recognition sequence may interfere with the pairing reactions should be taken under consideration. So, also if the detection rate is kept to a maximum by including all the 3 levels of mutational search, a full assessment of mutations is virtually impossible to reach, due to the likely, even if small, decrease in analytical sensitivity.

The practical application of this multistep approach changes depending on its use in subjects with disease suspect for diagnostic purposes or in general population subjects for genetic risk lowering. In the first case it is reasonable to progressively go through the levels up to the finding of 2 CFTR mutations on different alleles. If no mutation is found (or at least 1 mutation is not found) even at the III level, the genetic test contributes to a reasonable exclusion of the CF or CFTR-RD diagnosis. On the contrary, in the second case, since it can be difficult to apply all mutational search levels to each subject checking its carrier status, an appropriate genetic residual risk is usually chosen and the mutational search with the suitable detection rate is performed.

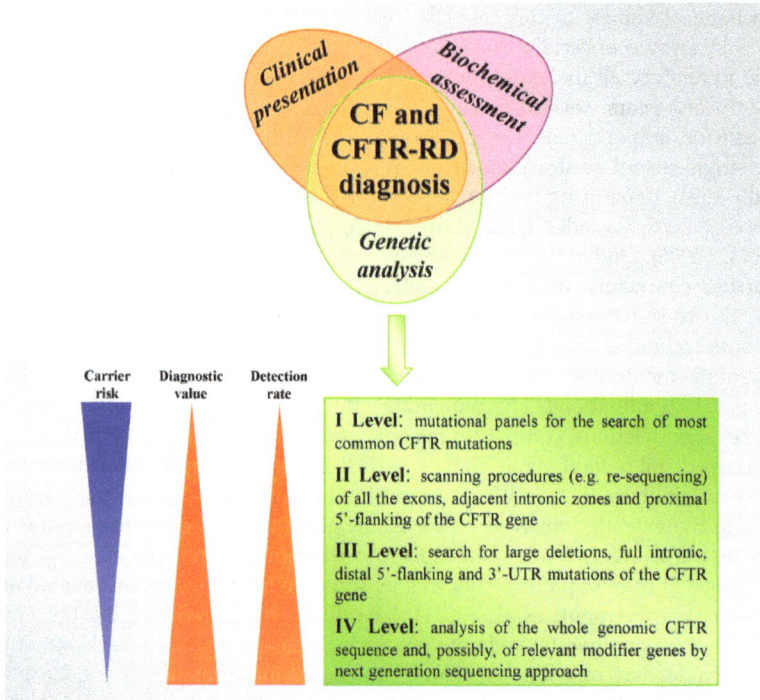

Fig. 2. The genetic analysis, biochemical assessment and clinical presentation contribute to the diagnosis of CF. The multistep genetic approach allows a progressive increase of detection rate and diagnostic value of the test in subjects with CF or CFTR-RD suspect, as well as a progressive decrease of carrier risk in general population subjects.

Usually, no scanning techniques are applied for genetic risk lowering , also because of the possibility to select sequence variations hardly valuable from a pathogenetic point of view. The use of the I level mutational panel approach to assess the genetic risk raises 4 possibilities. If both members of the couple are positive to the mutational search, the risk for an affected child is 1/4 (25%). If both members of the couple are negative the residual risk is so low that no other action is required, although it should be kept in mind that the risk is not zero and this should be made clear to the couple by the genetic counselling. For example, with a carrier frequency of 1/27 and a detection rate of the applied mutational panel of about 85%, the couple residual risk of having an affected child, with CFTR mutations different from those analyzed, if the genetic tests are both negative is about 1/120000. An intermediate residual risk arises when one member of the couple is carrier or CF. In these cases, considering the same above carrier frequency and detection rate, the risk is, respectively, of about 1/700 and 1/350. In these cases, in addition to the genetic counselling clarifying that a concrete risk exists, a possible extension of mutational search to further lower the genetic risk may be taken under consideration for the negative partner.

Following the above considerations, the often incomplete genetic characterization of CF and CFTR-RD patients is due to technical limitations; this constitute a further obstacle to our understanding of the genotype – phenotype relationship. An emblematic example of this are undetected complex alleles. Patients who do not undergo full mutational assessment, have discordant sweat test and/or clinical outcome, but show at a first mutational search apparently identical CFTR mutated genotypes, should undergo the search for complex alleles. The rising, within the last years, of parallel sequencing, also called next generation sequencing (NGS) (Su et al., 2011), allows to identify a possible IV level in the CFTR mutational search (Bell et al., 2011) (Figure 2 lower part). The possibility to study and analyze data of the whole genomic CFTR sequence (including introns, distal 5'-flanking and 3'-UTR zones) by massive re-sequencing, in an almost complete automated single run-based manner, will be a real possibility within next years. The NGS also has the potentiality to simultaneously study the genetics of modifier genes and, in general, of CFTR interactome to obtain a full assessment of genetic variability determining the final phenotype. If this kind of approach will be able to completely replace the multistep approach actually used is only matter of costs, investment and, finally, commercial choices. Several websites deal with CF and CFTR genetics, from diagnostic and quality assessment point of view, for example those of the European CF thematic network and of the European CF society (links reported in website section).

5. Conclusion

The comprehension of the gene network involved in CF and CFTR-RD is increasing. This is coupled with the enhancement of mutational search methodologies that allow the search for a continuously increasing number of mutations and sequence variations in the CFTR gene and in several other CF-related genes. The huge amount of structural data has to be supported by proper functional studies of single mutations, sequence variations, complex alleles and haplotypes. Only this will produce a full comprehension of genes and their molecular lesions cooperating in the definition of the final CF and CFTR-RD phenotypes, allowing full diagnosis and prognosis. As well, this will also allow the actual clinical use of mutation-specific therapies. When, in the mid-term, this objectives will be reached, the effect-oriented therapy now used will be turned into a cause-oriented therapy (Figure 3).

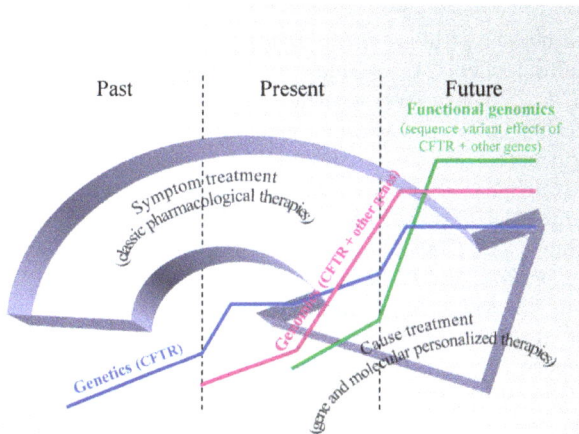

Fig. 3. A genetic-oriented view of CF and CFTR-RD therapy perspectives. The increasing knowledge about genetics, genomics and functional genomics change the therapy.

6. References

Amaral, M.D. & Kunzelmann, K. (2007). Molecular targeting of CFTR as a therapeutic approach to cystic fibrosis. *Trends Pharmacol.Sci.*, Vol.28, No.7, pp. 334-341.

Auerbach, S.D.; Loftus, R.W.; Itani, O.A. & Thomas, C.P. (2000). Human amiloride-sensitive epithelial Na$^+$ channel gamma subunit promoter: functional analysis and identification of a polypurine-polypyrimidine tract with the potential for triplex DNA formation. *Biochem.J.*, Vol.347 Pt 1, pp. 105-114.

Augusto, J.F.; Sayegh, J.; Malinge, M.C.; Illouz, F.; Subra, J.F. & Ducluzeau, P.H. (2008). Severe episodes of extra cellular dehydration: an atypical adult presentation of cystic fibrosis. *Clin.Nephrol.*, Vol.69, No.4, pp. 302-305.

Auriche, C.; Di Domenico, E.G.; Pierandrei, S.; Lucarelli, M.; Castellani, S.; Conese, M.; Melani, R.; Zegarra-Moran, O. & Ascenzioni, F. (2010). CFTR expression and activity from the human CFTR locus in BAC vectors, with regulatory regions, isolated by a single-step procedure. *Gene Ther.*, Vol.17, No.11, pp. 1341-1354.

Azad, A.K.; Rauh, R.; Vermeulen, F.; Jaspers, M.; Korbmacher, J.; Boissier, B.; Bassinet, L.; Fichou, Y.; Des, G.M.; Stanke, F.; De, B.K.; Dupont, L.; Balascakova, M.; Hjelte, L.; Lebecque, P.; Radojkovic, D.; Castellani, C.; Schwartz, M.; Stuhrmann, M.; Schwarz, M.; Skalicka, V.; de, M., I; Girodon, E.; Ferec, C.; Claustres, M.; Tummler, B.; Cassiman, J.J.; Korbmacher, C. & Cuppens, H. (2009). Mutations in the amiloride-sensitive epithelial sodium channel in patients with cystic fibrosis-like disease. *Hum.Mutat.*, Vol.30, No.7, pp. 1093-1103.

Bangel, N.; Dahlhoff, C.; Sobczak, K.; Weber, W.M. & Kusche-Vihrog, K. (2008). Upregulated expression of ENaC in human CF nasal epithelium. *J.Cyst.Fibros.*, Vol.7, No.3, pp. 197-205.

Becq, F.; Mall, M.A.; Sheppard, D.N.; Conese, M. & Zegarra-Moran, O. (2011). Pharmacological therapy for cystic fibrosis: from bench to bedside. *J.Cyst.Fibros.*, Vol.10 Suppl 2, pp. S129-S145.

Belcher, C.N. & Vij, N. (2010). Protein processing and inflammatory signaling in Cystic Fibrosis: challenges and therapeutic strategies. *Curr.Mol.Med.*, Vol.10, No.1, pp. 82-94.

Bell, C.J.; Dinwiddie, D.L.; Miller, N.A.; Hateley, S.L.; Ganusova, E.E.; Mudge, J.; Langley, R.J.; Zhang, L.; Lee, C.C.; Schilkey, F.D.; Sheth, V.; Woodward, J.E.; Peckham, H.E.; Schroth, G.P.; Kim, R.W. & Kingsmore, S.F. (2011). Carrier testing for severe childhood recessive diseases by next-generation sequencing. *Sci.Transl.Med.*, Vol.3, No.65, pp. 65ra4.

Berdiev, B.K.; Qadri Y.J. & Benos, D.J. (2009). Assessment of the CFTR and ENaC association. *Mol. Biosyst.*, Vol.5, No.2, pp. 123-127.

Bhalla, V. & Hallows, K.R. (2008). Mechanisms of ENaC regulation and clinical implications. *J.Am.Soc.Nephrol.*, Vol.19, No.10, pp. 1845-1854.

Bilan, F.; Thoreau, V.; Nacfer, M.; Derand, R.; Norez, C.; Cantereau, A.; Garcia, M.; Becq, F. & Kitzis, A. (2004). Syntaxin 8 impairs trafficking of cystic fibrosis transmembrane conductance regulator (CFTR) and inhibits its channel activity. *J.Cell Sci.*, Vol.117, No.Pt 10, pp. 1923-1935.

Bobadilla, J.L.; Macek, M., Jr.; Fine, J.P. & Farrell, P.M. (2002). Cystic fibrosis: a worldwide analysis of CFTR mutations--correlation with incidence data and application to screening. *Hum.Mutat.*, Vol.19, No.6, pp. 575-606.

Bombieri, C.; Benetazzo, M.; Saccomani, A.; Belpinati, F.; Gile, L.S.; Luisetti, M. & Pignatti, P.F. (1998). Complete mutational screening of the CFTR gene in 120 patients with pulmonary disease. *Hum.Genet.*, Vol.103, No.6, pp. 718-722.

Bombieri, C.; Claustres, M.; De, B.K.; Derichs, N.; Dodge, J.; Girodon, E.; Sermet, I.; Schwarz, M.; Tzetis, M.; Wilschanski, M.; Bareil, C.; Bilton, D.; Castellani, C.; Cuppens, H.; Cutting, G.R.; Drevinek, P.; Farrell, P.; Elborn, J.S.; Jarvi, K.; Kerem, B.; Kerem, E.; Knowles, M.; Macek, M., Jr.; Munck, A.; Radojkovic, D.; Seia, M.; Sheppard, D.N.; Southern, K.W.; Stuhrmann, M.; Tullis, E.; Zielenski, J.; Pignatti, P.F. & Ferec, C. (2011). Recommendations for the classification of diseases as CFTR-related disorders. *J.Cyst.Fibros.*, Vol.10 Suppl 2, pp. S86-102.

Bombieri, C.; Luisetti, M.; Belpinati, F.; Zuliani, E.; Beretta, A.; Baccheschi, J.; Casali, L. & Pignatti, P.F. (2000). Increased frequency of CFTR gene mutations in sarcoidosis: a case/control association study. *Eur.J.Hum.Genet.*, Vol.8, No.9, pp. 717-720.

Boucher, D.; Creveaux, I.; Grizard, G.; Jimenez, C.; Hermabessiere, J. & Dastugue, B. (1999). Screening for cystic fibrosis transmembrane conductance regulator gene mutations in men included in an intracytoplasmic sperm injection programme. *Mol.Hum.Reprod.*, Vol.5, No.6, pp. 587-593.

Boyne, J.; Evans, S.; Pollitt, R.J.; Taylor, C.J. & Dalton, A. (2000). Many deltaF508 heterozygote neonates with transient hypertrypsinaemia have a second, mild CFTR mutation. *J.Med.Genet.*, Vol.37, No.7, pp. 543-547.

Buchanan, P.J.; Ernst, R.K.; Elborn, J.S. & Schock, B. (2009). Role of CFTR, Pseudomonas aeruginosa and Toll-like receptors in cystic fibrosis lung inflammation. *Biochem.Soc.Trans.*, Vol.37, No.Pt 4, pp. 863-867.

Burrows, E.; Southern, K.W. & Noone, P. (2006). Sodium channel blockers for cystic fibrosis. *Cochrane.Database.Syst.Rev.*, Vol.3, pp. CD005087.

Butterworth, M.B. (2010). Regulation of the epithelial sodium channel (ENaC) by membrane trafficking. *Biochim.Biophys.Acta*, Vol.1802, No.12, pp. 1166-1177.

Caci, E.; Melani, R.; Pedemonte, N.; Yueksekdag, G.; Ravazzolo, R.; Rosenecker, J.; Galietta, L.J. & Zegarra-Moran, O. (2009). Epithelial sodium channel inhibition in primary human bronchial epithelia by transfected siRNA. *Am.J.Respir.Cell Mol.Biol.*, Vol.40, No.2, pp. 211-216.

Campodonico, V.L.; Gadjeva, M.; Paradis-Bleau, C.; Uluer, A. & Pier, G.B. (2008). Airway epithelial control of Pseudomonas aeruginosa infection in cystic fibrosis. *Trends Mol.Med.*, Vol.14, No.3, pp. 120-133.

Castellani, C.; Benetazzo, M.G.; Tamanini, A.; Begnini, A.; Mastella, G. & Pignatti, P. (2001a). Analysis of the entire coding region of the cystic fibrosis transmembrane regulator gene in neonatal hypertrypsinaemia with normal sweat test. *J.Med.Genet.*, Vol.38, No.3, pp. 202-205.

Castellani, C.; Cuppens, H.; Macek, M., Jr.; Cassiman, J.J.; Kerem, E.; Durie, P.; Tullis, E.; Assael, B.M.; Bombieri, C.; Brown, A.; Casals, T.; Claustres, M.; Cutting, G.R.; Dequeker, E.; Dodge, J.; Doull, I.; Farrell, P.; Ferec, C.; Girodon, E.; Johannesson, M.; Kerem, B.; Knowles, M.; Munck, A.; Pignatti, P.F.; Radojkovic, D.; Rizzotti, P.; Schwarz, M.; Stuhrmann, M.; Tzetis, M.; Zielenski, J. & Elborn, J.S. (2008). Consensus on the use and interpretation of cystic fibrosis mutation analysis in clinical practice. *J.Cyst.Fibros.*, Vol.7, No.3, pp. 179-196.

Castellani, C.; Gomez Lira, M.; Frulloni, L.; Delmarco, A.; Marzari, M.; Bonizzato, A.; Cavallini, G.; Pignatti, P. & Mastella, G. (2001b). Analysis of the entire coding region of the cystic fibrosis transmembrane regulator gene in idiopathic pancreatitis. *Hum.Mutat.*, Vol.18, No.2, pp. 166.

Castellani, C. & Massie, J. (2010). Emerging issues in cystic fibrosis newborn screening. *Curr.Opin.Pulm.Med.*, Vol.16, No.6, pp. 584-590.

Castellani, C.; Picci, L.; Scarpa, M.; Dechecchi, M.C.; Zanolla, L.; Assael, B.M. & Zacchello, F. (2005). Cystic fibrosis carriers have higher neonatal immunoreactive trypsinogen values than non-carriers. *Am.J.Med.Genet.A*, Vol.135, No.2, pp. 142-144.

Castellani, C.; Southern, K.W.; Brownlee, K.; Dankert, R.J.; Duff, A.; Farrell, M.; Mehta, A.; Munck, A.; Pollitt, R.; Sermet-Gaudelus, I.; Wilcken, B.; Ballmann, M.; Corbetta, C.; de, M., I; Farrell, P.; Feilcke, M.; Ferec, C.; Gartner, S.; Gaskin, K.; Hammermann, J.; Kashirskaya, N.; Loeber, G.; Macek, M., Jr.; Mehta, G.; Reiman, A.; Rizzotti, P.; Sammon, A.; Sands, D.; Smyth, A.; Sommerburg, O.; Torresani, T.; Travert, G.; Vernooij, A. & Elborn, S. (2009). European best practice guidelines for cystic fibrosis neonatal screening. *J.Cyst.Fibros.*, Vol.8, No.3, pp. 153-173.

Chang, S.S.; Grunder, S.; Hanukoglu, A.; Rosler, A.; Mathew, P.M.; Hanukoglu, I.; Schild, L.; Lu, Y.; Shimkets, R.A.; Nelson-Williams, C.; Rossier, B.C. & Lifton, R.P. (1996). Mutations in subunits of the epithelial sodium channel cause salt wasting with hyperkalaemic acidosis, pseudohypoaldosteronism type 1. *Nat.Genet.*, Vol.12, No.3, pp. 248-253.

Chen, J.H.; Stoltz, D.A.; Karp, P.H.; Ernst, S.E.; Pezzulo, A.A.; Moninger, T.O.; Rector, M.V.; Reznikov, L.R.; Launspach, J.L.; Chaloner, K.; Zabner, J. & Welsh, M.J. (2010). Loss of anion transport without increased sodium absorption characterizes newborn porcine cystic fibrosis airway epithelia. *Cell,* Vol.143, No.6, pp. 911-923.

Cheng, J.; Moyer, B.D.; Milewski, M.; Loffing, J.; Ikeda, M.; Mickle, J.E.; Cutting, G.R.; Li, M.; Stanton, B.A. & Guggino, W.B. (2002). A Golgi-associated PDZ domain protein modulates cystic fibrosis transmembrane regulator plasma membrane expression. *J.Biol.Chem.*, Vol.277, No.5, pp. 3520-3529.

Chillon, M.; Casals, T.; Mercier, B.; Bassas, L.; Lissens, W.; Silber, S.; Romey, M.C.; Ruiz-Romero, J.; Verlingue, C.; Claustres, M. & . (1995). Mutations in the cystic fibrosis gene in patients with congenital absence of the vas deferens. *N.Engl.J.Med.*, Vol.332, No.22, pp. 1475-1480.

Clain, J.; Fritsch, J.; Lehmann-Che, J.; Bali, M.; Arous, N.; Goossens, M.; Edelman, A. & Fanen, P. (2001). Two mild cystic fibrosis-associated mutations result in severe cystic fibrosis when combined in cis and reveal a residue important for cystic fibrosis transmembrane conductance regulator processing and function. *J.Biol.Chem.*, Vol.276, No.12, pp. 9045-9049.

Clain, J.; Lehmann-Che, J.; Girodon, E.; Lipecka, J.; Edelman, A.; Goossens, M. & Fanen, P. (2005). A neutral variant involved in a complex CFTR allele contributes to a severe cystic fibrosis phenotype. *Hum.Genet.*, Vol.116, No.6, pp. 454-460.

Claustres, M. (2005). Molecular pathology of the CFTR locus in male infertility. *Reprod.Biomed.Online.*, Vol.10, No.1, pp. 14-41.

Collaco, J.M. & Cutting, G.R. (2008). Update on gene modifiers in cystic fibrosis. *Curr.Opin.Pulm.Med.*, Vol.14, No.6, pp. 559-566.

Collardeau-Frachon, S.; Bouvier, R.; Le, G.C.; Rivet, C.; Cabet, F.; Bellon, G.; Lachaux, A. & Scoazec, J.Y. (2007). Unexpected diagnosis of cystic fibrosis at liver biopsy: a report of four pediatric cases. *Virchows Arch.*, Vol.451, No.1, pp. 57-64.

Conese, M.; Ascenzioni, F.; Boyd, A.C.; Coutelle, C.; De, F., I; De, S.S.; Rejman, J.; Rosenecker, J.; Schindelhauer, D. & Scholte, B.J. (2011). Gene and cell therapy for cystic fibrosis: from bench to bedside. *J.Cyst.Fibros.*, Vol.10 Suppl 2, pp. S114-S128.

Costes, B.; Fanen, P.; Goossens, M. & Ghanem, N. (1993). A rapid, efficient, and sensitive assay for simultaneous detection of multiple cystic fibrosis mutations. *Hum.Mutat.*, Vol.2, No.3, pp. 185-191.

Cuppens, H. & Cassiman, J.J. (2004). CFTR mutations and polymorphisms in male infertility. *Int.J.Androl,* Vol.27, No.5, pp. 251-256.

Cutting, G.R. (2010). Modifier genes in Mendelian disorders: the example of cystic fibrosis. *Ann.N.Y.Acad.Sci.,* Vol.1214, pp. 57-69.

D'Apice, M.R.; Gambardella, S.; Bengala, M.; Russo, S.; Nardone, A.M.; Lucidi, V.; Sangiuolo, F. & Novelli, G. (2004). Molecular analysis using DHPLC of cystic fibrosis: increase of the mutation detection rate among the affected population in Central Italy. *BMC.Med.Genet.,* Vol.5, pp. 8.

Davies, J.C. & Alton, E.W. (2011). Design of gene therapy trials in CF patients. *Methods Mol.Biol.,* Vol.741, pp. 55-68.

de Prada, M.A.; Butschi, F.N.; Bouchardy, I.; Beckmann, J.S.; Morris, M.A.; Hafen, G.M. & Fellmann, F. (2010). [R74W;R1070W;D1270N]: a new complex allele responsible for cystic fibrosis. *J.Cyst.Fibros.,* Vol.9, No.6, pp. 447-449.

Del Porto, P.; Cifani, N.; Guarnieri, S.; Di Domenico, E.G.; Mariggio, M.A.; Spadaro, F.; Guglietta, S.; Anile, M.; Venuta, F.; Quattrucci, S. & Ascenzioni, F. (2011). Dysfunctional CFTR alters the bactericidal activity of human macrophages against Pseudomonas aeruginosa. *PLoS.ONE.,* Vol.6, No.5, pp. e19970.

Dequeker, E.; Stuhrmann, M.; Morris, M.A.; Casals, T.; Castellani, C.; Claustres, M.; Cuppens, H.; Des, G.M.; Ferec, C.; Macek, M.; Pignatti, P.F.; Scheffer, H.; Schwartz, M.; Witt, M.; Schwarz, M. & Girodon, E. (2009). Best practice guidelines for molecular genetic diagnosis of cystic fibrosis and CFTR-related disorders--updated European recommendations. *Eur.J.Hum.Genet.,* Vol.17, No.1, pp. 51-65.

Di, A.; Brown, M.E.; Deriy, L.V.; Li, C.; Szeto, F.L.; Chen, Y.; Huang, P.; Tong, J.; Naren, A.P.; Bindokas, V.; Palfrey, H.C. & Nelson, D.J. (2006). CFTR regulates phagosome acidification in macrophages and alters bactericidal activity. *Nat.Cell Biol.,* Vol.8, No.9, pp. 933-944.

Dohle, G.R.; Halley, D.J.; Van Hemel, J.O.; van den Ouwel, A.M.; Pieters, M.H.; Weber, R.F. & Govaerts, L.C. (2002). Genetic risk factors in infertile men with severe oligozoospermia and azoospermia. *Hum.Reprod.,* Vol.17, No.1, pp. 13-16.

Donaldson, S.H.; Poligone, E.G. & Stutts, M.J. (2002). CFTR regulation of ENaC. *Methods Mol.Med.,* Vol.70, pp. 343-364.

Dork, T.; Wulbrand, U.; Richter, T.; Neumann, T.; Wolfes, H.; Wulf, B.; Maass, G. & Tummler, B. (1991). Cystic fibrosis with three mutations in the cystic fibrosis transmembrane conductance regulator gene. *Hum.Genet.,* Vol.87, No.4, pp. 441-446.

Duarte, A.; Amaral, M.; Barreto, C.; Pacheco, P. & Lavinha, J. (1996). Complex cystic fibrosis allele R334W-R1158X results in reduced levels of correctly processed mRNA in a pancreatic sufficient patient. *Hum.Mutat.,* Vol.8, No.2, pp. 134-139.

Dube, E.; Hermo, L.; Chan, P.T. & Cyr, D.G. (2008). Alterations in gene expression in the caput epididymides of nonobstructive azoospermic men. *Biol.Reprod.,* Vol.78, No.2, pp. 342-351.

Eaton, D.C.; Malik, B.; Bao, H.F.; Yu, L. & Jain, L. (2010). Regulation of epithelial sodium channel trafficking by ubiquitination. *Proc.Am.Thorac.Soc.*, Vol.7, No.1, pp. 54-64.

Edinger, R.S.; Yospin, J.; Perry, C.; Kleyman, T.R. & Johnson, J.P. (2006). Regulation of epithelial Na+ channels (ENaC) by methylation: a novel methyltransferase stimulates ENaC activity. *J.Biol.Chem.*, Vol.281, No.14, pp. 9110-9117.

Elia, J.; Delfino, M.; Imbrogno, N.; Capogreco, F.; Lucarelli, M.; Rossi, T. & Mazzilli, F. (2009). Human semen hyperviscosity: prevalence, pathogenesis and therapeutic aspects. *Asian J.Androl*, Vol.11, No.5, pp. 609-615.

Estivill, X. (1996). Complexity in a monogenic disease. *Nat.Genet.*, Vol.12, No.4, pp. 348-350.

Fanen, P.; Clain, J.; Labarthe, R.; Hulin, P.; Girodon, E.; Pagesy, P.; Goossens, M. & Edelman, A. (1999). Structure-function analysis of a double-mutant cystic fibrosis transmembrane conductance regulator protein occurring in disorders related to cystic fibrosis. *FEBS Lett.*, Vol.452, No.3, pp. 371-374.

Fanen, P.; Ghanem, N.; Vidaud, M.; Besmond, C.; Martin, J.; Costes, B.; Plassa, F. & Goossens, M. (1992). Molecular characterization of cystic fibrosis: 16 novel mutations identified by analysis of the whole cystic fibrosis conductance transmembrane regulator (CFTR) coding regions and splice site junctions. *Genomics*, Vol.13, No.3, pp. 770-776.

Farmen, S.L.; Karp, P.H.; Ng, P.; Palmer, D.J.; Koehler, D.R.; Hu, J.; Beaudet, A.L.; Zabner, J. & Welsh, M.J. (2005). Gene transfer of CFTR to airway epithelia: low levels of expression are sufficient to correct Cl- transport and overexpression can generate basolateral CFTR. *Am.J.Physiol Lung Cell Mol.Physiol*, Vol.289, No.6, pp. L1123-L1130.

Farrell, P.M.; Rosenstein, B.J.; White, T.B.; Accurso, F.J.; Castellani, C.; Cutting, G.R.; Durie, P.R.; Legrys, V.A.; Massie, J.; Parad, R.B.; Rock, M.J. & Campbell, P.W., III (2008). Guidelines for diagnosis of cystic fibrosis in newborns through older adults: Cystic Fibrosis Foundation consensus report. *J.Pediatr.*, Vol.153, No.2, pp. S4-S14.

Feldmann, D.; Couderc, R.; Audrezet, M.P.; Ferec, C.; Bienvenu, T.; Desgeorges, M.; Claustres, M.; Mittre, H.; Blayau, M.; Bozon, D.; Malinge, M.C.; Monnier, N.; Bonnefont, J.P.; Iron, A.; Bieth, E.; Dumur, V.; Clavel, C.; Cazeneuve, C. & Girodon, E. (2003). CFTR genotypes in patients with normal or borderline sweat chloride levels. *Hum.Mutat.*, Vol.22, No.4, pp. 340.

Ferraguti, G.; Pierandrei, S.; Bruno, S.M.; Ceci, F.; Strom, R. & Lucarelli, M. (2011). A template for mutational data analysis of the CFTR gene. *Clin.Chem.Lab Med.*, Vol.49, No.9, pp.1447-1451

Fichou, Y.; Genin, E.; Le, M.C.; Audrezet, M.P.; Scotet, V. & Ferec, C. (2008). Estimating the age of CFTR mutations predominantly found in Brittany (Western France). *J.Cyst.Fibros.*, Vol.7, No.2, pp. 168-173.

Frischmeyer, P.A. & Dietz, H.C. (1999). Nonsense-mediated mRNA decay in health and disease. *Hum.Mol.Genet.*, Vol.8, No.10, pp. 1893-1900.

Gadsby, D.C.; Vergani, P. & Csanady, L. (2006). The ABC protein turned chloride channel whose failure causes cystic fibrosis. *Nature*, Vol.440, No.7083, pp. 477-483.

Gaillard, E.A.; Kota, P.; Gentzsch, M.; Dokholyan, N.V.; Stutts, M.J. & Tarran, R. (2010). Regulation of the epithelial Na+ channel and airway surface liquid volume by serine proteases. *Pflugers Arch.*, Vol.460, No.1, pp. 1-17.

Gallegos-Orozco, J.F.; Yurk, E.; Wang, N.; Rakela, J.; Charlton, M.R.; Cutting, G.R. & Balan, V. (2005). Lack of association of common cystic fibrosis transmembrane conductance regulator gene mutations with primary sclerosing cholangitis. *Am.J.Gastroenterol.*, Vol.100, No.4, pp. 874-878.

Gentzsch, M.; Dang, H.; Dang, Y.; Garcia-Caballero, A.; Suchindran, H.; Boucher, R.C. & Stutts, M.J. (2010). The cystic fibrosis transmembrane conductance regulator impedes proteolytic stimulation of the epithelial Na+ channel. *J.Biol.Chem.*, Vol.285, No.42, pp. 32227-32232.

Gervais, R.; Dumur, V.; Letombe, B.; Larde, A.; Rigot, J.M.; Roussel, P. & Lafitte, J.J. (1996). Hypofertility with thick cervical mucus: another mild form of cystic fibrosis? *JAMA*, Vol.276, No.20, pp. 1638.

Gillen, A.E.; Gosalia, N.; Leir, S.H. & Harris, A. (2011). microRNA regulation of expression of the cystic fibrosis transmembrane conductance regulator gene. *Biochem.J.*, Vol.438, No.1, pp. 25-32.

Girodon, E.; Cazeneuve, C.; Lebargy, F.; Chinet, T.; Costes, B.; Ghanem, N.; Martin, J.; Lemay, S.; Scheid, P.; Housset, B.; Bignon, J. & Goossens, M. (1997). CFTR gene mutations in adults with disseminated bronchiectasis. *Eur.J.Hum.Genet.*, Vol.5, No.3, pp. 149-155.

Girodon, E.; Sternberg, D.; Chazouilleres, O.; Cazeneuve, C.; Huot, D.; Calmus, Y.; Poupon, R.; Goossens, M. & Housset, C. (2002). Cystic fibrosis transmembrane conductance regulator (CFTR) gene defects in patients with primary sclerosing cholangitis. *J.Hepatol.*, Vol.37, No.2, pp. 192-197.

Gomez Lira, M.; Benetazzo, M.G.; Marzari, M.G.; Bombieri, C.; Belpinati, F.; Castellani, C.; Cavallini, G.C.; Mastella, G. & Pignatti, P.F. (2000). High frequency of cystic fibrosis transmembrane regulator mutation L997F in patients with recurrent idiopathic pancreatitis and in newborns with hypertrypsinemia. *Am.J.Hum.Genet.*, Vol.66, No.6, pp. 2013-2014.

Green, A. & Kirk, J. (2007). Guidelines for the performance of the sweat test for the diagnosis of cystic fibrosis. *Ann.Clin.Biochem.*, Vol.44, No.Pt 1, pp. 25-34.

Griesenbach, U. & Alton, E.W. (2011). Current status and future directions of gene and cell therapy for cystic fibrosis. *BioDrugs.*, Vol.25, No.2, pp. 77-88.

Groman, J.D.; Meyer, M.E.; Wilmott, R.W.; Zeitlin, P.L. & Cutting, G.R. (2002). Variant cystic fibrosis phenotypes in the absence of CFTR mutations. *N.Engl.J.Med.*, Vol.347, No.6, pp. 401-407.

Gruenert, D.C.; Bruscia, E.; Novelli, G.; Colosimo, A.; Dallapiccola, B.; Sangiuolo, F. & Goncz, K.K. (2003). Sequence-specific modification of genomic DNA by small DNA fragments. *J.Clin.Invest*, Vol.112, No.5, pp. 637-641.

Hallows, K.R.; Raghuram, V.; Kemp, B.E.; Witters, L.A. & Foskett, J.K. (2000). Inhibition of cystic fibrosis transmembrane conductance regulator by novel interaction with the metabolic sensor AMP-activated protein kinase. *J.Clin.Invest*, Vol.105, No.12, pp. 1711-1721.

Hanukoglu, A.; Bistritzer, T.; Rakover, Y. & Mandelberg, A. (1994). Pseudohypoaldosteronism with increased sweat and saliva electrolyte values and frequent lower respiratory tract infections mimicking cystic fibrosis. *J.Pediatr.*, Vol.125, No.5 Pt 1, pp. 752-755.

Hayslip, C.C.; Hao, E. & Usala, S.J. (1997). The cystic fibrosis transmembrane regulator gene is expressed in the human endocervix throughout the menstrual cycle. *Fertil.Steril.*, Vol.67, No.4, pp. 636-640.

Hojo, S.; Fujita, J.; Miyawaki, H.; Obayashi, Y.; Takahara, J. & Bartholomew, D.W. (1998). Severe cystic fibrosis associated with a deltaF508/R347H + D979A compound heterozygous genotype. *Clin.Genet.*, Vol.53, No.1, pp. 50-53.

Huber, R.; Krueger, B.; Diakov, A.; Korbmacher, J.; Haerteis, S.; Einsiedel, J.; Gmeiner, P.; Azad, A.K.; Cuppens, H.; Cassiman, J.J.; Korbmacher, C. & Rauh, R. (2010). Functional characterization of a partial loss-of-function mutation of the epithelial sodium channel (ENaC) associated with atypical cystic fibrosis. *Cell Physiol Biochem.*, Vol.25, No.1, pp. 145-158.

Hummler, E.; Barker, P.; Gatzy, J.; Beermann, F.; Verdumo, C.; Schmidt, A.; Boucher, R. & Rossier, B.C. (1996). Early death due to defective neonatal lung liquid clearance in alpha-ENaC-deficient mice. *Nat.Genet.*, Vol.12, No.3, pp. 325-328.

Jakubiczka, S.; Bettecken, T.; Stumm, M.; Nickel, I.; Musebeck, J.; Krebs, P.; Fischer, C.; Kleinstein, J. & Wieacker, P. (1999). Frequency of CFTR gene mutations in males participating in an ICSI programme. *Hum.Reprod.*, Vol.14, No.7, pp. 1833-1834.

Jarvi, K.; McCallum, S.; Zielenski, J.; Durie, P.; Tullis, E.; Wilchanski, M.; Margolis, M.; Asch, M.; Ginzburg, B.; Martin, S.; Buckspan, M.B. & Tsui, L.C. (1998). Heterogeneity of reproductive tract abnormalities in men with absence of the vas deferens: role of cystic fibrosis transmembrane conductance regulator gene mutations. *Fertil.Steril.*, Vol.70, No.4, pp. 724-728.

Johnson, L.G.; Olsen, J.C.; Sarkadi, B.; Moore, K.L.; Swanstrom, R. & Boucher, R.C. (1992). Efficiency of gene transfer for restoration of normal airway epithelial function in cystic fibrosis. *Nat.Genet.*, Vol.2, No.1, pp. 21-25.

Joo N.S.; Irokawa T.; Robbins R.C. & Wine J.J. (2006). Hyposecretion, not hyperabsorption, is the basic defect of cystic fibrosis airway glands. *J. Biol. Chem.*, Vol.281, No.11, pp. 7392-7398.

Kalin, N.; Dork, T. & Tummler, B. (1992). A cystic fibrosis allele encoding missense mutations in both nucleotide binding folds of the cystic fibrosis transmembrane conductance regulator. *Hum.Mutat.*, Vol.1, No.3, pp. 204-210.

Karijolich, J. & Yu, Y.T. (2011). Converting nonsense codons into sense codons by targeted pseudouridylation. *Nature*, Vol.474, No.7351, pp. 395-398.

Kerem, B.; Rommens, J.M.; Buchanan, J.A.; Markiewicz, D.; Cox, T.K.; Chakravarti, A.; Buchwald, M. & Tsui, L.C. (1989). Identification of the cystic fibrosis gene: genetic analysis. *Science*, Vol.245, No.4922, pp. 1073-1080.

Kerem, E. (2005). Pharmacological induction of CFTR function in patients with cystic fibrosis: mutation-specific therapy. *Pediatr.Pulmonol.*, Vol.40, No.3, pp. 183-196.

Kerem, E. (2006). Atypical CF and CF related diseases. *Paediatr.Respir.Rev.*, Vol.7 Suppl 1, pp. S144-S146.

Kiesewetter, S.; Macek, M., Jr.; Davis, C.; Curristin, S.M.; Chu, C.S.; Graham, C.; Shrimpton, A.E.; Cashman, S.M.; Tsui, L.C.; Mickle, J. & . (1993). A mutation in CFTR produces different phenotypes depending on chromosomal background. *Nat.Genet.*, Vol.5, No.3, pp. 274-278.

Kim, D. & Steward, M.C. (2009). The role of CFTR in bicarbonate secretion by pancreatic duct and airway epithelia. *J.Med.Invest*, Vol.56 Suppl, pp. 336-342.

Lai, H.J.; Cheng, Y. & Farrell, P.M. (2005). The survival advantage of patients with cystic fibrosis diagnosed through neonatal screening: evidence from the United States Cystic Fibrosis Foundation registry data. *J.Pediatr.*, Vol.147, No.3 Suppl, pp. S57-S63.

Laroche, D. & Travert, G. (1991). Abnormal frequency of delta F508 mutation in neonatal transitory hypertrypsinaemia. *Lancet*, Vol.337, No.8732, pp. 55.

Le Marechal, C.; Audrezet, M.P.; Quere, I.; Raguenes, O.; Langonne, S. & Ferec, C. (2001). Complete and rapid scanning of the cystic fibrosis transmembrane conductance regulator (CFTR) gene by denaturing high-performance liquid chromatography (D-HPLC): major implications for genetic counselling. *Hum.Genet.*, Vol.108, No.4, pp. 290-298.

Legrys, V.A.; Yankaskas, J.R.; Quittell, L.M.; Marshall, B.C. & Mogayzel, P.J., Jr. (2007). Diagnostic sweat testing: the Cystic Fibrosis Foundation guidelines. *J.Pediatr.*, Vol.151, No.1, pp. 85-89.

Leoni, G.B.; Pitzalis, S.; Podda, R.; Zanda, M.; Silvetti, M.; Caocci, L.; Cao, A. & Rosatelli, M.C. (1995). A specific cystic fibrosis mutation (T338I) associated with the phenotype of isolated hypotonic dehydration. *J.Pediatr.*, Vol.127, No.2, pp. 281-283.

Lucarelli, M.; Grandoni, F.; Rossi, T.; Mazzilli, F.; Antonelli, M. & Strom, R. (2002). Simultaneous cycle sequencing assessment of (TG)m and Tn tract length in CFTR gene. *Biotechniques*, Vol.32, No.3, pp. 540-547.

Lucarelli, M.; Narzi, L.; Pierandrei, S.; Bruno, S.M.; Stamato, A.; d'Avanzo, M.; Strom, R. & Quattrucci, S. (2010). A new complex allele of the CFTR gene partially explains the variable phenotype of the L997F mutation. *Genet.Med.*, Vol.12, No.9, pp. 548-555.

Lucarelli, M.; Narzi, L.; Piergentili, R.; Ferraguti, G.; Grandoni, F.; Quattrucci, S. & Strom, R. (2006). A 96-well formatted method for exon and exon/intron boundary full sequencing of the CFTR gene. *Anal.Biochem.*, Vol.353, No.2, pp. 226-235.

Ludwig, M.; Bolkenius, U.; Wickert, L.; Marynen, P. & Bidlingmaier, F. (1998). Structural organisation of the gene encoding the alpha-subunit of the human amiloride-sensitive epithelial sodium channel. *Hum.Genet.*, Vol.102, No.5, pp. 576-581.

Maire, F.; Bienvenu, T.; Ngukam, A.; Hammel, P.; Ruszniewski, P. & Levy, P. (2003). [Frequency of CFTR gene mutations in idiopathic pancreatitis]. *Gastroenterol.Clin.Biol.*, Vol.27, No.4, pp. 398-402.

Mak, V.; Zielenski, J.; Tsui, L.C.; Durie, P.; Zini, A.; Martin, S.; Longley, T.B. & Jarvi, K.A. (2000). Cystic fibrosis gene mutations and infertile men with primary testicular failure. *Hum.Reprod.*, Vol.15, No.2, pp. 436-439.

Mall, M.; Bleich, M.; Greger, R.; Schreiber, R. & Kunzelmann, K. (1998). The amiloride-inhibitable Na+ conductance is reduced by the cystic fibrosis transmembrane conductance regulator in normal but not in cystic fibrosis airways. *J.Clin.Invest*, Vol.102, No.1, pp. 15-21.

Massie, R.J.; Poplawski, N.; Wilcken, B.; Goldblatt, J.; Byrnes, C. & Robertson, C. (2001). Intron-8 polythymidine sequence in Australasian individuals with CF mutations R117H and R117C. *Eur.Respir.J.*, Vol.17, No.6, pp. 1195-1200.

Massie, R.J.; Wilcken, B.; Van, A.P.; Dorney, S.; Gruca, M.; Wiley, V. & Gaskin, K. (2000). Pancreatic function and extended mutation analysis in DeltaF508 heterozygous infants with an elevated immunoreactive trypsinogen but normal sweat electrolyte levels. *J.Pediatr.*, Vol.137, No.2, pp. 214-220.

Matsui, H.; Grubb, B.R.; Tarran, R.; Randell, S.H.; Gatzy, J.T.; Davis, C.W. & Boucher, R.C. (1998). Evidence for periciliary liquid layer depletion, not abnormal ion composition, in the pathogenesis of cystic fibrosis airways disease. *Cell*, Vol.95, No.7, pp. 1005-1015.

Mattoscio, D.; Evangelista, V.; De, C.R.; Recchiuti, A.; Pandolfi, A.; Di, S.S.; Manarini, S.; Martelli, N.; Rocca, B.; Petrucci, G.; Angelini, D.F.; Battistini, L.; Robuffo, I.; Pensabene, T.; Pieroni, L.; Furnari, M.L.; Pardo, F.; Quattrucci, S.; Lancellotti, S.; Davi, G. & Romano, M. (2010). Cystic fibrosis transmembrane conductance regulator (CFTR) expression in human platelets: impact on mediators and mechanisms of the inflammatory response. *FASEB J.*, Vol.24, No.10, pp. 3970-3980.

Mayell, S.J.; Munck, A.; Craig, J.V.; Sermet, I.; Brownlee, K.G.; Schwarz, M.J.; Castellani, C. & Southern, K.W. (2009). A European consensus for the evaluation and management of infants with an equivocal diagnosis following newborn screening for cystic fibrosis. *J.Cyst.Fibros.*, Vol.8, No.1, pp. 71-78.

McGinniss, M.J.; Chen, C.; Redman, J.B.; Buller, A.; Quan, F.; Peng, M.; Giusti, R.; Hantash, F.M.; Huang, D.; Sun, W. & Strom, C.M. (2005). Extensive sequencing of the CFTR gene: lessons learned from the first 157 patient samples. *Hum.Genet.*, Vol.118, No.3-4, pp. 331-338.

Mekus, F.; Ballmann, M.; Bronsveld, I.; Dork, T.; Bijman, J.; Tummler, B. & Veeze, H.J. (1998). Cystic-fibrosis-like disease unrelated to the cystic fibrosis transmembrane conductance regulator. *Hum.Genet.*, Vol.102, No.5, pp. 582-586.

Mercier, B.; Verlingue, C.; Lissens, W.; Silber, S.J.; Novelli, G.; Bonduelle, M.; Audrezet, M.P. & Ferec, C. (1995). Is congenital bilateral absence of vas deferens a primary form of cystic fibrosis? Analyses of the CFTR gene in 67 patients. *Am.J.Hum.Genet.*, Vol.56, No.1, pp. 272-277.

Merlo, C.A. & Boyle, M.P. (2003). Modifier genes in cystic fibrosis lung disease. *J.Lab Clin.Med.*, Vol.141, No.4, pp. 237-241.

Mutesa, L.; Azad, A.K.; Verhaeghe, C.; Segers, K.; Vanbellinghen, J.F.; Ngendahayo, L.; Rusingiza, E.K.; Mutwa, P.R.; Rulisa, S.; Koulischer, L.; Cassiman, J.J.; Cuppens, H. & Bours, V. (2008). Genetic Analysis of Rwandan Patients With Cystic Fibrosis-Like Symptoms: Identification of Novel Cystic Fibrosis Transmembrane Conductance Regulator and Epithelial Sodium Channel Gene Variants. *Chest,*

Nagel G.; Barbry P.; Chabot H.; Brochiero E.; Hartung K. & Grygorczyk R. (2005). CFTR fails to inhibit the epithelial sodium channel ENaC expressed in Xenopus laevis oocytes. *J. Physiol.*, Vol.564, No.3, pp. 671-682.

Narzi, L.; Ferraguti, G.; Stamato, A.; Narzi, F.; Valentini, S.B.; Lelli, A.; Delaroche, I.; Lucarelli, M.; Strom, R. & Quattrucci, S. (2007). Does cystic fibrosis neonatal screening detect atypical CF forms? Extended genetic characterization and 4-year clinical follow-up. *Clin.Genet.*, Vol.72, No.1, pp. 39-46.

Narzi, L.; Lucarelli, M.; Lelli, A.; Grandoni, F.; Lo, C.S.; Ferraro, A.; Matarazzo, P.; Delaroche, I.; Quattrucci, S.; Strom, R. & Antonelli, M. (2002). Comparison of two different protocols of neonatal screening for cystic fibrosis. *Clin.Genet.*, Vol.62, No.3, pp. 245-249.

Niel, F.; Legendre, M.; Bienvenu, T.; Bieth, E.; Lalau, G.; Sermet, I.; Bondeux, D.; Boukari, R.; Derelle, J.; Levy, P.; Ruszniewski, P.; Martin, J.; Costa, C.; Goossens, M. & Girodon, E. (2006). A new large CFTR rearrangement illustrates the importance of searching for complex alleles. *Hum.Mutat.*, Vol.27, No.7, pp. 716-717.

Noone, P.G. & Knowles, M.R. (2001). 'CFTR-opathies': disease phenotypes associated with cystic fibrosis transmembrane regulator gene mutations. *Respir.Res.*, Vol.2, No.6, pp. 328-332.

O'Sullivan, B.P. & Freedman, S.D. (2009). Cystic fibrosis. *Lancet,* Vol.373, No.9678, pp. 1891-1904.

Padoan, R.; Bassotti, A.; Seia, M. & Corbetta, C. (2002). Negative sweat test in hypertrypsinaemic infants with cystic fibrosis carrying rare CFTR mutations. *Eur.J.Pediatr.,* Vol.161, No.4, pp. 212-215.

Pallares-Ruiz, N.; Carles, S.; Des, G.M.; Guittard, C.; Arnal, F.; Humeau, C. & Claustres, M. (1999). Complete mutational screening of the cystic fibrosis transmembrane conductance regulator gene: cystic fibrosis mutations are not involved in healthy men with reduced sperm quality. *Hum.Reprod.,* Vol.14, No.12, pp. 3035-3040.

Pallares-Ruiz, N.; Carles, S.; Des, G.M.; Guittard, C.; Claustres, M.; Larrey, D. & Pageaux, G. (2000). Is isolated idiopathic pancreatitis associated with CFTR mutations? *Gut,* Vol.46, No.1, pp. 141.

Parad, R.B. & Comeau, A.M. (2005). Diagnostic dilemmas resulting from the immunoreactive trypsinogen/DNA cystic fibrosis newborn screening algorithm. *J.Pediatr.,* Vol.147, No.3 Suppl, pp. S78-S82.

Patrizio, P. & Salameh, W.A. (1998). Expression of the cystic fibrosis transmembrane conductance regulator (CFTR) mRNA in normal and pathological adult human epididymis. *J.Reprod.Fertil.Suppl,* Vol.53, pp. 261-270.

Pawankar, R. (2003). Nasal polyposis: an update: editorial review. *Curr.Opin.Allergy Clin.Immunol.,* Vol.3, No.1, pp. 1-6.

Peckham, D.; Conway, S.P.; Morton, A.; Jones, A. & Webb, K. (2006). Delayed diagnosis of cystic fibrosis associated with R117H on a background of 7T polythymidine tract at intron 8. *J.Cyst.Fibros.,* Vol.5, No.1, pp. 63-65.

Peters, K.W.; Qi, J.; Johnson, J.P.; Watkins, S.C. & Frizzell, R.A. (2001). Role of snare proteins in CFTR and ENaC trafficking. *Pflugers Arch.,* Vol.443 Suppl 1, pp. S65-S69.

Pier, G.B.; Grout, M. & Zaidi, T.S. (1997). Cystic fibrosis transmembrane conductance regulator is an epithelial cell receptor for clearance of Pseudomonas aeruginosa from the lung. *Proc.Natl.Acad.Sci.U.S.A,* Vol.94, No.22, pp. 12088-12093.

Pignatti, P.F.; Bombieri, C.; Marigo, C.; Benetazzo, M. & Luisetti, M. (1995). Increased incidence of cystic fibrosis gene mutations in adults with disseminated bronchiectasis. *Hum.Mol.Genet.,* Vol.4, No.4, pp. 635-639.

Prince, L.S.; Peter, K.; Hatton, S.R.; Zaliauskiene, L.; Cotlin, L.F.; Clancy, J.P.; Marchase, R.B. & Collawn, J.F. (1999). Efficient endocytosis of the cystic fibrosis transmembrane conductance regulator requires a tyrosine-based signal. *J.Biol.Chem.,* Vol.274, No.6, pp. 3602-3609.

Priou-Guesdon, M.; Malinge, M.C.; Augusto, J.F.; Rodien, P.; Subra, J.F.; Bonneau, D. & Rohmer, V. (2010). Hypochloremia and hyponatremia as the initial presentation of cystic fibrosis in three adults. *Ann.Endocrinol.(Paris),* Vol.71, No.1, pp. 46-50.

Raman, V.; Clary, R.; Siegrist, K.L.; Zehnbauer, B. & Chatila, T.A. (2002). Increased prevalence of mutations in the cystic fibrosis transmembrane conductance regulator in children with chronic rhinosinusitis. *Pediatrics,* Vol.109, No.1, pp. E13.

Ratjen, F. & Doring, G. (2003). Cystic fibrosis. *Lancet,* Vol.361, No.9358, pp. 681-689.

Ravnik-Glavac, M.; Atkinson, A.; Glavac, D. & Dean, M. (2002). DHPLC screening of cystic fibrosis gene mutations. *Hum.Mutat.,* Vol.19, No.4, pp. 374-383.

Ravnik-Glavac, M.; Glavac, D.; Chernick, M.; di, S.P. & Dean, M. (1994). Screening for CF mutations in adult cystic fibrosis patients with a directed and optimized SSCP strategy. *Hum.Mutat.,* Vol.3, No.3, pp. 231-238.

Riordan, J.R. (2008). CFTR function and prospects for therapy. *Annu.Rev.Biochem.*, Vol.77, pp. 701-726.

Rogan, M.P.; Stoltz, D.A. & Hornick, D.B. (2011). Cystic fibrosis transmembrane conductance regulator intracellular processing, trafficking, and opportunities for mutation-specific treatment. *Chest*, Vol.139, No.6, pp. 1480-1490.

Rohlfs, E.M.; Zhou, Z.; Sugarman, E.A.; Heim, R.A.; Pace, R.G.; Knowles, M.R.; Silverman, L.M. & Allitto, B.A. (2002). The I148T CFTR allele occurs on multiple haplotypes: a complex allele is associated with cystic fibrosis. *Genet.Med.*, Vol.4, No.5, pp. 319-323.

Romey, M.C.; Guittard, C.; Chazalette, J.P.; Frossard, P.; Dawson, K.P.; Patton, M.A.; Casals, T.; Bazarbachi, T.; Girodon, E.; Rault, G.; Bozon, D.; Seguret, F.; Demaille, J. & Claustres, M. (1999). Complex allele [-102T>A+S549R(T>G)] is associated with milder forms of cystic fibrosis than allele S549R(T>G) alone. *Hum.Genet.*, Vol.105, No.1-2, pp. 145-150.

Rommens, J.M.; Iannuzzi, M.C.; Kerem, B.; Drumm, M.L.; Melmer, G.; Dean, M.; Rozmahel, R.; Cole, J.L.; Kennedy, D.; Hidaka, N. & . (1989). Identification of the cystic fibrosis gene: chromosome walking and jumping. *Science*, Vol.245, No.4922, pp. 1059-1065.

Rossi, T.; Grandoni, F.; Mazzilli, F.; Quattrucci, S.; Antonelli, M.; Strom, R. & Lucarelli, M. (2004). High frequency of (TG)mTn variant tracts in the cystic fibrosis transmembrane conductance regulator gene in men with high semen viscosity. *Fertil.Steril.*, Vol.82, No.5, pp. 1316-1322.

Rubenstein, R.C.; Lockwood, S.R.; Lide, E.; Bauer, R.; Suaud, L. & Grumbach, Y. (2011). Regulation of endogenous ENaC functional expression by CFTR and DeltaF508-CFTR in airway epithelial cells. *Am.J.Physiol Lung Cell Mol.Physiol*, Vol.300, No.1, pp. L88-L101.

Salvatore, D.; Buzzetti, R.; Baldo, E.; Forneris, M.P.; Lucidi, V.; Manunza, D.; Marinelli, I.; Messore, B.; Neri, A.S.; Raia, V.; Furnari, M.L. & Mastella, G. (2011). An overview of international literature from cystic fibrosis registries. Part 3. Disease incidence, genotype/phenotype correlation, microbiology, pregnancy, clinical complications, lung transplantation, and miscellanea. *J.Cyst.Fibros.*, Vol.10, No.2, pp. 71-85.

Salvatore, D.; Tomaiuolo, R.; Abate, R.; Vanacore, B.; Manieri, S.; Mirauda, M.P.; Scavone, A.; Schiavo, M.V.; Castaldo, G. & Salvatore, F. (2004). Cystic fibrosis presenting as metabolic alkalosis in a boy with the rare D579G mutation. *J.Cyst.Fibros.*, Vol.3, No.2, pp. 135-136.

Salvatore, F.; Scudiero, O. & Castaldo, G. (2002). Genotype-phenotype correlation in cystic fibrosis: the role of modifier genes. *Am.J.Med.Genet.*, Vol.111, No.1, pp. 88-95.

Sangiuolo, F.; Bruscia, E.; Serafino, A.; Nardone, A.M.; Bonifazi, E.; Lais, M.; Gruenert, D.C. & Novelli, G. (2002). In vitro correction of cystic fibrosis epithelial cell lines by small fragment homologous replacement (SFHR) technique. *BMC.Med.Genet.*, Vol.3, pp. 8.

Sangiuolo, F.; Scaldaferri, M.L.; Filareto, A.; Spitalieri, P.; Guerra, L.; Favia, M.; Caroppo, R.; Mango, R.; Bruscia, E.; Gruenert, D.C.; Casavola, V.; De, F.M. & Novelli, G. (2008). Cftr gene targeting in mouse embryonic stem cells mediated by Small Fragment Homologous Replacement (SFHR). *Front Biosci.*, Vol.13, pp. 2989-2999.

Savov, A.; Angelicheva, D.; Balassopoulou, A.; Jordanova, A.; Noussia-Arvanitakis, S. & Kalaydjieva, L. (1995). Double mutant alleles: are they rare? *Hum.Mol.Genet.*, Vol.4, No.7, pp. 1169-1171.

Schroeder, T.H.; Lee, M.M.; Yacono, P.W.; Cannon, C.L.; Gerceker, A.A.; Golan, D.E. & Pier, G.B. (2002). CFTR is a pattern recognition molecule that extracts Pseudomonas aeruginosa LPS from the outer membrane into epithelial cells and activates NF-kappa B translocation. *Proc.Natl.Acad.Sci.U.S.A*, Vol.99, No.10, pp. 6907-6912.

Scotet, V.; De Braekeleer, M.; Audrezet, M.P.; Lode, L.; Verlingue, C.; Quere, I.; Mercier, B.; Dugueperoux, I.; Codet, J.P.; Moineau, M.P.; Parent, P. & Ferec, C. (2001). Prevalence of CFTR mutations in hypertrypsinaemia detected through neonatal screening for cystic fibrosis. *Clin.Genet.*, Vol.59, No.1, pp. 42-47.

Seidler, U.; Singh, A.K.; Cinar, A.; Chen, M.; Hillesheim, J.; Hogema, B. & Riederer, B. (2009). The role of the NHERF family of PDZ scaffolding proteins in the regulation of salt and water transport. *Ann.N.Y.Acad.Sci.*, Vol.1165, pp. 249-260.

Sermet-Gaudelus, I.; Mayell, S.J. & Southern, K.W. (2010). Guidelines on the early management of infants diagnosed with cystic fibrosis following newborn screening. *J.Cyst.Fibros.*, Vol.9, No.5, pp. 323-329.

Sharma, M.; Benharouga, M.; Hu, W. & Lukacs, G.L. (2001). Conformational and temperature-sensitive stability defects of the delta F508 cystic fibrosis transmembrane conductance regulator in post-endoplasmic reticulum compartments. *J.Biol.Chem.*, Vol.276, No.12, pp. 8942-8950.

Sheridan, M.B.; Fong, P.; Groman, J.D.; Conrad, C.; Flume, P.; Diaz, R.; Harris, C.; Knowles, M. & Cutting, G.R. (2005). Mutations in the beta-subunit of the epithelial Na+ channel in patients with a cystic fibrosis-like syndrome. *Hum.Mol.Genet.*, Vol.14, No.22, pp. 3493-3498.

Sheth, S.; Shea, J.C.; Bishop, M.D.; Chopra, S.; Regan, M.M.; Malmberg, E.; Walker, C.; Ricci, R.; Tsui, L.C.; Durie, P.R.; Zielenski, J. & Freedman, S.D. (2003). Increased prevalence of CFTR mutations and variants and decreased chloride secretion in primary sclerosing cholangitis. *Hum.Genet.*, Vol.113, No.3, pp. 286-292.

Shimkets, R.A.; Warnock, D.G.; Bositis, C.M.; Nelson-Williams, C.; Hansson, J.H.; Schambelan, M.; Gill, J.R., Jr.; Ulick, S.; Milora, R.V.; Findling, J.W. & . (1994). Liddle's syndrome: heritable human hypertension caused by mutations in the beta subunit of the epithelial sodium channel. *Cell*, Vol.79, No.3, pp. 407-414.

Slieker, M.G.; Sanders, E.A.; Rijkers, G.T.; Ruven, H.J. & van der Ent, C.K. (2005). Disease modifying genes in cystic fibrosis. *J.Cyst.Fibros.*, Vol.4 Suppl 2, pp. 7-13.

Southern, K.W. (2007). Cystic fibrosis and formes frustes of CFTR-related disease. *Respiration*, Vol.74, No.3, pp. 241-251.

Southern, K.W.; Munck, A.; Pollitt, R.; Travert, G.; Zanolla, L.; nkert-Roelse, J. & Castellani, C. (2007). A survey of newborn screening for cystic fibrosis in Europe. *J.Cyst.Fibros.*, Vol.6, No.1, pp. 57-65.

Steiner, B.; Rosendahl, J.; Witt, H.; Teich, N.; Keim, V.; Schulz, H.U.; Pfutzer, R.; Luhr, M.; Gress, T.M.; Nickel, R.; Landt, O.; Koudova, M.; Macek, M., Jr.; Farre, A.; Casals, T.; Desax, M.C.; Gallati, S.; Gomez-Lira, M.; Audrezet, M.P.; Ferec, C.; Des, G.M.; Claustres, M. & Truninger, K. (2011). Common CFTR haplotypes and susceptibility to chronic pancreatitis and congenital bilateral absence of the vas deferens. *Hum.Mutat.*, Vol.32, No.8, pp. 912-920.

Steiner, B.; Truninger, K.; Sanz, J.; Schaller, A. & Gallati, S. (2004). The role of common single-nucleotide polymorphisms on exon 9 and exon 12 skipping in nonmutated CFTR alleles. *Hum.Mutat.*, Vol.24, No.2, pp. 120-129.

Stuhrmann, M. & Dork, T. (2000). CFTR gene mutations and male infertility. *Andrologia,* Vol.32, No.2, pp. 71-83.

Stutts, M.J.; Canessa, C.M.; Olsen, J.C.; Hamrick, M.; Cohn, J.A.; Rossier, B.C. & Boucher, R.C. (1995). CFTR as a cAMP-dependent regulator of sodium channels. *Science,* Vol.269, No.5225, pp. 847-850.

Su, Z.; Ning, B.; Fang, H.; Hong, H.; Perkins, R.; Tong, W. & Shi, L. (2011). Next-generation sequencing and its applications in molecular diagnostics. *Expert.Rev.Mol.Diagn.,* Vol.11, No.3, pp. 333-343.

Tang, B.L.; Gee, H.Y. & Lee, M.G. (2011). The cystic fibrosis transmembrane conductance regulator's expanding SNARE interactome. *Traffic.,* Vol.12, No.4, pp. 364-371.

Teem, J.L.; Berger, H.A.; Ostedgaard, L.S.; Rich, D.P.; Tsui, L.C. & Welsh, M.J. (1993). Identification of revertants for the cystic fibrosis delta F508 mutation using STE6-CFTR chimeras in yeast. *Cell,* Vol.73, No.2, pp. 335-346.

Thomas, C.P.; Loftus, R.W.; Liu, K.Z. & Itani, O.A. (2002). Genomic organization of the 5' end of human beta-ENaC and preliminary characterization of its promoter. *Am.J.Physiol Renal Physiol,* Vol.282, No.5, pp. F898-F909.

Tomaiuolo, A.C.; Alghisi, F.; Petrocchi, S.; Surace, C.; Roberti, M.C.; Bella, S.; Lucidi, V. & Angioni, A. (2010). Clinical hallmarks and genetic polymorphisms in the CFTR gene contribute to the disclosure of the A1006E mutation. *Clin.Invest Med.,* Vol.33, No.4, pp. E234-E239.

Tomaiuolo, R.; Spina, M. & Castaldo, G. (2003). Molecular diagnosis of cystic fibrosis: comparison of four analytical procedures. *Clin.Chem.Lab Med.,* Vol.41, No.1, pp. 26-32.

Trezise, A.E.; Chambers, J.A.; Wardle, C.J.; Gould, S. & Harris, A. (1993a). Expression of the cystic fibrosis gene in human foetal tissues. *Hum.Mol.Genet.,* Vol.2, No.3, pp. 213-218.

Trezise, A.E.; Linder, C.C.; Grieger, D.; Thompson, E.W.; Meunier, H.; Griswold, M.D. & Buchwald, M. (1993b). CFTR expression is regulated during both the cycle of the seminiferous epithelium and the oestrous cycle of rodents. *Nat.Genet.,* Vol.3, No.2, pp. 157-164.

van der Ven, K.; Messer, L.; van, d., V; Jeyendran, R.S. & Ober, C. (1996). Cystic fibrosis mutation screening in healthy men with reduced sperm quality. *Hum.Reprod.,* Vol.11, No.3, pp. 513-517.

Vankeerberghen, A.; Cuppens, H. & Cassiman, J.J. (2002). The cystic fibrosis transmembrane conductance regulator: an intriguing protein with pleiotropic functions. *J.Cyst.Fibros.,* Vol.1, No.1, pp. 13-29.

Voilley, N.; Bassilana, F.; Mignon, C.; Merscher, S.; Mattei, M.G.; Carle, G.F.; Lazdunski, M. & Barbry, P. (1995). Cloning, chromosomal localization, and physical linkage of the beta and gamma subunits (SCNN1B and SCNN1G) of the human epithelial amiloride-sensitive sodium channel. *Genomics,* Vol.28, No.3, pp. 560-565.

Voilley, N.; Lingueglia, E.; Champigny, G.; Mattei, M.G.; Waldmann, R.; Lazdunski, M. & Barbry, P. (1994). The lung amiloride-sensitive Na^+ channel: biophysical properties, pharmacology, ontogenesis, and molecular cloning. *Proc.Natl.Acad.Sci.U.S.A,* Vol.91, No.1, pp. 247-251.

Wagner, K.; Greil, I.; Schneditz, P.; Pommer, M. & Rosenkranz, W. (1994). A cystic fibrosis patient with delta F508, G542X and a deletion at the D7S8 locus. *Hum.Mutat.,* Vol.3, No.3, pp. 327-329.

Wang, S.; Yue, H.; Derin, R.B.; Guggino, W.B. & Li, M. (2000a). Accessory protein facilitated CFTR-CFTR interaction, a molecular mechanism to potentiate the chloride channel activity. *Cell*, Vol.103, No.1, pp. 169-179.

Wang, X.; Moylan, B.; Leopold, D.A.; Kim, J.; Rubenstein, R.C.; Togias, A.; Proud, D.; Zeitlin, P.L. & Cutting, G.R. (2000b). Mutation in the gene responsible for cystic fibrosis and predisposition to chronic rhinosinusitis in the general population. *JAMA*, Vol.284, No.14, pp. 1814-1819.

Wang, X.; Venable, J.; LaPointe, P.; Hutt, D.M.; Koulov, A.V.; Coppinger, J.; Gurkan, C.; Kellner, W.; Matteson, J.; Plutner, H.; Riordan, J.R.; Kelly, J.W.; Yates, J.R., III & Balch, W.E. (2006). Hsp90 cochaperone Aha1 downregulation rescues misfolding of CFTR in cystic fibrosis. *Cell*, Vol.127, No.4, pp. 803-815.

Wei, L.; Vankeerberghen, A.; Jaspers, M.; Cassiman, J.; Nilius, B. & Cuppens, H. (2000). Suppressive interactions between mutations located in the two nucleotide binding domains of CFTR. *FEBS Lett.*, Vol.473, No.2, pp. 149-153.

Weixel, K.M. & Bradbury, N.A. (2000). The carboxyl terminus of the cystic fibrosis transmembrane conductance regulator binds to AP-2 clathrin adaptors. *J.Biol.Chem.*, Vol.275, No.5, pp. 3655-3660.

Xu, W.; Hui, C.; Yu, S.S.; Jing, C. & Chan, H.C. (2011a). MicroRNAs and cystic fibrosis--an epigenetic perspective. *Cell Biol.Int.*, Vol.35, No.5, pp. 463-466.

Xu, W.M.; Chen, J.; Chen, H.; Diao, R.Y.; Fok, K.L.; Dong, J.D.; Sun, T.T.; Chen, W.Y.; Yu, M.K.; Zhang, X.H.; Tsang, L.L.; Lau, A.; Shi, Q.X.; Shi, Q.H.; Huang, P.B. & Chan, H.C. (2011b). Defective CFTR-dependent CREB activation results in impaired spermatogenesis and azoospermia. *PLoS.ONE.*, Vol.6, No.5, pp. e19120.

Xu, W.M.; Shi, Q.X.; Chen, W.Y.; Zhou, C.X.; Ni, Y.; Rowlands, D.K.; Yi, L.G.; Zhu, H.; Ma, Z.G.; Wang, X.F.; Chen, Z.H.; Zhou, S.C.; Dong, H.S.; Zhang, X.H.; Chung, Y.W.; Yuan, Y.Y.; Yang, W.X. & Chan, H.C. (2007). Cystic fibrosis transmembrane conductance regulator is vital to sperm fertilizing capacity and male fertility. *Proc.Natl.Acad.Sci.U.S.A*, Vol.104, No.23, pp. 9816-9821.

Yoshimura, K.; Nakamura, H.; Trapnell, B.C.; Chu, C.S.; Dalemans, W.; Pavirani, A.; Lecocq, J.P. & Crystal, R.G. (1991a). Expression of the cystic fibrosis transmembrane conductance regulator gene in cells of non-epithelial origin. *Nucleic Acids Res.*, Vol.19, No.19, pp. 5417-5423.

Yoshimura, K.; Nakamura, H.; Trapnell, B.C.; Dalemans, W.; Pavirani, A.; Lecocq, J.P. & Crystal, R.G. (1991b). The cystic fibrosis gene has a "housekeeping"-type promoter and is expressed at low levels in cells of epithelial origin. *J.Biol.Chem.*, Vol.266, No.14, pp. 9140-9144.

Yueksekdag, G.; Drechsel, M.; Rossner, M.; Schmidt, C.; Kormann, M.; Illenyi, M.C.; Rudolph, C. & Rosenecker, J. (2010). Repeated siRNA application is a precondition for successful mRNA gammaENaC knockdown in the murine airways. *Eur.J.Pharm.Biopharm.*, Vol.75, No.3, pp. 305-310.

Zhang, L.; Button, B.; Gabriel, S.E.; Burkett, S.; Yan, Y.; Skiadopoulos, M.H.; Dang, Y.L.; Vogel, L.N.; McKay, T.; Mengos, A.; Boucher, R.C.; Collins, P.L. & Pickles, R.J. (2009). CFTR delivery to 25% of surface epithelial cells restores normal rates of mucus transport to human cystic fibrosis airway epithelium. *PLoS.Biol.*, Vol.7, No.7, pp. e1000155.

Zhang, L.N.; Karp, P.; Gerard, C.J.; Pastor, E.; Laux, D.; Munson, K.; Yan, Z.; Liu, X.; Godwin, S.; Thomas, C.P.; Zabner, J.; Shi, H.; Caldwell, C.W.; Peluso, R.; Carter, B.

& Engelhardt, J.F. (2004). Dual therapeutic utility of proteasome modulating agents for pharmaco-gene therapy of the cystic fibrosis airway. *Mol.Ther.*, Vol.10, No.6, pp. 990-1002.

Zhou, Z.; Treis, D.; Schubert, S.C.; Harm, M.; Schatterny, J.; Hirtz, S.; Duerr, J.; Boucher, R.C. & Mall, M.A. (2008). Preventive but not late amiloride therapy reduces morbidity and mortality of lung disease in betaENaC-overexpressing mice. *Am.J.Respir.Crit Care Med.*, Vol.178, No.12, pp. 1245-1256.

Zielenski, J.; Rozmahel, R.; Bozon, D.; Kerem, B.; Grzelczak, Z.; Riordan, J.R.; Rommens, J. & Tsui, L.C. (1991). Genomic DNA sequence of the cystic fibrosis transmembrane conductance regulator (CFTR) gene. *Genomics*, Vol.10, No.1, pp. 214-228.

Websites

Consortium for CF genetic analysis database
    http://www.genet.sickkids.on.ca/cftr/Home.html
Ensembl
    http://www.ensembl.org/Homo_sapiens/Gene/Summary?db=core;g=ENSG0000
    0001626;r=7:117105838-117308719
European CF thematic network
    http://cf.eqascheme.org/info/public/index.xhtml
European CF society
    http://www.ecfs.eu/
Human gene mutation database (HGMD)
    http://www.hgmd.org/
OMIM
    http://omim.org/entry/602421
U.S. CF Foundation drug development pipeline
    http://www.cff.org/treatments/Pipeline/
U.S. National Institutes of Health Clinical Trials registry and database
    http://www.clinicaltrials.gov/ct2/results?term=Cystic+Fibrosis

6

Biochemical and Molecular Genetic Testing Used in the Diagnosis and Assessment of Cystic Fibrosis

Donovan McGrowder

*Department of Pathology, Faculty of Medical Sciences, University of the West Indies,
Mona Campus, Kingston,
Jamaica*

1. Introduction

1.1 Mutations in the CFTR gene

Cystic fibrosis (CF) is the most common life-threatening autosomal recessive genetic disease among the Caucasian population, with an estimated incidence throughout the world of between 0.25 - 5 per 10,000 live births (Lewis et al., 1995). It is caused by mutations on both CF transmembrane conductance regulator (CFTR) alleles, resulting in pancreatic exocrine insufficiency in 95% of patients, abnormal sweat electrolytes, sino-pulmonary disease and male infertility (MacCready, 1963). In its classic form, this multi-system disease is characterized by one or more of several features varying in severity, including a progressive decline of pulmonary function secondary to chronic lung infections, pancreatic exocrine insufficiency leading to malnutrition and growth impairment, liver disease, and decreased reabsorption of chloride ions from sweat (Zielenski et al., 2000). The disease is easily diagnosed early in life, through a combination of clinical evaluation and laboratory testing including sweat testing and CFTR mutation analysis (Ross, 2008). However, 7% of CF patients are not diagnosed until age 10 years, with a proportion not diagnosed until after age 15 years. Because the phenotype in these patients may vary widely some of these patients present a considerable challenge in establishing a diagnosis of CF (Wilcken et al., 1995; Hammond et al., 1991).

The heterogeneity of CF disease is partially explained by the identification of 1890 mutations in the CFTR gene (Cystic Fibrosis Mutation Database). The delta F508 (ΔF508) mutation, the most common CF allele is a 3-base pair deletion in exon 10 causing a loss of phenylalanine at the amino acid position 508 of the protein product (Kerem et al., 1989). The ΔF508 mutation reaches frequencies of 70% or more in northern European populations, with lower frequencies in southern European populations. In the United States of America (USA), two-thirds of patients carry at least one copy of the ΔF508 mutation, with approximately 50% of CF patients being homozygous for this mutation (Crossley et al., 1979). Other common mutations existing in most populations include G542X, G551D, R553X, W1282X and N1303K. These mutations have population frequencies of approximately 1 - 2% (De Boeck, 2006).

The CFTR gene consists of a TATA-less promoter and 27 exons spanning about 215 kb of genomic sequence (Zielenski et al., 1991). It encodes a transmembrane protein with a symmetrical, multi-domain structure, consisting of two nucleotide-binding domains (NBD1, NBD2), two membrane-spanning domains (MSD1, MSD2), and a central, highly charged regulatory domain (R) with multiple phosphorylation consensus sites (Riordan et al., 1989). The principal function of CFTR is that of cyclic adenosine-5'-monophosphate (cAMP)-regulated chloride transport at the apical membranes of epithelial cells. It has also been implicated in many other processes such as membrane trafficking regulation of other ion channels and pH, and apoptosis (Quinton, 1999; Sheppard & Welsh, 1999).

Mutations in CFTR may result in: (1) defective processing of CFTR, such as ΔF508 or G480C, where the mutant protein is not processed to its mature glycosylated form and is not correctly localised to the apical membrane, but is retained in the endoplasmic reticulum and degraded, (2) defective CFTR production, such as R553X, due to unstable messenger ribonucleic acid (mRNA) and/or premature protein truncation and/or (3) defective ion channel function, such as G551D or R117H, in which case some of the mutant protein becomes correctly localised but results in either very little residual function (in the case of G551D) or a substantially reduced level of ion transport (in the case of R117H). In each class of mutation the level of functional CFTR at the apical membrane of epithelial cells in CF patients falls below a critical level, resulting in the characteristic clinical abnormalities observed in the organs in which CFTR is expressed (Comeau et al., 2004).

Mutations in CFTR result in abnormalities in epithelial ion and water transport, which are associated with derangements in airway mucociliary clearance and other cellular functions related to normal cell biology (Sontag et al., 2005). Furthermore, mutations in the CFTR gene can alter the structure, function, or production of a cAMP-dependent trans-membrane chloride channel protein that is critical for normal functioning of multiple organs. The organs and systems that are affected in CF include: pancreas, liver, sweat glands, genitourinary and gastrointestinal tracts, the lungs and upper respiratory tract (Welsh et al., 2001). It is the involvement of the latter which leads to most morbidity and is the most common cause of death. A large retrospective cohort study of approximately 17,000 patients from the USA CF Foundation National Registry, confirmed that the CFTR genotype affects mortality (McKone et al., 2003).

Extensive genetic studies have produced both greater awareness of the spectrum of mutations in specific population groups (Alper et al., 2004) and increased the understanding of genotype-phenotype relationships (Groman et al., 2005; Mickle, 2000), illuminating distinctions between CFTR mutations with limited or no functional effects and those known or predicted to cause CF disease. Most classically diagnosed patients with CF carry severe loss-of-function mutations on both alleles and have evidence of pancreatic insufficiency (Kerem et al., 1999). Those with non-classic CF carry a mild CFTR gene mutation on at least one allele, and usually retain sufficient residual pancreatic function to confer pancreatic sufficiency (Cystic Fibrosis Genotype-Phenotype Consortium, 1993; Zielenski, 2000). Both pancreatic insufficiency and sufficiency are associated with specific CFTR mutations.

The CFTR gene mutations have been placed into five classes depending on their effect on the CFTR protein (Welsh et al., 2001). Classes I – III are associated with complete loss of cAMP-regulated chloride channel function and are identified as "severe" mutations. Class I mutations lead to defective protein production, class II to defective protein maturation and processing, and class III to defective channel regulation/gating. Mutations in classes IV - V might allow for residual CFTR function, and lead to altered channel conductance in class IV and altered protein stability in class V. They are usually associated with milder phenotypes and pancreatic sufficiency (Welsh et al., 2001; Ahmed et al., 2003). Persons who have two mutations from within classes I, II, or III almost invariably experience pancreatic insufficiency, and those with < 2 mutations from classes IV or V usually maintain pancreatic insufficiency. The common ΔF508 mutation is a class II mutation that is associated with pancreatic insufficiency (Ahmed et al., 2003).

The sensitivity of a given DNA mutation panel for detecting persons with CF varies by race and ethnicity as different populations have different mutation frequencies. The inclusion of mutations specific to racial and ethnic minority populations can improve detection of CF among those populations (Bobadilla et al., 2002). Data from US newborn screening programs showed that birth prevalence is 1/2,500 - 3,500 births among non-Hispanic whites, 1/4,000 - 10,000 births among Hispanics, and 1/15,000 - 20,000 births among non-Hispanic Blacks (Comeau et al., 2004; Parad & Comeau, 2003). Non-Hispanic Whites constituted >90% of USA patients who received a diagnosis of CF (Cystic Fibrosis Foundation, 2001).

The spectrum of CFTR mutation frequencies varies in populations of each ethnicity, and a large proportion of CFTR mutations is still unidentified in Hispanic and Black people. Heim and colleagues in their study used a 70- and 86-DNA mutation panel, and reported a detection rate of 62% in Black infants, 58% in Hispanic infants, 38% in Asian infants, and 81% in Native American infants in the USA compared with 85% in White infants and 95% in Ashkenazi Jewish infants (Heim et al., 2001). Identification of infants with CF can be enhanced by choosing an appropriate mutation panel. A 75% detection rate can be achieved in Black populations by screening for 16 "common white" mutations and 8 "common African" mutations (Macek et al., 1997).

This review will examine the advances in adult and newborn screening for CF that are reported in the literature such as the use of genetic testing techniques to identify CFTR gene mutations. It will also critically examine the use of biochemical tests capable of diagnosis, detecting and monitoring the end-organ disease processes in patients with CF. These tests include sweat test, immunoreactive trypsinogen (IRT), nasal potential difference (NPD), pancreatic associated protein (PAP) and intestinal current measurement (ICM).

2. Analysis of CFTR gene mutations for diagnostic purposes

2.1 Mutations within the CFTR gene

According to The Cystic Fibrosis Genetic Analysis Consortium (1994), the ΔF508 mutation, the most common CFTR defect identified among Caucasians accounted for 66% of 43,849 tested CF chromosomes (The Cystic Fibrosis Genetic Analysis Consortium, 1994). However its occurrence varies considerably between geographical locations and different populations with the lowest reported incidence in Tunisia (17.9%) and highest in Denmark (90%) (Messaoud et al., 1996; Schwartz et al., 1990). The spectrum of remaining CFTR mutations is highly variable and is represented by a large number of rare alleles. All types of mutations are represented (missense, frameshift, nonsense, splice, small and large in-frame deletions or insertions), and are distributed throughout the entire gene (The Cystic Fibrosis Genetic Analysis Consortium, 1994).

A mutation detection rate of 90% in a specific population signifies that a mutation will be identified on both CFTR genes in 81% of the typical CF patients; a mutation will be found on only one CFTR gene in 18%; and no mutation will be found on either CFTR gene in 1% (De Boeck et al., 2006). Although currently available mutation screening panels can identify 90% of CFTR mutations, 9.7% of genotyped individuals in the Cystic Fibrosis Foundation Patient Registry have at least 1 un-identified mutation (Cystic Fibrosis Foundation Patient Registry, 2005).

2.2 Techniques used to analyze and detect CFTR gene mutations

The analysis and interpretation of CF genotype information requires the use of appropriate testing techniques to identify CFTR mutations, standardized criteria for defining a CF-causing mutation, and an understanding of the contribution of the genetic background to the phenotypic variability of CF. Rapid accurate identification of CFTR gene mutations is important for confirming the clinical diagnosis, for cascade screening in families at risk for CF, for understanding the correlation between genotype and phenotype, and moreover it is also the only means for prenatal diagnosis (Kolesár et al., 2008). The scanning of the whole coding region of the CFTR gene permits to identify about 90% of alleles from patients bearing CF and a lower percentage in patients bearing atypical CF. Several techniques such as allele specific oligonucleotide (ASO) dot-blot, reverse dot-blot, amplification refractory mutation (ARMS), and an oligo-ligation assay, are available to detect the most common mutations (Eshaque & Dixon, 2006). The ARMS is routinely used for the identification of specific mutations within genomes. This polymerase chain reaction (PCR)-based assay, although simple, is performed at a low-throughput scale, usually requiring gel-electrophoresis for the identification of specific mutations (Eaker et al., 2005). An extensive mutation screening of both CFTR genes may be required with assays such as single strand conformation polymorphism (SSCP) assay, sequencing, denaturing gradient gel electrophoresis (DGGE) and denaturing high pressure liquid chromatography (DHPLC) (Cuppens et al., 1993; Le Maréchal et al., 2001). Sequencing approaches 100% sensitivity while the other techniques are indirect mutation scanning assays with sensitivities varying from close to 100% to as low as 90%. Other available commercial assays for CFTR mutation screening include the INNO-LiPA CFTR Assay (Innogenetics NV, Technologiepark, Gent, Belgium), oligonucleotide ligation assay (OLA) Cystic Fibrosis Assay (Abbott Laboratories, Abbott Park, Illinois, USA), and the Elucigene CF Assay (Tepnel Diagnostics Ltd, Oxon, UK). Most of these tests only screen for about 30 mutations, the majority of which are associated with classic CF (Dequeker et al., 2000).

A number of methods have been proposed for the detection of ΔF508. The multiplex ARMS analysis identified the ΔF508 mutation at an allele frequency of 24.0% in Indian CF cases (Ashavaid et al., 2005). Another study has reported that quantitative real-time PCR with melting curve analysis is a reliable and fast method for the detection of ΔF508 mutation. By using this method, the results are ready in 1 h following the DNA isolation. The applied primer-probe set with melting curve analysis gives additional information for the presence of other mutations in the ΔF508del region (Nagy et al., 2007). Furthermore, the ΔF508 mutation has been identified by PCR-SSCP. The appropriate 98 bp region of the CFTR gene was amplified by PCR and the reaction products were analysed by SSCP-electrophoresis using silver staining for band visualization. Single-strand DNA fragments gave a reproducible pattern of bands, characteristic for the ΔF508 mutation (Kakavas et al., 2006). However, detecting compound heterozygotes between ΔF508 and other mutations which are rare is difficult as some mutations are common only to particular ethnic groups. Therefore, diagnostic tests such as restriction enzyme assays and SSCP have been designed to recognize rare and population-specific mutations (Eshaque & Dixon, 2006).

2.3 Analysis, spectrum and frequency of CFTR mutations in different populations

One challenging aspect of genetic analysis as it relates to CF is the identification of CF mutations in some populations. There are a number of studies that have examined the spectrum and frequency of mutations in different countries. In a study conducted in Minas Gerais State, Brazil, the frequency of 8 mutations (ΔF508, G542X, R1162X, N1303K, W1282X, G85E, 3120+1G>A, and 711+1G>T) was analyzed using by ASO-PCR with specially designed primers in 111 newborn patients. An allele frequency of 48.2% was observed for the ΔF508 mutation, and allele frequencies of 5.41%, 4.50%, 4.05%, and 3.60% were found for the R1162X, G542X, 3120+1G>A, and G85E mutations, respectively (Perone et al., 2010). Mutational analysis of the CFTR gene was performed in 49 Lithuanian CF patients through a combined approach of ASO-PCR and DGGE analysis. A CFTR mutation was characterized in 62.2% of CF chromosomes and ΔF508 (52.0%) was the most frequent Lithuanian CF mutation. Seven CFTR mutations, N1303K (2.0%), R75Q (1.0%), G314R (1.0%), R553X (4.2%), W1282X (1.0%), and 3944delGT (1.0%), accounted for 10.1% of Lithuanian CF chromosomes (Giannattasio et al., 2006).

There is a reported high incidence of the CFTR mutations 3272-26A-->G and L927P in Belgian CF patients. The technique DGGE was used to extensively analyse the CFTR gene in those patients with at least one unknown mutation after preliminary screening. There was also the identification of three new CFTR mutations (186-2A-->G, E588V, and 1671insTATCA). The mutation, 3272-26A-->G has a frequency of 3.8%, while L927P, 2.4% (Storm et al., 2007). In another study, different methods, such as ARMS-PCR, SSCP analysis, restriction enzyme digestion analysis, direct sequencing, and MLPA (Multiplex Ligation-mediated Probe Amplification) were used to analyse mutations in the complete coding region, and its exon/intron junctions, of the CFTR gene in 69 Iranian CF patients. CFTR mutation analysis revealed the identification of 37 mutations with a CFTR mutation detection rate of 81.9% (Alibakhsh et al., 2007). The most common mutations were ΔF508 (18.1%), 2183AA>G (6.5%), S466X (5.8%), N1303K (4.3%), 2789+5G>A (4.3%), G542X (3.6%), 3120+1G>A (3.6%), R334W (2.9%) and 3130delA (2.9%). These 9 types of mutant CFTR genes accounted for 52.0% of all CFTR genes derived from the Iranian CF patients (Alibakhsh et al., 2007).

Extensive CFTR gene sequencing can detect rare mutations which are not found with other screening and diagnostic tests, and can thus establish a definitive diagnosis in symptomatic patients with previously negative results. This enables carrier detection and prenatal diagnosis in additional family members (McGinniss et al., 2005). Prenatal diagnosis and carrier screening of relatives can be performed by segregation analysis of polymorphisms within or linked to the CFTR gene. Most commercial tests screen for the T5 allele, a splicing error in intron 8 that is considered to be a mild mutation with an incomplete penetrance (Rave-Harel et al., 1997). The T5 polymorphism is found on about 5% of the CFTR genes in the general White ethnic population, but on about 21% of the CFTR genes derived from patients with congenital bilateral absence of the vas deferens (CBAVD) (Chillo'n et al., 1995) and it may even confer non-classic CF (Cuppens et al., 1998; Noone et al., 2000). In most cases the partial penetrance is explained by the polymorphic TGm locus (11, 12 or 13 TG repeats) in front of the T5 allele. Analysis of the TGm locus can be accurately determined by sequencing (De Boeck et al., 2006). A higher number of TG repeats also results in less efficient splicing of CFTR transcripts (Cuppens et al., 1998). In patients with CBAVD and non-classic CF, the milder TG11-T5 allele is infrequent while the TG12-T5 allele is most frequently found (Cuppens et al., 1998). The TG13-T5 is rarer but also more frequently found in patients with CBAVD and non-classic CF (Cuppens et al., 1998; Groman et al., 2004).

Mutation analysis of the CFTR gene in Slovak CF patients by DHPLC and subsequent sequencing resulted in the identified four novel mutations (G437D, H954P, H1375N, and 3120+33G>T). This was done by the gene scanning approach using DHPLC system for analysing specifically all CFTR exons. There was the identification of a total of 28 different mutations in Slovak CF patients, and 17 different polymorphisms (Kolesár et al., 2008). Elce et al. (2009) reported three novel CFTR polymorphic repeats (IVS3polyA, IVS4polyA, and IVS10CA repeats) which improve segregation analysis for CF. They also developed and validated a procedure based on PCR followed by capillary electrophoresis (CE) for large-scale analysis of these polymorphisms. The allelic distribution and heterozygosity results suggest that the 3 novel intragenic polymorphic repeats strongly contribute to carrier and prenatal diagnosis of CF in families in which 1 or both causal mutations have not been identified (Elce et al., 2009). A universal array-based multiplexed test for CF carrier screening using the Tag-It multiplex mutation platform and the Cystic Fibrosis Mutation Detection Kit have been introduced. The Tag-It CF assay is a multiplexed genotyping assay that detects a panel of 40 CFTR mutations including the 23 mutations recommended by the American College of Medical Genetics (ACMG) and American College of Obstetricians and Gynecologists (ACOG) for population screening. A total of 16 additional mutations detected by the Tag-It CF assay may also be common (Amos et al., 2006).

Methods that include genetic testing can be done using a single sample. The controversy is the appropriate number of mutations to include in the genetic test. The answer depends in part on the heterogeneity of the population. The ΔF508 mutation is found in 72% of the US Non-Hispanic Caucasian CF population, but in much lower percentages of patients with CF from other ethnicities (Hispanic Caucasian, 54%; African American, 44%; Asian American, 39%; Ashekenazi Jewish, 31%) (Watson et al., 2004). In 2001, the ACMG Cystic Fibrosis Carrier Screening Working Group recommended a panel of 25 mutations which would account for > 80% of CF alleles in the pan-ethnic US population with CF (Grody et al., 2001). This panel was updated in 2004 based on a larger more pan-ethnic CF data-base that finds six additional mutations with a frequency > 0.10% and another 14 that occurred at slightly lower frequency but would be useful for specific ethnic minority communities (Watson et al., 2004).

2.4 Detection of rearrangements in CFTR gene

Large rearrangements (deletions, duplications, or insertion/deletion mutations) have recently been reported to constitute 1-2% of CFTR mutations (Svensson et al., 2010). The developments in quantitative PCR technologies have greatly improved our ability to detect large genome rearrangements. In particular oligonucleotide-based array comparative genomic hybridisation has become a useful tool for appropriate and rapid detection of breakpoints (Ramos et al., 2010). Using quantitative PCR analysis of all coding regions, the occurrence of CFTR rearrangements in 130 alleles from classic CF patients bearing unidentified mutations after the scanning of CFTR were assessed in the Italian population. Seven rearrangements (i.e. dele1, dele2, dele23, dele 14b17b, dele17a18, dele2223, and dele2224) were identified in 26.0% of CF alleles bearing undetected mutations (Tomaiuolo et al., 2008).

Ramos et al. (2010) analysed 80 samples (42 unknown CF alleles) applying three quantitative technologies (MLPA, quantitative PCR and array-comparative genomic hybridization) to detect recurrent as well as novel large rearrangements in the Spanish CF population. They identified three deletions and one duplication in five alleles. The new duplication in this cohort, CFTRdupProm-3 mutation spans 35.7 kb involving the 5'-end of the CFTR gene. Additionally, RNA analysis revealed a cryptic sequence with a premature termination codon leading to a disrupted protein (Ramos et al. 2010). In another study, de Becdelièvre et al. determined the contribution of large CFTR gene rearrangements in fetuses with bowel anomalies using a semi-quantitative fluorescent multiplex PCR (QFM-PCR) assay. Deletions were found in 5/70 cases in which QFM-PCR was applied, dele19, dele22_23, dele2_6b, dele14b_15 and dele6a_6b, of which the last three remain un-described (de Becdelièvre et al. 2010).

Schneider et al. (2007) used the CFTR MLPA Kit (MRC-Holland, Amsterdam, Netherlands) that allows the exact detection of copy numbers from all 27 exons in the CFTR gene, to screen 50 patients with only one identified mutation for large deletions in the CFTR gene. Detected deletion in the CFTR gene was confirmed using real-time PCR assay and deletion-specific PCR reactions using junction fragment primers. Large deletions were detected in eight CF alleles belonging to four different deletion types (CFTRindel2, CFTRdele14b-17b, CFTRdele17a-17b and CFTRdele 2-9) (Schneider et al., 2006). The LightCycler assay allows reliable and rapid screening for large deletions in the CFTR gene and detects the copy number of all 27 exons (Schneider et al., 2007).

3. Diagnosis of CF using sweat test

3.1 Methods used for assessing sweat chloride

The report of the Consensus Conference initiated by the CF Foundation in the USA stated that the criteria for the diagnosis of CF should include the following: (1) one or more characteristic phenotypic features, or a history of CF in a sibling, or positive newborn screening test results; and (2) an elevated sweat chloride concentration by pilocarpine iontophoresis (>60 mmol/L) on two or more occasions, or identification of two CF mutations (Rosen & Cutting, 1998), or 3) *in vivo* demonstration of characteristic abnormalities in ion transport across the nasal epithelium (Welsh et al., 2001; Rosenstein & Cutting, 1998).

The chloride ion is most directly related to CFTR dysfunction. Chloride concentration measurement is the analysis of choice because the chloride ion concentration shows the greatest discrimination between normal individuals and CF subjects. Concurrent measurement of sodium acts as a quality control. The sweat test is based on the observation in 1953 by Darting et al. (1953) that stimulated sweat of CF patients contains elevated levels of sodium and chloride ions. The development of the quantitative pilocarpine iontophoresis by Gibson and Cooke dates from 1959 and is preferred method of sweat stimulation (Gibson & Cooke, 1959). The sweat test involves transdermal administration of pilocarpine by iontophoresis to stimulate sweat gland secretion, followed by collection and quantitation of sweat onto gauze or filter paper or into a Macroduct coil (Wescor Inc, Logan, Utah) and analysis of chloride concentration as described by Clinical Laboratory Standards Institute (2000). If carried out properly and with considerable care, this method is still the most specific biochemical test for CF (Shwachman, 1979). There is documentation in the literature of a semi-quantitative test, based on die production of a white silver chloride precipitate ring on a brown silver chromate background that was originally proposed by Shwachman and Gahm (1956) and adapted to die so-called paper patch test (Yeung et al., 1984). Although intended for the non-specialist centre, die method is very subjective and liable to misinterpretation and has not gained popularity.

One of the major consequences of mutations in the CFTR gene is a dysfunction of ion channels resulting in elevated sweat chloride concentrations, progressive lung disease and pancreatic insufficiency (Pilewski & Frizzell, 1999; Bals et al., 1999). In CF subjects the sweat chloride is usually higher than the sweat sodium, but the converse is true in normal persons. Normal sweat contains less than 60 mmol/L chloride and sodium (Association of Clinical Biochemistry, 2002). The 60 mmol/L value of sweat chloride concentrations has been used for a long time to discriminate between the populations of patients with CF and without CF (LeGrys, 1996). An elevated sweat chloride level has been the "gold standard" for diagnosis of CF (Gibson & Cooke, 1959). All patients with a sweat chloride level above 60 mmol/L and a clinical phenotype compatible with CF have a diagnosis of classic CF. However patients have been reported with characteristic manifestations of CF, and chloride levels, below 60 mmol/L (Highsmith et al., 1994; Cystic Fibrosis Genotype-Phenotype Consortium, 1993). Most of the studies exploring these patients with equivocal sweat tests have focused on the chloride range 40 - 60 mmol/L (Desmarquest et al., 2000). In the UK guidelines on sweat testing (Association of Clinical Biochemistry, 2000), 40 mmol/L is considered as the lower limit for equivocal sweat tests because this value represents the mean +2SD in carriers.

3.2 Intermediate sweat test results

The evidence that a proportion of CF patients with chloride concentrations of 30 - 60 mmol/L with two CFTR mutations following testing is documented in the literature (Lebecque et al., 2002). Sweat chloride concentrations of 30 - 60 mmol/L are seen in about 4% of sweat tests; 23% of these patients will subsequently be found to have two CFTR mutations. CF affected patients occur with similar frequency in the 30 - 40 mmol/L range as in the 40 - 60 mmol/L range (Lebecque et al., 2002). Furthermore, in the 2005 Cystic Fibrosis Foundation Patient Registry, only 3.5% of patients with a diagnosis of CF had a sweat chloride value <60 mmol/L, and only 1.2% had a value <40 mmol/L (Cystic Fibrosis Foundation Patient Registry, 2005). A Canadian study reported that sweat chloride values <60 mmol/L were observed in 21% with pancreatic-sufficient CF (Wilschanski et al., 2006).

Increasing recognition of the wide range of CF phenotypic variability (Nick & Rodman, 2005; Bishop et al., 2005) should lead to increasing diagnosis of CF in individuals with intermediate sweat chloride values. Farrell et al. (2008) recommends that sweat chloride values ≥40 mmol/L in individuals over age 6 months should be considered beyond the normal range and merit further evaluation, to include repeat sweat chloride testing and DNA analysis for CFTR mutations. A sweat chloride level above 60 mmol/L in the absence of CF is rare, although it has been reported in a number of unusual clinical conditions that can usually be readily distinguished from CF (Rosenstein, 2000). In patients with a sweat chloride level below 30 mmol/L the diagnosis of CF becomes very unlikely.

3.3 Sweat tests in infants

New born screening (NBS) of CF identifies only newborns at risk for CF. A positive screening result, indicating persistent hypertrypsinogenemia, should be followed by referral for direct diagnostic testing (i.e. sweat chloride test) to confirm a diagnosis of CF. With sufficient experience, sweat testing can be performed adequately in infants, but interpreting the results can be problematic. Studies of sweat chloride testing in infants have demonstrated most infants identified by NBS will undergo sweat testing after 2 weeks of age. Earlier testing could lead to misleading results, because sweat chloride concentrations in healthy newborns gradually decrease over the first weeks of life (Parad et al., 2005). A study in 103 infants without CF found a mean sweat chloride value of 23.3 ± 5.7 mmol/L at age 3 to 7 days, decreasing to 17.6 ± 5.6 mmol/L by age 8 to 14 days and then to 13.1 ± 7.4 mmol/L after age 6 weeks (Eng et al., 2005). This gradual early decline in sweat chloride values suggests that sweat test results are less likely to be difficult to interpret after age 2 weeks (Eng et al., 2005).

The Consensus Committee recommends based on the available data on sweat chloride test results in healthy and CF-affected infants, the following sweat chloride reference ranges for infants up to age 6 months: ≤29 mmol/L, CF unlikely; 30 to 59 mmol/L, intermediate; ≥60 mmol/L, indicative of CF (Farrell et al., 2008). A study of 725 infants identified as being at risk through NBS or based on clinical presentation who carried 0, 1, or 2 copies of the common CFTR gene mutation ΔF508, showed that all of the ΔF508 homozygous infants had sweat chloride concentrations >60 mmol/L. The findings from this study are in accordance with other studies from Australia (Massie et al., 2000; Parad et al., 2005). Although sweat chloride values are generally ≥60 mmol/L in infants with CF, lower values also can occur (Taceetti et al., 2004; Rock et al., 2005). In a 4-year cohort of infants in the Massachusetts NBS program in the USA who had clinician-diagnosed CF, 8.2% had a sweat chloride concentration of 30 to 59 mmol/L and 2.7% had a concentration <30 mmol/L (Parad & Comeau, 2005).

There are studies which support the recommendation that a sweat chloride value ≥ 30 mmol/L in infants <age 6 months should be considered abnormal and trigger further patient evaluation (Eng et al., 2005; Barben et al., 2005). A sweat chloride value ≤39 mmol/L after age 6 months generally is not consistent with a diagnosis of CF, although CF can occur in this group in rare cases (Lebecque et al., 2002; O'Sullivan et al., 2006). Some infants have been particularly difficult to classify, such as those with 2 CF mutations and a sweat chloride value <40 mmol/L and those with only 1 CF mutation and a slightly elevated sweat chloride value. Although such infants represent only a small fraction of patients, they may be at risk for developing complications of CF and thus should be identified and followed (Farrell et al., 2008). Sweat testing can be performed accurately on the majority of infants at age 2-3 weeks; however, not all infants have sufficient quantities of sweat for reliable testing (Boyle, 2003).

3.4 Limitations, advantages and disadvantages of sweat test

The sweat test is cheap and, in nearly all populations, will result in a greater diagnostic yield than a standard CFTR deoxyribonucleic acid (DNA) screening test. Sweat should be collected for 30 minutes onto pre-weighed gauze or filter paper low in sodium chloride. A minimum sweat rate of 1 g/m^2 body surface area/min is required; thus a sweat volume of 50 -100 mL is adequate. Testing can be carried out after the first 2 weeks of life in infants weighing more than 3 kg who are normally hydrated and without significant illness. Testing should be delayed in infants who are acutely ill or dehydrated, who have eczema or oedema, or who are receiving supplemental oxygen. Raised sweat electrolyte concentrations can be found in infants who are underweight or dehydrated.

Sweat electrolyte concentrations can be lowered by systemic steroids and oedema. Sweat electrolytes are not affected by administration of intravenous fluids, diuretics or intake of flucloxacillin (Association of Clinical Biochemistry, 2002; National Committee for Clinical Laboratory Standards, 2000). False negative results have been reported (LeGrys & Wood, 1988) as well as consistently borderline values (Canciam et al., 1988). False positive results can also occur (Smalley et al., 1979) often due to lack of care during sweat collection, resulting in evaporation of collected sweat prior to analysis. Consequently the test which is time-consuming should be done only by properly trained personnel. An additional problem is that in the very young and those with dry skin, sweat collection volumes may be too small for analysis.

As the appropriate performance of the sweat test is crucial for the accurate diagnosis of CF, the Cystic Fibrosis Foundation (2007) requires that sweat testing conducted at accredited CF care centers adheres to the standards recommended by a Cystic Fibrosis Foundation Committee comprising CF center directors (LeGrys et al., 2007). Laboratories accredited by the College of American Pathologists must follow the protocols and procedures outlined in the College's Laboratory Accreditation Program Inspection Checklist (College of American Pathologists, 2007). Because of the additional technical challenges involved in obtaining sweat from newborns, it is often recommended that NBS-positive newborns undergo sweat testing only at a Cystic Fibrosis Foundation certified laboratory.

4. Immunoreactive trypsinogen (IRT) in CF neonatal screening

4.1 The sensitivity and specificity of IRT

The purpose of CF newborn screening is identification of CF-affected infants. Strategies used by CF newborn screening programs have included measuring for elevated levels of IRT which is relatively inexpensive and adaptable to large numbers (Crossley et al., 1981). The IRT is an indirect measure of pancreatic injury that is present at birth in most newborns who have CF on serial dried blood spot specimens (Hammond et al., 1991) or measuring for elevated IRT followed by assaying for ΔF508 on the same dried blood spot (2-tier algorithm)

(Gregg et al., 1993). Increased IRT concentrations at birth are characteristic of newborns affected by CF, but can also be found in healthy infants. In 1979, Crossley et al. reported a two to threefold increase in IRT in blood from CF neonates, compared with normal (non-CF) infants. The test was based on a radioimmunoassay for serum trypsin, and was adapted for use on dried blood-spots.

The IRT levels tend to remain elevated for several months in newborns with CF, because pancreatic trypsinogen leaks back through interstitial fluid due to partial obstruction of pancreatic ducts (Crossley et al., 1979). The lack of specificity of IRT means, however, that they may also be false positives (Wilcken et al., 1983). The 'falsely' elevated IRT levels usually return to normal within the first weeks of life of the child's birth. This presents a diagnostic dilemma. CF should be confirmed or ruled out as quickly as possible in these situations to alleviate parental distress and allow earlier therapeutic intervention and genetic counseling. In most older CF children IRT levels are subnormal and there is considerable child to child variation (Chatfield et al., 1991). To improve the specificity of neonatal screening, a second blood sample is obtained in neonates with raised levels of IRT at birth, and only infants with persistently raised IRT values progress to a sweat test. Furthermore, standard diagnostic strategy calls for extensive analysis of the CFTR gene and repetition of the sweat Cl⁻ measurement (De Boeck et al., 2006; Rosenstein & Cutting, 1998).

Prospective studies have shown false positive incidence of 0.5% (from first blood spots) but the false negative incidence was very low if infants presenting with meconium ileus were excluded (Crossley et al., 1981; Heeley et al., 1982). The false positive incidence could be significantly reduced by repeating the test on a second blood spot (Travert, 1988). The results of routine screening from 16 centres around the world were correlated and it was found that false positive rate ranged from 0.2 - 0.5% although this was higher in those laboratories where a lower cut-off point was taken (Travert, 1988). There have been reports concerning improvement in sensitivity and specificity for the IRT test, by including the use of complementary tests (Pederzini et al., 1990) have suggested a combination of meconium screening by measurement of lactase, on those infants who are IRT positive. Sweat tests are done on those patients who test positive, either by the lactase test or where blood spots are above a certain value by IRT test. This approach achieved a marked drop in false negative incidence but it seems likely that the extra work and expense will be unacceptable (Pederzini et al., 1990).

In most neonatal screening protocols, IRT retesting in infants with an initially raised value has been replaced by analysis of a panel of CF causing mutations in the neonatal blood sample (Ranieri, 1994). Comeau et al. (2004) implemented statewide CF newborn screening in Massachusetts, USA using a 2-tier algorithm in which all specimens were assayed for IRT. Those with elevated IRT then had multiple- CFTR-mutation testing. Infants who screened positive by detection of 1 or 2 mutations or extremely elevated IRT (>99.8%; failsafe protocol) were then referred for definitive diagnosis by sweat testing. The authors reported that by using the multiple-CFTR-mutation panel, a screening result with a genetic "diagnosis" of CF was made in 75% of screened-positive CF-affected infants, compared with 50% had they used ΔF508 alone, thus facilitating more rapid referral and intervention (Comeau et al., 2004).

4.2 The use of the IRT/IRT method in neonatal screening

Multiple protocols and algorithms are used to screen newborns for CF. All protocols begin with a first-tier phenotypic test that measures IRT in dried blood spots. Different laboratory kits for IRT produce varying distributions of IRT measures, and screening programs set cut-offs on the basis of evaluations of specimens from their own populations and the screening protocols and algorithms used. Screening programs in five states in the USA (Colorado, Connecticut, Montana, New Jersey, and Wyoming) have set absolute cut-offs for a normal IRT value on the first newborn blood spot (range: 90 - 105 ng/mL) (Wilfond et al., 2003).

The IRT-IRT algorithm involves measurement of IRT during the first week on the Guthrie blood spot and repeating the measurement at 3 - 4 weeks in those with initial high levels. The sensitivity of a raised 3 - 5 day IRT is high, but the positive predictive value is low. Because blood levels of IRT decay slowly in CF infants, a second IRT at 3 - 4 weeks increases the specificity, but about 1 in 200 newborn infants progress to the second blood test (Price, 2006).

In the USA, because normal IRT reference values vary slightly, the individual NBS program in the state in which the newborn is being tested sets the specific cut-off value that defines an elevated IRT. After an abnormal IRT value is identified, most NBS programs perform DNA testing to identify known CFTR gene mutations (IRT/DNA strategy), while other programs repeat the IRT measurement in a second blood sample obtained from the infant at age approximately 2 weeks (IRT/IRT strategy) (Comeau et al., 2007). These strategies have been reported to provide approximately 90% to 95% sensitivity (Wilcken et al., 1995) and have identified newborns at risk for a wide spectrum of disease severity (Farrell et al., 1997). However, there are studies which have shown that IRT/DNA screening suggested better sensitivity than IRT/IRT (Gregg et al., 1997; Padoan et al., 2002), but relatively small populations were previously studied.

In the IRT/IRT algorithm, both the first and the second IRT values must be above the fixed cut-offs to recommend a sweat test; therefore, the initial IRT is the more crucial step. In the USA, a first IRT value of 100 or 105 ng/mL, and a second value of 70 ng/mL are used. These values have been set in an attempt to maximize sensitivity and positive predictive value. Although the initial cut-off for IRT/IRT algorithm decreased over time from 140 ng/mL (Hammond et al., 1991) to 100 or 105 ng/mL (Sontag et al., 2005) in attempts to decrease false negative results in the IRT/IRT, there are concerns regarding sub-optimal sensitivity and observations which have revealed that the second specimens of some patients with CF showed precipitous decreases which have led Wisconsin in the USA (Rock et al., 1990) and Australia (Gregg et al., 1993) to develop the 2-tier IRT/DNA (ΔF508) method.

4.3 IRT/DNA and IRT/DNA/IRT protocols in neonatal screening

According to Price (2006), IRT/DNA employs DNA analysis instead of a second IRT at 3 - 4 weeks. Infants with very high IRT in the first week undergo DNA analysis and those with at least one mutation have a sweat test. The advantage of the IRT/DNA protocol is that both tests can be done on the initial blood spot sample (Price, 2006). However, the sensitivity of the IRT/DNA protocol is, however, dependent on the gene frequency of common CFTR mutations in the population. Many programs that use an IRT/DNA methodology also recommend sweat testing on children with a very high IRT level without mutations in an attempt to capture children who have rare mutations. This safeguard will reduce the number of false negatives (Benhardtet et al., 1987).

If an IRT/DNA method is used, the number of carriers detected will depend on the number of mutations included in the screening test. The more mutations included, the more children will be identified with one common mutation. The screening panel should include more rather than less mutations to avoid disproportionate number of missed screened cases (false negatives) in USA ethnic minorities. In order to capture a high percentage of cases involving ethnic minorities, full sequencing of the CFTR gene is required (Ross, 2008). Kammesheidt et al. (2006) have shown the feasibility of temporal temperature gradient electrophoresis-based full sequence analysis and targeted sequencing from DNA in newborn blood specimens which can increase the identification of mutations in ethnic minorities. This method allowed a more comprehensive diagnosis on one blood sample because only children with two mutations and/or variants would need to undergo sweat testing. It should reduce the overall number of cases referred for sweat tests, unless questionable variants are more common than previously anticipated (Kammesheidt et al., 2006).

The IRT/DNA/IRT protocol use 2 IRT measurements and DNA testing. This method, applies a mutation panel to primary samples with an elevated IRT. Children whose sample has at least one mutation or whose sample has a very high initial IRT measurement are asked to provide a second sample for a second IRT measurement. Only those with an elevated IRT levels on the second sample undergo sweat testing (Ross, 2008). Corbetta et al. (2002) assessed the performance of IRT/DNA/IRT based on IRT followed by direct CFTR gene analysis (based on a panel of up to 31 mutations) in hypertrypsinaemic newborn infants in Italy. The screening strategy consisted of an IRT assay from dried blood spots, a PCR followed by an OLA (PCR-OLA), and a sequence code separation. The researchers reported that the IRT/DNA/IRT protocol with an OLA showed the identification of 94% of infants with CF. They concluded that PCR-OLA assay was a reliable, robust method to apply to the neonatal screening programme (Corbetta et al., 2002).

In the UK approximately 4% of children diagnosed with CF are non-Caucasian in origin. A DNA panel comprising the most common 31 CF mutations will detect 97% of mutations in a Caucasian population, but only just over 65% of mutations in a non-Caucasian population. The gene frequency of ΔF508 in the UK Indian sub-continent CF population is less than half that in the UK Caucasian CF population (McCormick et al., 2002). A three stage IRT/DNA/IRT protocol is reported to likely increase the chances of detecting CF in non-Caucasian infants (McCormick et al., 2002).

The main benefits of the IRT/DNA/IRT protocol over a single IRT/DNA methodology is that they reduce the number of children who need to undergo sweat testing, and the number of parents who are informed of their child's carrier status and need genetic counselling (Ross, 2008). However, the main disadvantage of the IRT/DNA/IRT protocol is its complexity and the anxiety generated for families who have to wait for the result of a second IRT (McCormick et al., 2002). Both the IRT/DNA/IRT and IRT/DNA protocols involve DNA testing, and may fail to detect ethnic minorities with rare mutations. Some ethnic minority children with rare mutations may still be detected to the extent that the IRT/DNA/IRT method employs the safeguard of recommending sweat testing of children with a very high IRT measurement even if no mutations are detected. Modeling in different ethnic communities using different DNA panels would be necessary to determine whether the costs of the extra laboratory testing are outweighed by the benefits achieved by reducing the number of children who need to undergo sweat testing and genetic counselling (Ross, 2008).

5. The use of the nasal potential difference (NPD) in aiding the diagnosis of CF

Genetic studies sometimes take several weeks and may find no useful information, neither confirming nor ruling out CF, such as when one or both mutant alleles remain unidentified or when the CF-causing nature of the mutations cannot be proven (Castellani et al., 2001). In addition, there are ancillary tests currently used by clinicians to clarify the diagnostic status of individuals with less CF-specific gastrointestinal or pulmonary symptomatology. The NPD test, which has been used in CF research for decades, has been introduced to clinical practice to aid diagnosis (Knowles et al., 1995). It may be particularly helpful in individuals with inconclusive sweat chloride values (Wilson et al., 1998). In *vivo* demonstration of abnormal CFTR-related ion transport across nasal epithelium could serve as an important diagnostic tool in these difficult situations.

Measurements of trans-epithelial NPD in adults accurately characterize CFTR-related ion transport. Nasal PD is determined by standard criteria as described by Knowles et al (1995). The PD is measured between a fluid filled exploring bridge on the nasal mucosa and a reference bridge on the skin of the forearm. The reference bridge may be applied to the skin by a thin needle inserted subcutaneously or placed directly on the skin after performing a small abrasion (Gelrud et al., 2004). After consistent baseline PD measurements have been obtained, the effect of amiloride superfusion through a second tube overriding the exploring catheter is evaluated. To study nasal chloride permeability and cAMP activation of chloride permeability, a large chloride chemical gradient is generated across the apical membrane by superfusion of the nasal mucosa for 3 minutes with a chloride free solution containing 10^{-4} M amiloride in Ringer's solution with gluconate substituted for chloride at a rate of 5 ml/min. Sodium (Na^+) transport and CFTR-related Cl^- transport is measured electrically by recording the changes in the nasal transepithelial PD (Knowles et al., 1995).

The nasal PD of a patient with classic CF is remarkably different from controls. The profile of classic CF patients is characterized by hyperpolarization of basal PD, increased Na^+ channel activity, an amiloride response that is exaggerated, and there is very little or no response to chloride free and isoproterenol solutions. In non-classic CF the nasal PD may be borderline and there is not yet a total consensus as to what exactly constitutes an abnormal result, but a formula which takes into account both sodium and chloride transport has been proposed by Wilschanski and colleagues (Wilschanski et al., 2001).

There have been several reports on the usefulness of NPD measurements for diagnosing CF (Hubert et al., 2004; Schüler et al., 2004). Nasal PD measurement has been widely validated in adults (Knowles et al., 1995) and provides an easy, quick and painless tool to discriminate between adults with atypical CF and those presenting some CF symptoms without CF (Delmarco et al., 1997; Wilschanski et al., 2001). Therefore a NPD test showing a significant response to zero-chloride perfusate containing isoproterenol may be useful in ruling out a diagnosis of CF. But the quantitative aspects of NPD results that are clearly indicative of CF are not defined consistently across all CF-testing centers. Moreover, some overlap likely occurs between CF and non-CF values for both the basal PD and response to zero-chloride and isoproterenol, analogous to the overlap in sweat chloride values. The NPD test's predictive capability improves somewhat when analyses of sodium and chloride channel abnormalities are combined (Standaert et al., 1997).

The NPD measurements in infants reported so far come mostly from case reports (Barker et al., 1997; Southern et al., 2001). These few studies used either the equipment already validated in adults, or specially designed one-of-a-kind devices. In a study, Sermet-Gaudelus et al. (2006) sought to validate NPD testing as a diagnostic tool for children with borderline results in neonatal screening. They adapted the standard NPD protocol for young children, designed a special catheter for them, used a slower perfusion rate, and shortened the protocol to include only measurement of basal PD, transepithelial sodium (Na^+) transport in response to amiloride, and CFTR-mediated Cl⁻ secretion in response to isoproterenol. The authors reported that the new protocol was well tolerated and produced NPD measurements that did not differ significantly from those obtained with the standard protocol. They conclude that this preliminary study will provide a basis for interpreting NPD measurements in patients with suspected CF after neonatal screening (Sermet-Gaudelus et al., 2005).

It is important however to standardize the protocol and to verify that the reference data and patterns in infants are similar to the values previously validated in adults. It is not yet known, for example, whether airway epithelium undergoes maturation during the first months of life, as renal and sweat gland epithelia do (Wilken and Travert, 1999). Therefore, before this test is implemented as a diagnostic tool for cases with borderline observations in neonatal screening, there is an urgent need to obtain and validate reference data for NPD measurements in infants and very young children with CF, and in healthy controls of the same age (Wilken and Travert, 1999). Properly conducted NPD testing at a research center can provide valuable information for diagnosis when clinical evidence is not clear-cut; however, access to the test is limited. Because there are no clear reference values, validation studies, or standardized technical protocols for NPD testing for diagnostic purposes, the test should be used only to provide contributory evidence in a diagnostic evaluation (Standaert et al., 2004).

6. The value of pancreatic associated protein (PAP) as a screening test for CF

Genetic analysis has certain drawbacks, the most important of which being the management of heterozygotes, and in France the requirement by law of previous informed consent (Barthellemy et al., 2001). In cases of CF, pancreatic alterations are already present in utero. Previous studies have demonstrated the value of PAP as a screening test for CF, and has indicated that a feasible two-stage strategy could involve the selection of infants with elevated PAP levels, and in this group of infants, subsequent detection of those with elevated IRT levels for direct CF diagnosis by the sweat test thereby avoiding the use of genetic analysis (Sarles et al., 1999; Sarles et al., 2005).

The IRT/PAP protocol can be done on one sample and preliminary data show comparable sensitivity and specificity with the other methods using the Guthrie cards (Sarles et al.,

2005). Barthellemy et al. (2001) evaluated PAP levels in a prospective study involving 47, 213 infants in the Provence region of France. In infants with a PAP > 7.5 ng/mL, 1.28% had an elevated IRT level > 700 ng/mL (0.37%). In this limited population sample (0.37% of the total), the sweat test diagnosed five cases of CF. The authors concluded that the PAP/IRT technique for CF detection seems to be suitable for mass screening, without the drawbacks of genetic testing (Barthellemy et al., 2001).

A recent study Sommerburg et al. (2010) used a prospective and sequential IRT/PAP strategy, and validated this biochemical approach against the widely used IRT/DNA protocol in a population-based NBS study in southwest Germany. The study involved the prospective quantitation of PAP and genetic analysis for the presence of four mutations in the CFTR gene most prevalent in southwest Germany (ΔF508, R553X, G551D, G542X) on all newborns with IRT >99.0th percentile. New born screening was rated positive when either PAP was ≥1.0 ng/mL and/or at least one CFTR mutation was detected. The results showed that out of 73,759 newborns tested, 0.13% were positive with IRT/PAP and 0.08% with IRT/DNA. In addition, after sweat testing of 135 CF NBS-positive infants, 13 were diagnosed with CF. The authors reported that the detection rates were similar for both IRT/PAP and IRT/DNA protocols (Sommerburg et al., 2010).

Sequential measurement of IRT/PAP provides good sensitivity and specificity and allows reliable and cost-effective CF NBS which circumvents the necessity of genetic testing with its inherent ethical problems. However, to-date it has not been tested outside of Europe and its benefits and harms in a pan-ethnic community have not been clarified.

7. Intestinal current measurement (ICM) as a diagnostic tool for CF

As many intestinal ion transport processes are electrogenic, measuring the electrical current that they generate (ICM) can be used to monitor their activity. Intestinal current measurements on rectal suction biopsies are a tool for the *ex vivo* diagnosis of classical and atypical CF. The ICM technique allows the registration of CF-induced changes in electrogenic transepithelial ion transport (Cl-, HCO$_3$-, K+) in a Cl- secretory epithelium, and on the basis of pharmacological criteria, is able to discriminate between CFTR-mediated Cl- secretion, and secretion through alternative anion channels. In CF, intestinal chloride secretion is impaired while absorptive processes remain unchanged and may even be enhanced. Furthermore, ICM is particularly useful for the classification of individuals with CF-like clinical features with equivocal sweat test values (De Jonge et al., 2004).

There is a clear difference between ICM measurement in classic CF and in normal individuals. There is information in the literature about the use of ICM as a clinical diagnostic tool (De Jonge et al., 2004; Hug et al., 2004). Derichs et al. (2010) described reference values and validated ICM for the diagnostic classification of questionable CF at all patient ages. The ICM method was performed in 309 rectal biopsies from 130 infants, children and adults including patients with known pancreatic-insufficient, pancreatic-sufficient, patients with an unclear diagnosis with mild CF symptoms, intermediate sweat test and/or *CFTR* mutation screening and healthy controls. The researchers found that the cumulative chloride secretory response of $\Delta I_{sc,carbachol}$, $\Delta I_{sc,cAMP/forskolin}$ and $\Delta I_{sc,histamine}$ was the best diagnostic ICM parameter, differentiating patients with questionable CF into pancreatic-sufficient-CF and 'CF unlikely' groups. The study underlines the diagnostic value of ICM, especially for confirmation of CF in the absence of two disease-causing *CFTR* mutations, exclusion of CF despite intermediate sweat test and age groups unsuitable for NPD measurements (Derichs et al., 2010). They conclude that ICM is an important tool for functional assessment in *CFTR* mutations of unknown clinical relevance (Derichs et al., 2010). However at present the technique has remained mainly in the research setting, so it is not yet included in the diagnostic algorithms.

8. Conclusion

Cystic fibrosis, a recessively inherited condition caused by mutation of the CFTR gene is a disease with the complex, multi-faceted clinical phenotype and is one of the most investigated monogenic disorders. More than 1800 different disease-causing mutations within the CFTR gene have been described. Mutations affect CFTR through a variety of molecular mechanisms, which can produce little or no functional gene product at the apical membrane. This results in abnormal viscous mucoid secretions in multiple organs and the main clinical features are chronic infection and progressive obstruction of the respiratory tract, pancreatic insufficiency and intestinal disease. Disease severity, to some extent, correlates with organ sensitivity to CFTR dysfunction and to the amount of functional protein, which is influenced by the type of mutation.

CFTR gene studies are now one of the most frequent activities in clinical molecular genetics laboratories and with advances in DNA analysis there is an increased knowledge of the mutational spectrum for cystic fibrosis. Genetic testing can confirm a clinical diagnosis of CF and can be used for infants with meconium ileus, for carrier detection in individuals with positive family history and partners of proven CF carriers, and for prenatal diagnostic testing if both parents are carriers. A growing number of tests capable of simultaneously detecting several frequent CF mutations are being developed, and commercial kits are now available.

The sweat chloride test remains the gold standard for CF diagnosis but does not always give a clear answer. For patients in whom sweat chloride concentrations are normal or borderline and in whom two CF mutations are not identified, an abnormal NPD measurement recorded on 2 separate days can be used as evidence of CFTR dysfunction. Newborn infants with CF have raised levels of IRT in their serum. Measurement of IRT in the first week of life has enabled CF to be incorporated into existing NBS blood spot protocols. The IRT detection test is practical, adaptable to large scale screening of dried neonatal blood spots, relatively inexpensive, and promising for the detection of newborns with CF who have pancreatic insufficiency. However, IRT is not a specific test for CF and NBS therefore requires a further tier of tests to avoid unnecessary referral for diagnostic testing. DNA analysis for common CF-associated mutations has been increasingly used as a second tier test. The sequential measurement of IRT/PAP provides good sensitivity and specificity and allows reliable and cost-effective CF newborn screening which circumvents the necessity of genetic testing. ICM is particularly useful for the classification of individuals with CF-like clinical features with equivocal sweat test values However, standardization of international programs for newborns has not yet been achieved. The significant advances in our understanding of CF and the development of new technologies now allow prenatal diagnosis. However, despite steady improvements in prenatal diagnosis, NBS and adult, CF remains a serious disease which places a heavy burden on affected families.

9. References

Ahmed, N., Corey, M., Forstner, G., Zielenski, J., Tsui, L.C., Ellis, L., Tullis, E. & Durie P. (2003). Molecular consequences of Cystic Fibrosis Transmembrane Regulator (CFTR) gene mutations in the exocrine pancreas. *Gut,* Vol. 52, pp. 1159-1164.

Alibakhshi, R., Kianishirazi, R., Cassiman, J.J., Zamani, M. & Cuppens H. (2008). Analysis of the CFTR gene in Iranian cystic fibrosis patients: identification of eight novel mutations. J Cyst Fibros Vol. 7, pp. 102-109.

Alper, O.M., Wong, L.J., Young, S., Pearl, M., Graham, S., Sherwin, J., Nussbaum, E., Nielson, D., Platzker, A., Davies, Z., Lieberthal, A., Chin, T., Shay, G., Hardy, K. & Kharrazi, M. (2004). Identification of novel and rare mutations in California Hispanic and African-American cystic fibrosis patients. *Hum Mutat* Vol. 24, pp. 353.

Amos, J.A., Bridge-Cook, P., Ponek, V. & Jarvis M.R. (2006). A universal array-based multiplexed test for cystic fibrosis carrier screening. Expert Rev Mol Diagn Vol. 6, pp. 15-22.

Ashavaid, T.F., Kondkar, A.A., Dherai, A.J., Raghavan, R., Udani, S.V., Udwadia, Z.F. & Desai, D. (2005). Application of multiplex ARMS and SSCP/HD analysis in molecular diagnosis of cystic fibrosis in Indian patients. Mol Diagn Vol. 9, pp. 59-66.

Association of Clinical Biochemistry. Guidelines for the performance of the sweat test for the investigation of cystic fibrosis in the UK, Report from the Multidisciplinary Working Group, 2002. Available at http://www.acb.org.uk.

Bals, R., Weiner, D. & Wilson J. (1999). The innate immune system in cystic fibrosis lung disease. *J Clin Invest* Vol. 103, pp.303-307.

Barben, J., Ammann, R.A., Metlagel, A. & Schoeni, M.H. (2005). Conductivity determined by a new sweat analyzer compared to chloride concentrations for the diagnosis of cystic fibrosis. *J Pediatr* Vol. 146, pp. 183-188.

Barker, P.M., Gowen, C.W., Lawson, E.E. & Knowles, M.R. (1997). Decreased sodium ion absorption across nasal epithelium of very premature infants with respiratory distress syndrome. *J Pediatr* Vol. 130, pp. 373-377.

Barthellemy, S., Maurin, N., Roussey, M., Férec, C., Murolo, S., Berthézène, P., Iovanna, J.L., Dagorn, J.C. & Sarles J. (2001). Evaluation of 47,213 infants in neonatal screening for cystic fibrosis, using pancreatitis-associated protein and immunoreactive trypsinogen assays. *Arch Pediatr* Vol. 8, pp.275-281.

Bernhardt, B.A., Weiner, J., Foster, E.C., Tumpson, J.E. & Pyeritz RE. (1987). The economics of clinical genetics services. II. A time analysis of a medical genetics clinic. *American Journal of Human Genetics* Vol. 41, pp. 559-565.

Bishop, M.D., Freedman, S.D., Zielenski, J., Ahmed, N., Dupuis, A., Martin, S., Ellis, L., Shea, J., Hopper, I., Corey, M., Kortan, P., Haber, G., Ross, C., Tzountzouris, J., Steele, L. Ray, P.N., Tsui, L.C. & Durie, P.R. (2005). The cystic fibrosis transmembrane conductance regulator gene and ion channel function in patients with idiopathic pancreatitis. *Hum Genet* Vol. 118, pp.372-381.

Bobadilla, J.L., Macek, M. Jr., Fine, J.P. & Farrell, P.M. (2002). Cystic fibrosis: a worldwide analysis of CFTR mutations-correlation with incidence data and application to screening. *Hum Mutat* Vol. 19, pp. 575-606.

Boyle, M.P. (2003). Nonclassic cystic fibrosis and CFTR-related diseases. *Curr Opin Pulm Med* Vol. 9, pp. 498-503.

Canciam, M., Fomo, S. & Mastella, G. (1988). Borderline sweat test Criteria for cystic fibrosis diagnosis. *Scand J Gastroenterol* Vol. 143, pp. 19-27.

Castellani, C., Benetazzo, M.G., Tamanini, A., Begnini, A., Mastella, G. & Pignatti, P. (2001). Analysis of the entire coding region of the cystic fibrosis transmembrane regulator gene in neonatal. hypertrypsinaemia with normal sweat test. *J Med Genet* Vol. 38, pp. 202-205.

Castellani, C., Tamanini, A. & Mastella, G. (2000). Protracted neonatal hypertrypsinogenaemia, normal sweat chloride, and cystic fibrosis. *Arch Dis Child* Vol. 82, pp. 481-482.

Chatfield, S., Owen, G., Ryley, H.C., *Williams, J., Alfaham, M., Weller, P.H., Goodchild, M.C., Carter, R.A., Bradley, D. & Dodge, J.A. (1991).* Neonatal Screening for cystic fibrosis in Wales and the West Midlands Clinical assessment after five years of screening. *Arch Dis Child* Vol. 66, pp. 29-33.

Cheillan, D., Vercherat, M., Cheavlier-Porst, F., Charcosset, M., Rolland, M.O. & Dorche, C. (2005). False positive results in neonatal screening for cystic fibrosis based on a three-stage protocol (IRT/DNA/IRT): Should we adjust IRT cut-off to ethnic origin? *Journal of Inherited Metabolic Disease* Vol. 28, pp. 813-818.

Chillo'n, M., Casals, T., Mercier, B., Bassas, L., Lissens, W., Silber, S., Romey, M.C., Ruiz-Romero, J., Verlingue, C., Claustres, M., Nunes, D.V., Férec, C. & Estivill, X. (1995). Mutations in the cystic fibrosis gene in patients with congenital absence of the vas deferens. *N Engl J Med* Vol. 332, pp. 1475-1480.

Clinical Laboratory Standards Institute (formerly National Committee for Clinical Laboratory Standards) Approved guideline. National Committee for Clinical Laboratory Standards; 2000. Sweat testing: sample collection and quantitative analysis. Document, pp. C34-A2.

College of American Pathologists. Chemistry checklist, laboratory accreditation program. [Accessed August 10, 2011]. Available from: http://www.cap.org/apps/docs/laboratory_accreditation/checklists/chemistry_and_toxic ology_april2006.pdf

Comeau, A.M., Accurso, F.J., White, T.B., Campbell, P.W., III, Hoffman, G., Parad, R.B., Wilfond, B.S., Rosenfeld, M., Sontag, M.K., Massie, J., Farrell, P.M. & O'Sullivan, B.P. (2007). Cystic Fibrosis Foundation. Guidelines for implementation of cystic fibrosis newborn screening programs: Cystic Fibrosis Foundation workshop report. *Pediatrics* Vol. 119, pp. 495-518.

Comeau, A.M., Parad, R.B., Dorkin, H.L., Dovey, M., Gerstle, R., Haver, K., Lapey, A., O'Sullivan, B.P., Waltz, D.A., Zwerdling, R.G. & Eaton, R.B. (2004). Population-based newborn screening for genetic disorders when multiple mutation DNA testing is incorporated: a cystic fibrosis newborn screening model demonstrating increased sensitivity but more carrier detections. *Pediatrics* Vol. 113:1573-1581.

Corbetta, C., Seia, M., Bassotti, A., Ambrosioni, A., Giunta, A. & Padoan, R. (2002). Screening for cystic fibrosis in newborn infants: results of a pilot programme based on a two tier protocol (IRT/DNA/IRT) in the Italian population. *J Med Screen* Vol. 9, pp. 60-63.

Crossley, J.R., Smith, P.A., Edgar, B.W., Gluckman, P.D. & Elliott, R.B. (1981). Neonatal screening for cystic fibrosis using lmmunoreactive trypsin assay in dried blood spots. *Clin Chim Acta* Vol. 113, pp. 111-121.

Crossley, J.R., Elliott, R.B. & Smith, P.A. (1979). Dried blood spot screening for cystic fibrosis in the newborn *Lancet* Vol. 1, pp. 472-474.

Crossley, J.R., Smith P.A., Edgar, B.W., Gluckman, P.D. & Elliott, R.B. (1981). Neonatal screening for cystic fibrosis, using immunoreactive trypsin assay dried blood spots. *Clin Chim Acta* Vol. 113, pp. 111-121.

Cuppens, H., Lin, W., Jaspers, M., Costes, B., Teng, H., Vankeerberghen, A., Jorissen, M., Droogmans, G., Reynaert, I., Goossens, M., Nilius, B. & Cassiman, J.J. (1998). Polyvariant mutant cystic fibrosis transmembrane conductance regulator genes: the polymorphic (TG)m locus explains the partial penetrance of the T5 polymorphism as a disease mutation. *J Clin Invest* Vol. 101, pp. 487-496.

Cuppens, H., Marynen, P., De Boeck, K. & Cassiman, J.J. (1993). Detection of 98.5% of the mutations in 200 Belgian cystic fibrosis alleles by reverse dot blot and sequencing of the complete coding regin and exon/intron junctions of the CFTR gene. *Genomics* Vol. 18, pp.693-697.

Cystic Fibrosis Foundation. Patient registry 2001 annual report. Bethesda, MD: Cystic Fibrosis Foundation, 2002.

Cystic Fibrosis Foundation Patient Registry. Annual Data Report to the Center Directors. Bethesda, MD: Cystic Fibrosis Foundation, 2005.

Cystic Fibrosis Genotype-Phenotype Consortium. (1993). Correlation between genotype and phenotype in patients with cystic fibrosis. *N Engl J Med* Vol. 329, pp. 1308-1313.

Cystic Fibrosis Mutation Database. [www.genet.sickkids.on.ca/cftr]. Accessed 10 August 2011.

Darting, R.C., di Sant'Agnese, P.A., Perera, G.A. & Anderson, D.H. (1953). Electrolyte abnormalities of sweat in fibrocysic disease of the pancreas. *Am J Med Sci* Vol. 225, pp. 67-70.

De Boeck, K., Wilschanski, M., Castellani, C., Taylor, C., Cuppens, H., Dodge, J. & Sinaasappel, M. (2006). Cystic fibrosis: terminology and diagnostic algorithms. *Thorax* Vol. 61, pp. 627-635.

de Becdelièvre, A., Costa, C., LeFloch, A., Legendre, M., Jouannic, J.M., Vigneron, J., Bresson, J.L., Gobin, S., Martin, J., Goossens, M. & Girodon, E. (2010). Notable contribution of large CFTR gene rearrangements to the diagnosis of cystic fibrosis in fetuses with bowel anomalies. *Eur J Hum Genet* Vol. 18, pp. 1166-1169.

De Jonge, H.R., Ballmann, M., Veeze, H., Bronsveld, I., Stanke, F., Tümmler, B. & Sinaasappel, M. (2004). Ex vivo CF diagnosis by intestinal current measurements (ICM) in small aperture, circulating Ussing chambers. *J Cyst Fibros* Vol. 3, pp. 159-163.

Delmarco, A., Pradal, U., Cabrini, G., Bonizzato, A. & Mastella G. (1997). Nasal potential difference in cystic fibrosis patients presenting borderline sweat test. *Eur Respir J* Vol. 10, pp. 1145-1149.

Dequeker, E., Cuppens, H., Dodge, J., Estivill, X., Goossens, M., Pignatti, P.F., Scheffer, H., Schwartz, M., Schwarz, M., Tümmler, B. & Cassiman, J.J. (2000). Recommendations for quality improvement in genetic testing for cystic fibrosis. European Concerted Action on Cystic Fibrosis. *Eur J Hum Genet* Vol. 8, pp. S1-S24.

Derichs, N., Sanz, J., Von Kanel, T., Stolpe, C., Zapf, A., Tümmler, B., Gallati, S. & Ballmann, M. (2010). Intestinal current measurement for diagnostic classification of patients with questionable cystic fibrosis: validation and reference data. *Thorax* Vol. 65, pp. 594-599.

Desmarquest, P., Feldman, D., Tamalat, A., Estivill, X., Goossens, M., Pignatti, P.F., Scheffer, H., Schwartz, M., Schwarz, M., Tümmler, B. & Cassiman, J.J. (2000). Genotype analysis and phenotypic manifestation of children with intermediate sweat chloride test results. *Chest* Vol. 118, pp. 1591-1597.

Eaker, S., Johnson, M., Jenkins, J., Bauer, M. & Little, S. (2005). Detection of CFTR mutations using ARMS and low-density microarrays. Biosens Bioelectron Vol. 21, pp. 933-939.

Elce, A., Boccia, A., Cardillo, G., Giordano, S., Tomaiuolo, R., Paolella, G. & Castaldo, G. (2009). Three novel CFTR polymorphic repeats improve segregation analysis for cystic fibrosis. *Clin Chem* Vol. 55, pp. 1372-1379.

Eng, W., LeGrys, V.A., Schechter, M.S., Laughon, M.M. & Barker, P.M. (2005). Sweat-testing in preterm and full-term infants less than 6 weeks of age. *Pediatr Pulmonol* Vol. 40, pp. 64-67.

Eshaque, B. & Dixon, B. (2006). Technology platforms for molecular diagnosis of cystic fibrosis. Biotechnol Adv Vol. 24, pp. 86-93.

Farrell, P.M., Kosorok, M.R., Laxova, A., Shen, G., Koscik, R.E., Bruns, W.T., Splaingard, M. & Mischler, E.H. (1997). Nutritional benefits of neonatal screening for cystic fibrosis. Wisconsin Cystic Fibrosis Neonatal Screening Study Group. *N Engl J Med* Vol. 337, pp. 963-969.

Farrell, P.M., Rosenstein, B.J., White, T.B., Accurso, F.J., Castellani, C., Cutting, G.R., Durie, P.R., Legrys, V.A., Massie, J., Parad, R.B., Rock, M.J. & Campbell, P.W. (2008). 3rd; Cystic Fibrosis Foundation. Guidelines for diagnosis of cystic fibrosis in newborns through older adults: Cystic Fibrosis Foundation consensus report. J Pediatr Vol. 153, pp. S4-S14.

Gelrud, A., Sheth, S., Banerjee, S., Weed, D., Shea,, J., Chuttani, R., Howell, D.A., Telford, J.J., Carr-Locke, D.L., Regan, M.M., Ellis, L., Durie, P.R. & Freedman, S.D. (2004). Analysis of CFTR function in patients with pancreas divisum and recurrent acute pancreatitis. *Am J Gastroenterol* Vol. 99, pp. 1557-1562.

Giannattasio, S., Bobba, A., Jurgelevicius, V., Vacca, R.A., Lattanzio, P., Merafina, R.S., Utkus, A., Kucinskas, V. & Marra, E. (2006). Molecular basis of cystic fibrosis in Lithuania: incomplete CFTR mutation detection by PCR-based screening protocols. Genet Test Vol. 10, pp. 169-173.

Gibson, L.E. & Cooke, R.E. (1959). A test for concentration of electrolytes in sweat in cystic fibrosis of the pancreas utilizing pilocarpine by iontophoresis. *Pediatrics* Vol. 23, pp. 545-549.

Gregg, R.G., Simantel, A., Farrell, P.M., Koscik, R., Kosorok, M.R., Laxova, A., Laessig, R., Hoffman, G., Hassemer, D., Mischler, E.H. & Splaingard M. (1997). Newborn screening for cystic fibrosis in Wisconsin: comparison of biochemical and molecular methods. *Pediatrics* Vol. 99, pp. 819-824.

Gregg, R.G., Wilfond, B.S., Farrell, P.M., Laxova, A., Hassemer, D. & Mischler EH. (1993). Application of DNA analysis in a population screening program for neonatal diagnosis of cystic fibrosis: comparison of screening protocols. *Am J Hum Genet* Vol. 52, pp. 616-626.

Grody, W.W., Cutting, G.R., Klinger, K.W., Richards, C.S., Watson, M.S. & Desnick, R.J. (2001). Laboratory standards and guidelines for population-based cystic fibrosis carrier screening. *Genetics in Medicine* Vol. 3, pp. 149-154.

Groman, J.D., Hefferon, T.W., Casals, T., Bassas, L., Estivill, X., Des Georges, M., Guittard, C., Koudova, M., Fallin, M.D., Nemeth, K., Fekete, G., Kadasi, L., Friedman, K., Schwarz, M., Bombieri, C., Pignatti, P.F., Kanavakis, E., Tzetis, M., Schwartz, M., Novelli, G., D'Apice, M.R., Sobczynska-Tomaszewska, A., Bal, J., Stuhrmann, M., Macek, M. Jr., Claustres, M. & Cutting, G.R. (2004). Variation in a repeat sequence determines whether a common variant of the cystic fibrosis transmembrane conductance regulator gene is pathogenic or benign. *Am J Hum Genet* Vol. 74, pp. 176-179.

Groman, J.D., Karczeski, B., Sheridan, M., Robinson, T.E., Fallin, M.D. & Cutting, G.R. (2005). Phenotypic and genetic characterization of patients with features of "nonclassic" forms of cystic fibrosis. *J Pediatr* Vol. 146, pp. 675-680.

Hammond, K.B., Abman, S.H., Sokol, R.J. & Accurso, F.J. (1991). Efficacy of statewide neonatal screening for cystic fibrosis by assay of trypsinogen concentrations. *New Engl J Med* Vol. 325, pp. 769-774.

Heim, R., Sugarman, E. & Allitto B. (2001). Improved detection of cystic fibrosis mutations in the heterogeneous U.S. population using an expanded, pan-ethnic mutation panel. *Genet Med* Vol. 3, pp. 168-176.

Highsmith, W.E., Burch, L.H., Zhou, Z., Olsen, J.C., Boat, T.E., Spock, A., Gorvoy, J.D., Quittel, L., Friedman, K.J. & Silverman, L.M. (1994). A novel mutation in the cystic fibrosis gene in patients with pulmonary disease but normal sweat chloride concentrations. *N Engl J Med* Vol. 331, pp. 97-80.

Heeley, A.F., Heeley, M.E., King, D.N., Kuzemko, J.A. & Walsh, M.P. (1982). Screening for cystic fibrosis by dried blood spot trypsin assay. *Arch Dis Child* Vol. 57, pp. 18-21.

Hubert, D., Jajac, I., Bienvenu, T., Desmazes-Dufeu, N., Ellaffi, M., Dall'ava-Santucci, J. & Dusser, D. (2004). Diagnosis of cystic fibrosis in adults with diffuse bronchiectasis. *J Cyst Fibros* Vol. 3, pp. 15-22.

Hug, M.J. & Tummler, B. (2004). Ex vivo CF diagnosis by intestinal current measurement (ICM) in small aperture, circulating Ussing chambers. *J Cyst Fibros* Vol. 3(Suppl 2), pp. 157-158.

Kakavas, K.V., Noulas, A.V., Kanakis, I., Bonanou, S. & Karamanos, N.K. (2006). Identification of the commonest cystic fibrosis transmembrane regulator gene DeltaF508 mutation: evaluation of PCR-single-strand conformational polymorphism and polyacrylamide gel electrophoresis. Biomed Chromatogr Vol. 20, pp. 1120-1125.

Kammesheidt, A., Kharrazi, M., Graham, S., Young, S., Pearl, M., Dunlop, C. & Keiles S. (2006). Comprehensive genetic analysis of the cystic fibrosis transmembrane conductance regulator from dried blood specimens - Implications for newborn screening. *Genetics in Medicine* Vol. 8, pp. 557-562.

Kerem, B., Rommens, J.M., Buchanan, J.A., Markiewicz, D., Cox, T.K., Chakravarti, A., Buchwald, M. & Tsui, L.C. (1989). Identification of the cystic fibrosis gene: Genetic analysis. *Science* Vol. 245, pp. 1073-1080.

Kerem, E., Corey, M., Kerem, B.S., Rommens, J., Markiewicz, D., Levison, H., Tsui, L.C. & Durie, P. (1990). The relation between genotype and phenotype in cystic fibrosis: analysis of the most common mutation (delta F508). *N Engl J Med* Vol. 323, pp. 1517-1522.

Knowles, M.R., Paradiso, A.M. & Boucher, R.C. (1995). In vivo nasal potential difference: techniques and protocols for assessing efficacy of gene transfer in cystic fibrosis. *Hum Gene Ther* Vol. 6, pp. 445-455.

Kolesár, P., Minárik, G., Baldovic, M., Ficek, A., Kovács, L. & Kádasi L. (2008). Mutation analysis of the CFTR gene in Slovak cystic fibrosis patients by DHPLC and subsequent sequencing: identification of four novel mutations. Gen Physiol Biophys Vol. 27, pp. 299-305.

Kristidis, P., Bozon, D., Corey, M., Markiewicz, D., Rommens, J., Tsui, L.C. & Durie P. (1992). Genetic determination of exocrine pancreatic function in cystic fibrosis. *Am J Hum Genet* Vol. 50, pp. 1178-1184.

Lebecque, P., Leal, T., De Boeck, C., Jaspers, M., Cuppens, H. & Cassiman, J.J. (2002). Mutations of the cystic fibrosis gene and intermediate sweat chloride levels in children. *Am J Respir Crit Care Med* Vol. 165, pp. 757-761.

LeGrys, V.A. & Wood, R.E. (1988). Incidence and implications of false negative sweat test reports in patients with cystic fibrosis. *Pediatr Pulmonol* Vol. 4, pp. 169-172.

LeGrys, V. (1996). Sweat testing for the diagnosis of cystic fibrosis: practical considerations. *J Pediatr* Vol. 129, pp. 892-897.

LeGrys, V.A., Yankaskas, J.R., Quittell, L.M., Marshall, B.C. & Mogayzel, P.J. Jr. (2007). Diagnostic sweat testing: the Cystic Fibrosis Foundation guidelines. *J Pediatr* Vol. 151, pp. 85-89.

Le Mare´chal, C., Audrezet, M.P., Quere, I., Quéré, I., Raguénès, O., Langonné, S. & Férec, C. (2001). Complete and rapid scanning of the cystic fibrosis conductance regulator (CFTR) gene by denaturing high performance liquid chromatography (D-HPLC): major implications for genetic counselling. *Hum Genet* Vol. 108, pp.290-298.

Lewis, P.A. (1995). The epidemiology of cystic fibrosis. In: Hodson ME, Geddes DM, editor(s). Cystic Fibrosis. London: Chapman & Hall Medical, pp. 1-5.

MacCready, R. (1963). Phenylketonuria screening program. *N Engl J Med* Vol. 269, pp. 52-56.

Macek, M. Jr., Mackova, A., Hamosh, A., Hilman, B.C., Selden, R.F., Lucotte, G., Friedman, K.J., Knowles, M.R., Rosenstein, B.J. & Cutting, G.R. (1997). Identification of common cystic fibrosis mutations in African-Americans with cystic fibrosis increases the detection rate to 75%. *Am J Hum Genet* Vol. 60, pp. 1122-1127.

Massie, J., Gaskin, K., Van Asperen, P. & Wilcken, B. (2000). Sweat testing following newborn screening for cystic fibrosis. *Pediatr Pulmonol* Vol. 29, pp. 452-456.

Messaoud, T., Verlingue, C., Denamur, E., Pascaud, O., Quere, I., Fattoum, S., Elion, J. & Ferec, C. (1996). Distribution of CFTR mutations in cystic fibrosis patients of Tunisian origin: Identification of two novel mutations. *Eur J Hum Genet* Vol. 4, pp. 20-24.

McCormick, J., Green, M., Mehta, G., Culross, F. & Mehta, A. (2002). Demographics of the UK cystic fibrosis population: implications for neonatal screening. *Eur J Hum Genet* Vol. 10, pp. 583-590.

McGinniss, M.J., Chen, C., Redman, J.B., Buller, A., Quan, F., Peng, M., Giusti, R., Hantash, F.M., Huang, D., Sun, W. & Strom, C.M. (2005). Extensive sequencing of the CFTR gene: lessons learned from the first 157 patient samples. Hum Genet Vol. 118, pp. 331-338.

McKone, E.F., Emerson, S.S., Edwards, K.L. & Aitken, M.L. (2003). Effect of genotype on phenotype and mortality in cystic fibrosis: a retrospective cohort study. *Lancet* Vol. 361, pp. 1671-1676.

Mickle, J.E. & Cutting, G.R. (2000). Genotype-phenotype relationships in cystic fibrosis. *Med Clin North Am* Vol. 84, pp. 597-607.

Nagy, B., Nagy, G.R., Lázár, L., Bán, Z. & Papp, Z. (2007). Detection of DeltaF508del using quantitative real-time PCR, comparison of the results obtained by fluorescent PCR. Fetal Diagn Ther Vol. 22, pp. 63-67.

National Committee for Clinical Laboratory Standards (NCCLS). (2000). Sweat testing: sample collection and quantitative analysis, Approved guideline C34-A2. Wayne, PA: NCCLS.

Nick, J.A. & Rodman, D.M. (2005). Manifestations of cystic fibrosis diagnosed in adulthood. *Curr Opin Pulm Med* Vol. 11, pp. 513-518.

Noone, P.G., Pue, C.A., Zhou, Z., Friedman, K.J., Wakeling, E.L., Ganeshananthan, M., Simon, R.H., Silverman, L.M. & Knowles, M.R. (2000). Lung disease associated with the IVS8 5T allele of the CFTR gene. *Am J Respir Crit Care Med* Vol. 162, pp. 1919-1924.

O'Sullivan, B.P., Zwerdling, R.G., Dorkin, H.L., Comeau, A.M. & Parad R. (2006). Early pulmonary manifestation of cystic fibrosis in children with the deltaF508/R117H-7T genotype. *Pediatrics* Vol. 118, pp. 1260-1265.

Padoan, R., Genoni, S., Moretti, E., Seia, M., Giunta, A. & Corbetta, C. (2002). Genetic and clinical features of false-negative infants in a neonatal screening programme for cystic fibrosis. *Acta Paediatr* Vol. 91, pp. 82-87.

Parad, R.B. & Comeau, A.M. (2003). Newborn screening for cystic fibrosis. *Pediatr Ann* Vol. 32, pp. 528-535.

Parad, R.B. & Comeau, A.M. (2005). Diagnostic dilemmas resulting from the immunoreactive trypsinogen/DNA cystic fibrosis newborn screening algorithm. *J Pediatr* Vol. 147(Suppl), pp. S78-S82.

Parad, R.B., Comeau, A.M., Dorkin, H.L., Dovey, M., Gerstle, R., Martin, T. & O'Sullivan, B.P. (2005). Sweat testing newborn infants detected by cystic fibrosis newborn screening. *J Pediatr* Vol. 147(Suppl), pp. S69-S72.

Pederziru, F., Faraguna, D., Giglio, L., Pedrotti, D., Perobelh, L. & Mastella, G. (1990). Development of a screening system for cystic fibrosis meconium or blood spot trypsin assay or both? *Acta Paediatr* Scand Vol. 79, pp. 935-942.

Perone, C., Medeiros, G.S., del Castillo, D.M., de Aguiar, M.J., Januário, J.N. (2010). Frequency of 8 CFTR gene mutations in cystic fibrosis patients in Minas Gerais, Brazil, diagnosed by neonatal screening. *Braz J Med Biol Res* Vol. 43, pp. 134-138.

Pilewski, J. & Frizzell, R. (1999). Role of CFTR in airway disease. *Physiol Rev* Vol. 79(1 Suppl), pp. S215-S255.

Price, J.F. (2006). Newborn screening for cystic fibrosis: do we need a second IRT? *Arch Dis Child* Vol. 91, pp. 209-210.

Quinton, P.M. (1999). Physiological basis of cystic fibrosis: A historical perspective. *Physiol Rev* Vol. 79, pp. S3-S22.

Ramos, M.D., Masvidal, L., Giménez, J., Bieth, E., Seia, M., des Georges, M., Armengol, L. Casals, T. (2010). CFTR rearrangements in Spanish cystic fibrosis patients: first new duplication (35kb) characterised in the Mediterranean countries. *Ann Hum Genet* Vol. 74, pp. 463-469.

Ranieri, E., Lewis, B.D., Gerase, R.L., Ryall, R.G., Morris, C.P., Nelson, P.V., Carey, W.F. & Robertson, E.F. (1994). Neonatal screening for cystic fibrosis using immunoreactive trypsinogen and direct gene analysis: four years' experience. *BMJ* Vol. 308, pp. 1469-1472.

Rave-Harel, N., Kerem, E., Nissim-Rafinia, M., Madjar, I., Goshen, R., Augarten, A., Rahat, A., Hurwitz, A., Darvasi, A. & Kerem. (1997). The molecular basis of partial penetrance of splicing mutations in cystic fibrosis. *Am J Hum Genet* Vol. 60, pp. 87-94.

Riordan, J.R., Rommens, J.M., Kerem, B., Alon, N., Rozmahel, R., Grzelczak, Z., Zielenski, J., Lok, S., Plavsic, N. & Chou, J.L. (1989). Identification of the cystic fibrosis gene: Cloning and characterization of complementary DNA. *Science* Vol. 245, pp. 1066-1073.

Rock, M.J., Mischler, E.H., Farrell, P.M., Wei, L.J., Bruns, W.T., Hassemer, D.J. Laessig, R.H. (1990). Newborn screening for cystic fibrosis is complicated by age-related decline in immunoreactive trypsinogen levels. *Pediatrics* Vol. 85, pp. 1001-1007.

Rock, M.J., Hoffman, G., Laessig, R.H., Kopish, G.J., Litsheim, T.J. & Farrell, P.M. (2005). Newborn screening for cystic fibrosis in Wisconsin: nine years experience with routine trypsinogen/DNA testing. *J Pediatr* Vol. 147(Suppl), pp. S73-S77.

Rock, M.J., Mischler, E.H., Farrell, P.M., Bruns, W.T., Hassemer, D.J. & Laessig R.H. (1989). Immunoreactive Trypsinogen Screening for Cystic Fibrosis: Characterization of Infants with a False-Positive Screening Test. *Pediatric Pulmonology* Vol. 6, pp. 42-48.

Ross, L.F. (2008). Newborn screening for cystic fibrosis: a lesson in public health disparities. *Pediatr* Vol. 153, pp. 308-313.

Rosenstein, B.J. (2000). Diagnostic methods. In: Hodson M, Geddes D, eds. Cystic fibrosis. 2nd ed. Arnold Publishers, pp. 177-188.

Rosenstein, B.J. & Cutting, G.R. (1998) for the Cystic Fibrosis Foundation Consensus Panel. The diagnosis of cystic fibrosis: a consensus statement. *J Pediatr* Vol. 132, pp. 589-595.

Sarles, J., Berthezene. P,, Le Louarn, C., Somma, C., Perini, J.M., Catheline, M., Mirallie, S., Luzet, K., Roussey, M., Farriaux, J.P., Berthelot, J. & Dagorn, J.C. (2005). Combining immunoreactive trypsinogen and pancreatitisassociated protein assays, a method of newborn screening for cystic fibrosis that avoids DNA analysis. *Journal of Pediatrics* Vol. 147, pp. 302-305.

Sarles, J., Barthellemy, S., Ferec, C., Iovanna, J., Roussey, M., Farriaux, J.P., Toutain, A., Berthelot, J., Maurin, N., Codet, J.P., Berthezene, P. & Dagorn, J.C. (1999). Blood concentrations of pancreatitis associated protein in neonates: relevance to neonatal screening for cystic fibrosis. *Archives of Disease in Childhood Fetal & Neonatal Edition* Vol. 80, pp. F118-F122.

Schneider, M., Joncourt, F., Sanz, J., von Känel, T. & Gallati, S. (2006). Detection of exon deletions within an entire gene (CFTR) by relative quantification on the Light Cycler. Clin Chem Vol. 52, pp. 2005-2012.

Schneider, M., Hirt, C., Casaulta, C., Barben, J., Spinas, R., Bühlmann, U., Spalinger, J., Schwizer, B., Chevalier-Porst, F., Gallati, S. (2007). Large deletions in the CFTR gene: clinics and genetics in Swiss patients with CF. Clin Genet Vol. 72, pp. 30-38.

Schüler, D., Sermet-Gaudelus, I., Wilschanski, M., Ballmann, M., Dechaux, M., Edelman, A., Hug, M., Leal, T., Lebacq, J., Lebecque, P., Lenoir, G., Stanke, F., Wallemacq, P., Tümmler, B. & Knowles, M.R. (2004). Basic protocol for transepithelial potential difference measurements. J Cyst Fibros Vol. 3, pp. 151-156.

Schwartz, M., Johansen, H.K., Koch, C. & Brandt, N.J. (1990). Frequency of the delta F508 mutation on cystic fibrosis chromosomes in Denmark. Hum Genet Vol. 85, pp. 427-428.

Sermet-Gaudelus, I., Roussel, D., Bui, S., Deneuville, E., Huet, F., Reix, P., Bellon, G., Lenoir, G. & Edelman, A. (2006). The CF-CIRC study: a French collaborative study to assess the accuracy of cystic fibrosis diagnosis in neonatal screening. BMC Pediatr Vol. 6:25.

Sermet-Gaudelus, I., Dechaux, M., Vallee, B., Fajac, A., Girodon, E., Nguyen-Khoa, T., Marianovski, R., Hurbain, I., Bresson, J.L., Lenoir, G. & Edelman, A. (2005). Chloride transport in nasal ciliated cells of cystic fibrosis heterozygotes. Am J Respir Crit Care Med Vol. 171, pp. 1026-1031.

Sheppard, D.N. & Welsh, M.J. (1999). Structure and function of the CFTR chloride channel. Physiol Rev Vol. 79, pp. S23-S45.

Shwachman, H. & Gahm, N. (1956). Studies in cystic fibrosis of the pancreas. A simple test for the detection of excess chloride on the skin. N Eng J Med Vol. 255, pp. 999-1001.

Smalley, C.A., Addy, D.P. & Anderson, C.M. (1978). Does that child really have cystic fibrosis? Lancet Vol. n, pp. 415-416.

Sommerburg, O., Lindner, M., Muckenthaler, M., Kohlmueller, D., Leible, S., Feneberg, R., Kulozik, A.E., Mall, M.A. & Hoffmann, G.F. (2010). Initial evaluation of a biochemical cystic fibrosis newborn screening by sequential analysis of immunoreactive trypsinogen and pancreatitis-associated protein (IRT/PAP) as a strategy that does not involve DNA testing in a Northern European population. J Inherit Metab Dis Vol. 33(Suppl 2), pp. S263-S271.

Sontag, M.K., Hammond, K.B., Zielenski, J., Wagener, J.S. & Accurso, F.J. (2005). Two-tiered immunoreactive trypsinogen-based newborn screening for cystic fibrosis in Colorado: screening efficacy and diagnostic outcomes. J Pediatr Vol. 147(3 Suppl), pp. S83-S88.

Southern, K.W., Noone, P.G., Bosworth, D.G., Legrys, V.A., Knowles, M.R. & Barker PM. (2001). A modified technique for measurement of nasal transepithelial potential difference in infants. J Pediatr Vol. 139, pp. 353-358.

Standaert, T.A., Boitano, L., Emerson, J., Milgram, L.J., Konstan, M.W., Hunter, J., Hunter, J., Berclaz, P.Y., Brass, L., Zeitlin, P.L., Hammond, K., Davies, Z., Foy, C., Noone, P.G., Knowles, M.R. (2004). Standardized procedure for measurement of nasal potential difference: an outcome measure in multi-center cystic fibrosis clinical trials. Pediatr Pulmonol Vol. 37, pp. 385-392.

Stewart, B., Zabner, J., Shuber, A., Welsh, M.J. & McCray, P.B. (1995). Normal sweat chloride values do not exclude the diagnosis of cystic fibrosis. Am J Respir Crit Care Med Vol. 151, pp. 899-903.

Storm, K., Moens, E., Vits, L., De Vlieger, H., Delaere, G., D'Hollander, M., Wuyts, W., Biervliet, M., Van Schil, L., Desager, K. & Nöthen, M.M. (2007). High incidence of the CFTR mutations 3272-26A-->G and L927P in Belgian cystic fibrosis patients, and identification of three new CFTR mutations (186-2A-->G, E588V, and 1671insTATCA). J Cyst Fibros Vol. 6, pp. 371-375.

Svensson, A.M., Chou, L.S., Miller, C.E., Robles, J.A., Swensen, J.J., Voelkerding, K.V., Mao, R. & Lyon, E. (2010). Detection of large rearrangements in the cystic fibrosis transmembrane conductance regulator gene by multiplex ligation-dependent probe amplification assay when sequencing fails to detect two disease-causing mutations. *Genet Test Mol Biomarkers* Vol. 14, pp. 171-174.

Taccetti, G., Festini, F., Braccini, G., Campana, S. & deMartino, M. (2004). Sweat testing in newborns positive to neonatal screening for cystic fibrosis. *Arch Dis Child Fetal Neonatal Ed* Vol. 89, pp. F463-F464.

The Cystic Fibrosis Genetic Analysis Consortium: Population variation of common cystic fibrosis mutations. (1994). The Cystic Fibrosis Genetic Analysis Consortium. *Hum Mutat* Vol. 4, pp. 167-177.

Tomaiuolo, R., Sangiuolo, F., Bombieri, C., Bonizzato, A., Cardillo, G., Raia, V., D'Apice, M.R., Bettin, M.D., Pignatti, P.F., Castaldo, G. & Novelli, G. (2008). Epidemiology and a novel procedure for large scale analysis of CFTR rearrangements in classic and atypical CF patients: a multicentric Italian study. J Cyst Fibros Vol. 7, pp. 347-351.

Travert G. (1988). Analyse de l'expenence mondiale de depistage neonatal de la mucoviscidose par dosage de la trypsirje immunoreactive (Conference Internationale Mucoviscidose- Deistage neonatal et pnse en charge precore). *Caen,* pp. 1-23.

Watson, M.S., Cutting, G.R., Desnick, R.J., Driscoll, D.A., Klinger, K., Mennuti, M., Palomaki, G.E., Popovich, B.W., Pratt, V.M., Rohlfs, E.M., Strom, C.M., Richards, C.S., Witt, D.R. & Grody, W.W. (2004). Cystic fibrosis population carrier screening: 2004 revision of American College of Medical Genetics mutation panel. *Genetics in Medicine* Vol. 6, pp. 387-391.

Welsh, M.J., Ramsey, B.W., Accurso, F. & Cutting, G.R. (2001). Cystic fibrosis. In: Scriver AB, Sly WS, Valle D, eds. The Molecular and Metabolic Basis of Inherited Disease. New York: McGraw-Hill, pp. 5121-5188.

Wilcken, B. & Travert, G. (1999). Neonatal screening for cystic fibrosis: present and future. *Acta Paediatr Suppl* Vol. 88, pp. 33-35.

Wilcken, B., Wiley, V., Sherry, G. & Bayliss, U. (1995). Neonatal screening for cystic fibrosis: a comparison of two strategies for case detection in 1.2 million babies. *J Pediatr* Vol. 127, pp. 965-970.

Wilcken, B., Brown, A.R., Urwin, R. & Brown, D.A. (1983). Cystic fibrosis screening by dried blood spot trypsin assay: results in 75,000 newborn infants. *J Pediatr* Vol. 102, pp. 383-387.

Wilfond, B.S. & Gollust, S.E. (2003). Policy issues for expanding newborn screening programs: a look "behind the curtain" at cystic fibrosis newborn screening programs in the United States [presentation]. Newborn Screening for Cystic Fibrosis Meeting; November 21, 2003; Atlanta, GA.

Wilschanski, M., Dupuis, A., Ellis, L., Jarvi, K., Zielenski, J., Tullis, E., Martin, S., Corey, M., Tsui, L.C. & Durie P. (2006). Mutations in the cystic fibrosis transmembrane regulator gene and in vivo transepithelial potentials. *Am J Respir Crit Care Med* Vol. 174, pp. 787-794.

Wilschanski, M., Famini, H., Strauss-Liviatan, N., Rivlin, J., Blau, H., Bibi, H., Bentur, L., Yahav, Y., Springer, H., Kramer, M.R., Klar, A., Ilani, A., Kerem, B. & Kerem E. (2001). Nasal potential difference measurements in patients with atypical cystic fibrosis. *Eur Respir J* Vol. 17, pp. 1208-1215.

Wilson, D.C., Ellis, L., Zielenski, J., Corey, M., Ip, W.F., Tsui, L.C., Tullis, E., Knowles, M.R. & Durie, P.R. (1998). Uncertainty in the diagnosis of cystic fibrosis: possible role of *in vivo* nasal potential difference measurements. *J Pediatr* Vol. 132, pp. 596-599.

Yeung, W.H., Palmer, J., Schidlow, D., Bye, M.R. & Huang, N.N. (1984). Evaluation of a paper patch test for sweat chloride determination *Clin Pediatr* Vol. 23, pp. 603-607.

Zielenski, J. (2000). Genotype and phenotype in cystic fibrosis. *Respiration* Vol. 67, pp. 117-133.

Zielenski, J., Rozmahel, R., Bozon, D., Kerem, B., Grzelczak, Z., Riordan, J.R., Rommens, J. & Tsui, L.C. (1991). Genomic DNA sequence of the cystic fibrosis transmembrane conductance regulator (CFTR) gene. *Genomics* Vol. 10, pp. 214-228.

Part 3

Microbiology and Immunology

7

Infection by Non-Tuberculous Mycobacteria in Cystic Fibrosis

María Santos[1], Ana Gil-Brusola[1] and Pilar Morales[2]
[1]Microbiology Department,
[2]Lung Transplant Unit, University Hospital La Fe, Valencia,
Spain

1. Introduction

Cystic fibrosis (CF) is a common autosomal recessive genetic condition affecting white population with an approximate incidence of 1 per 2500 live births (Davis et al., 1996), nearly 30,000 people in the USA (Olivier et al., 2003). Patients with this life-shortening disease have abnormally thickened secretions that facilitate chronic infection of the airways, bronchiectasis and early death. The respiratory pathogens most frequently isolated in these patients are *Staphylococcus aureus* and *Pseudomonas aeruginosa*.

As the survival of this group of patients has been improved by better nutrition, intensive therapy to clear airway secretions and more aggressive use of antibiotics (FitzSimmons, 1993, Ramsey, 1996), new pathogens such as *Stenotrophomonas maltophilia, Burkholderia cepacia, Alkaligenes xylosoxidans, Nocardia* spp., fungi and non tuberculous mycobacteria (NTM) are evolving (Burns et al., 1998; Burns & Saiman, 1999; Olivier et al., 1996)

NTM have increasingly been reported in the world as pulmonary pathogens not only in immunosuppressed but also in non immunocompromised persons, mainly in patients with lung disease (bronchiectasis, hypersensitivity, pneumonitis, chest wall disorders, previous mycobacteriosis and CF) (Huang et al., 1999; Prince et al., 1989; Hjelte et al., 1990; Fauroux et al., 1997)

Two important issues to consider are: 1) the clinical significance of isolation of a NTM (contamination, colonization or disease) (Hayes, 2005); and 2) bacterial overgrowth, especially with *P. aeruginosa*, leading to difficulty in the isolation of the mycobacterium from sputum samples.

NTM produce insidious infections that require several months of combined antibiotic therapy, difficult eradication and frequent relapses with progressive lung function deterioration (Esther et al., 2010). They represent an important social and health problem (Olivier et al., 2003), with not well defined and unsolved aspects, such as mode of infection, pathogenic role, standardized treatment or prophylaxis.

In this chapter we will review the main epidemiological, clinical, diagnostic, therapeutic and prophylactic aspects of NTM infections in CF patients.

2. Epidemiology and pathogenesis

2.1 General aspects

The term NTM refers to *Mycobacterium* spp. different to *M. tuberculosis complex* and *M. leprae*. These microorganisms are widely distributed in the environment (water, soil, dust, animals and food). Almost all NTM are less virulent and contagious than *M. tuberculosis* (Runyon, 1959; Brown-Elliot et al., 2002). There are more than 100 described species, of which only 15-20 produce infections in humans.

NTM are resistant to chlorination and ozonation (Prim et al., 2004) and to multiple antiseptics and antibiotics. They are opportunistic microorganisms capable of causing disease in a different range of locations (skin and soft tissues, lymph nodes and lung) as well as disseminated diseases.

The extent and severity of infection depends on the anatomic and immune integrity of the host. These bacteria can adhere to biomedical materials (catheters, prosthesis, filters or membranes of inhalation systems) forming a biofilm that may complicate the pharmacological treatment of such infections (Williams et al., 2009).

Infection by NTM was first reported in a patient with CF in 1980 (Boxerbaum, 1980). Few infections were described before 1990, but in the last 20 years, NTM have emerged as new pathogens in CF (Griffith, 2003; Olivier et al., 1996). This increase may be due to several factors: greater survival of patients with CF, increasing their environmental exposure; more aggressive therapies, which facilitate susceptibility to infection; improved microbiological diagnostic methods; and better interaction between clinicians and microbiologists. In 1997, the American Thoracic Society (ATS) published a Consensus Statement that identified CF as a risk factor for NTM pulmonary disease in HIV-seronegative patients and provided recommendations for laboratory and clinical diagnosis of NTM infection (Official Statement ATS, 1997).

In summary, NTM are common in patients with CF but neither person to person nor nosocomial acquisition explain their high prevalence. Clinical significance of NTM is incompletely defined but patients with these organisms should be monitored with repeated sample cultures (Olivier et al., 2003).

2.2 Pathogenesis

Patients with CF have abnormally viscous and thickened airway and gastrointestinal secretions as a result of a defect or decrease in the transmembrane conductance regulator protein or gene product which regulates chloride and liquid secretions across epithelial surfaces and resorption of sodium and liquid. These thick respiratory secretions occlude the airways and ductal lumens leading to recurrent pulmonary infections, pancreatic insufficiency and intestinal obstruction (Welsh, 1990).

NTM, which enter mainly through the respiratory tract, are phagocytosed by macrophages and survive and reproduce within patients until symptomatic infection occurs. The disease manifestations depend on the immune cellular response and the possible granulome formation; hence, its difficult eradication and its tendency to persistence or recurrence (Morales et al., 2011).

2.3 Frequency and distribution

Prevalence rates of NTM infections in patients with CF are variable, due mainly to the few multicenter studies (Olivier et al., 2003; Roux et al., 2009; Mussaffi, et al., 2005; Levy et al., 2008) and their diversity in the methodology used, since some refer to patients who had at least one positive culture and others to those who met disease criteria following the ATS recommendations from 1997 (Official Statement ATS, 1997) or 2007 (Griffith et al., 2007), obtaining fewer cases.

Infection data vary between 2 and 30%, with an average of 13 to 15%. These differences are due to the number of cases reported in each study - the most numerous being Olivier et al, 1186 and Roux et al, 1582-, the geographical location - with differences between continents (America greater reports) and within countries (the highest prevalence values were those reported for coastal states) - and the age of the patients included. In general, more isolates may be found in teenagers (10-20%) and young adults with CF (American Academy of Paediatrics, 2006).

Regarding age, both multicenter studies and general observations, suggest that NTM infections occur as a complication in adolescents and young adults (10 to 25 years old) although with small differences between mycobacteria, since the rapidly growing can be acquired at almost any age and *M. avium complex* (MAC) in older patients (Roux et al., 2009). Some do not find significant differences among sex (Olivier et al., 2003), while as others describe more cases in women than men (Roux et al., 2009).

2.4 Isolated NTM

In relation to the isolated species of NTM, most authors agree that both, MAC and the rapidly growing mycobacteria (RGM), are the most frequent, accounting around 80% (Roux et al., 2009). Infection is usually caused by a single species and exceptionally by a mixture of two mycobacteria.

MAC is composed of a group of slow, fastidiously growing mycobacteria that includes *M. avium*, *M. intracellulare* and unnamed genetically related species. It ranks first in North America with 72% of the isolates, mainly *M. avium* (Olivier et al., 2003) but is second and third in frequency in other series. *M. abscessus*, a member of the RGM (culture growth in less than 7 days) seems to prevail in Western Europe (Roux et al., 2009; Jönsson et al., 2007; Sermet-Gaudelus et al., 2003) and Israel (Levy et al., 2008), where *M. simiae* is also frequent. (Figure 1).

M. abscessus may be confused due to its different classification in time, since it was first included within *M. chelonae* group, then as a different species by itself, and more recently as part of the *M. abscessus complex* (MABSC), together with *M. massiliense* (Adékambi et al., 2004) and *M. bolletii* (Adékambi et al., 2006).

The prevalence of these two groups - MAC and MABSC - varies with age. MABSC may appear at any age, but most frequently in teenagers age 11 to 15 years old, while as MAC is more common in young adults aged 20 to 25 (Pierre-Audigier et al., 2005; Rodman et al., 2005). In all series, there is a minority group of varied mycobacteria named "others", which includes *M. gordonae* (possible contaminant), *M. fortuitum*, *M. kansasii*, *M. simiae*, *M. peregrinum*, *M. malmoense*, all of them infrequent and poorly representative.

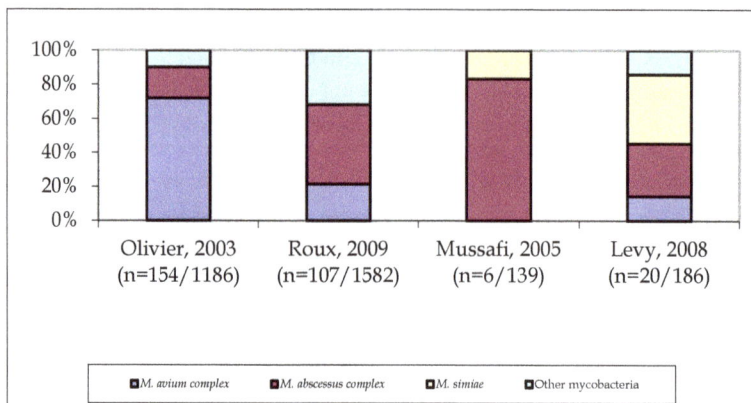

Fig. 1. Frequency of NTM species isolated in CF patients according to several studies (Olivier et al., 2003; Roux et al., 2009; Mussaffi et al., 2005; Levy et al., 2008).

2.5 Transmission

Given the ubiquitous nature of NTM, the port of entry for infection may be diverse: cutaneous, oropharyngeal mucosa, digestive or respiratory. NTM are frequently present in tap water and shower heads, where they remain viable in aerosols (Parker et al., 1983). Some, such as MAC, are resistant to chlorine and ozone, as already mentioned. Most infections remain near the port of entry but may also disseminate to other organs if the patient is immunocompromised. There is no evidence of person-to-person transmission of NTM infection. Therefore, no patient isolation but only universal precautions are necessary. Infections usually present as single cases, but outbreaks have also been reported, some of them by molecular techniques, secondary to a common focus neither identified nor corrected (Wallace et al., 1998; Kim et al., 2007; Viana-Niero et al, 2008).

2.6 Risk factors

In the last ten years, several authors have sought the relationship between NTM infection and different aspects of the patients, the disease or the microorganisms involved, describing some predisposing or risk factors (Table 1). (Olivier et al., 2003; Roux et al., 2009; Mussafi et al., 2005; Levy et al., 2008).

Age	Sweat chloride	*P. aeruginosa*
Race	Insulin-requiring diabetes	*S. aureus*
Sex	Pancreatic enzymes use	*Aspergillus spp.*
BMI	Steroids	Sputums cultured
Place of residence	Severe genotypes	FEV1

BMI, body mass index; FEV1, forced espiratory volume in the 1st second.

Table 1. Predictors of NTM infection in CF patients

Olivier et al, compared CF patients with and without positive culture for NTM. The culture-positive patients were significantly older (26 versus 22, p<0,001), had higher FEV1 (60% versus 54%), higher frequency of *S. aureus* (43% versus 31%) and lower frequency of *P. aeruginosa* co-infection (71% versus 82%). Another related factor was the body mass index (BMI). There were no significant differences between *M. abscessus* and *MAC*. When several risk factors are present (for example, age, FEV1 and *S. aureus* co-infection) the probability of having NTM is 50-fold higher.

Roux et al, found nuances in age between the two groups of mycobacteria, as previously mentioned, suggesting that this difference may be due to the different degree of virulence of these mycobacteria. Women were more frequently affected, a fact not previously referenced. Little is known about the clinical significance and the risk factors of the new species of RGM, apart from their tendency to produce cutaneous lesions. A recent study has also found clinical differences between *M. maxiliense* and *M. abscessus* infection (Zelazny et al., 2009).

Levy et al, found that the presence of *Aspergillus* spp. in sputum and the number of the sputum specimens processed for mycobacteria were the most significant predictors for isolation of NTM.

Mussafi et al, have found a relationship between pulmonary *M. abscessus* disease and allergic bronchopulmonary aspergillosis and corticosteroid therapy. Eradication of infection was more difficult in these circumstances.

In addition to the risk factors analyzed, we must not forget that, back in 1997, the ATS published a consensus document identifying CF as a risk factor itself for NTM infection, providing extensive information about it.

3. Clinical manifestations and radiology

Clinical manifestations, together with radiological findings and the microbiological cultures that will be commented further on, constitute the three basic pillars for the diagnosis of NTM disease (Table 2) (Griffith et al., 2007).

CATEGORY	REQUIREMENTS
Clinical findings	Pulmonary symptoms Exclusion of other diagnoses
Radiological findings	Chest X-ray: nodular or cavitary images; or HRCT: multifocal bronchiectasis with multiple small nodules.
Bacteriological findings	Sputum: 2 or more positive cultures or BAS or BAL: ≥ 1 positive culture or lung biopsy: granulomatous inflammation or positive staining for AFB together with one or more positive cultures (biopsy, sputum, BAS; BAL)

Table 2. ATS / IDSA criteria for the diagnosis of lung disease caused by NTM

Diagnosis requires: all the clinical criteria + 1 radiological criterion + 1 bacteriological criterion. ATS: American Thoracic Society; IDSA: Infectious Diseases Society of America; NTM: Non-tuberculous Mycobacteria; HRCT: high-resolution computerized tomography; BAS: bronchoalveolar secretions (aspirate); BAL: bronchoalveolar lavage; AFB: acid-alcohol resistant bacilli.

Lung infections in general tend to have non specific symptoms (cough, dyspnea, weight loss, increased expectoration, sometimes hemoptysis) and chest radiographic findings that vary from innocuous or no findings, to infiltrates or nodules, sometimes cavitated, (Morales et al., 2007) with HRCT scanning chest abnormalities - nodules and/or multifocal bronchiectasis (Hayes, 2005).

The chest radiography in NTM pulmonary disease caused by RGM is likely to show multilobular, patchy, reticulonodular or mixed interstitial and alveolar infiltrates with upper lobe predominance and cavitation in only 15% of cases (Griffith et al., 1993, Daley & Griffith, 2002) (Figure 2).

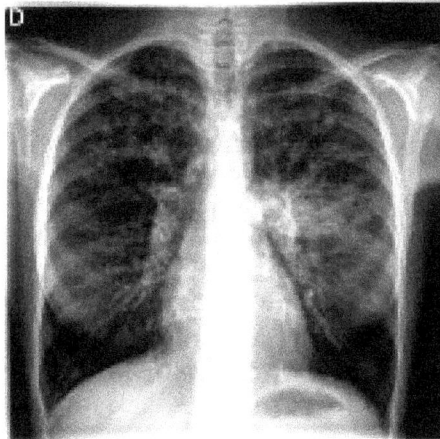

Fig. 2. Chest radiography of *M. abscessus* infection in CF patient.

The most common radiographic changes in MAC infection are cavitary disease and fibronodular bronchiectasis (Goo & Im, 2002). Cavities are finer and surrounded by less parenchymal opacification than in the case of tuberculosis (TB) (Erasmus et al., 1999). Bronchiectasis appear preferentially in the middle lobe and lingula (Lynch et al., 1995). Pleural effusion is not common. In HRCT scanning, the presence of bronchiectasis and multiple small nodules are predictive of MAC lung disease (Maycher et al., 2000).

Cutaneous manifestations may vary from small single nodes to ulcers, sometimes coincident with skin disruptions such as wounds, burns, surgical incisions, catheter implantation sites and so forth. These cutaneous lesions are very important in lung transplant recipients (LTx), since they can be the first sign of dissemination (Taylor & Palmer, 2006, Morales et al., 2007).

In isolated cases and, especially, in immunossuppressed patients, including transplant recipients, infection may diseminate to other organs, like from skin to lungs, intestine or other sites.

3.1 Clinical course and evolution

Clinical course is similar to that of TB, with insidious and slow progression that requires combined treatment for various months. This is difficult to comply due to its adverse effects and interactions with other drugs. Initial clinical and microbiological response is usually good but, even after complete compliance, with apparently successful therapy, there is a tendency to persistance and relapse (Mussaffi et al., 2005). NTM affects pulmonary function and chronic lung infection in CF patients is the main cause of morbidity and mortality (Esther et al., 2010). There is no data of mortality directly associated to mycobaterial infection, since these patients usually suffer simultaneous infections by different microorganisms (Figure 3).

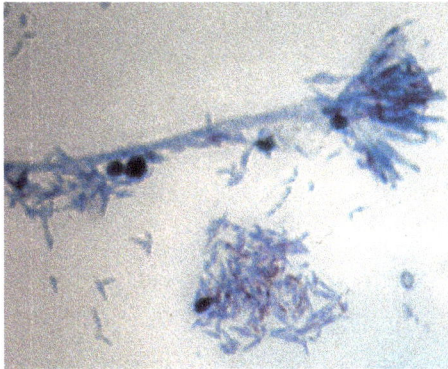

Fig. 3. Modified Ziehl-Neelsen stain showing co-infection of *Mycobacterium* spp. with *Aspergillus* spp. in a CF patient.

4. Microbiological diagnosis

Samples that reach the laboratory are mainly of respiratory origin (sputum, pleural fluid or its biopsy specimen, BAL and lung biopsy specimen). They can also be from skin or other locations if infection is disseminated.

With the staining methods - Ziehl-Neelsen or auramine fluorescence -, there are features on the AFB in terms of their number, shape, and grouping, that characterize the different NTM.

Bacterial overgrowth, especially with *P. aeruginosa*, is problematic and leads to difficulties in isolating mycobacteria from respiratory secretions and sputum. Therefore, together with the classical decontamination process using 0.25% N-acetylcysteine and 1% NaOH, addition of 5% oxalic acid is recommended (Whittier et al., S. 1997)

Samples are cultured in solid (Löwenstein-Jenssen or other) and liquid media (radiometric BACTEC 460 and nonradiometric BACTEC 9050 and 960, Becton Dickinson, or other). Some NTM have specific requirements for culture, such as temperature (MAC 42°C) and time (RGM grow in less than 7 days, whereas others in 10-14 days).

Colonies may be identified phenotypically in most cases (Kent & Kubica, 1983, Metchock et al., 1999) and be confirmed by molecular typing methods, using commercial RNA/DNA probes (AccuProbe, GenProbe, San Diego, Ca) (Cousins et al.,1996, Wallace et al., 1998) and other techniques (Zhang et al., 1997). The different species included in the MABSC are distinguished by *rpoB* sequencing (AdéKambi et al., 2003). Molecular identification of the mycobacteria also helps in differentiating between relapse and reinfection, and in determining whether an outbreak is secondary to a common origin or not.

Chromatography techniques (Butler & Guthertz, 2001) are less used, since they are more complex and less precise (Leite et al., 2005). Serologic diagnosis, such as determining the presence of IgG immunoglobulin against antigen A 60 (Oliver et al., 2001), has been discarded due to its low sensitivity and specificity (Pottumarthy et al., 2000). Tuberculin skin testing may be positive in patients infected with NTM, since *M. tuberculosis* shares antigens with various species, but generally the induration induced is less than 10 mm in diameter (Field & Cowie, 2006). Techniques based on lymphocyte interferon gamma (IFN-γ) production have been developed and can be useful in distinguishing between infection by *M. tuberculosis*, NTM, or BCG vaccination (Scholvink et al., 2004).

There is controversy over the systematic use of susceptibility testing of NTM, since there is no clear correlation to the clinical therapeutic response. At least for clarithromycin in the case of MAC disease there are some recommendations (Wayne, 2000). RGM are intrinsically resistant to classic antituberculous drugs and have variable antimicrobial susceptibility profile. Clinically significant isolates should be tested against amikacin, cefoxitine, ciprofloxacin, clarithromycin, doxycycline, imipenem, trimethoprim/sulfamethoxazole and recently, linezolid (Woods, 2000). Synergy studies with two or more antibiotics can also be done. Methods used include dilution, diffussion (E-test) and automated techniques.

5. Treatment and evolution

5.1 General aspects

No guidelines exist for the treatment of NTM pulmonary diseases in the CF population. Given the natural tendency of these bacteria to seek refuge in macrophages and to the fact that *in vitro* susceptibility tests do not show true antibiotic concentration, combined therapy may favour synergy and minimize the appearance of resistance. It is difficult to determine a treatment of choice since experience is limited and results are variable, and *in vitro* tests do not always correlate to *in vivo* response. Duration of treatment is also variable, depending on the NTM to be treated, the severity and extent of disease, and the clinical and immune status of the patient. In any case, treatment compliance is difficult since it is long lasting, antibiotics have adverse effects and interactions with other drugs, in particular with immunesuppressors in the case of transplant recipients. A close clinical and microbiological surveillance of the patients is necessary, to watch out for possible relapses, dissemination or risk of graft rejection in the case of transplantation (Morales et al, 2007; Morales et al., 2011).

We will focus on the treatment of MAC and *M. abscessus*, the most frequent NTM in CF patients. Treatment of the less common mycobacteria requires individualized considerations, keeping as a basic principle the combination of two or three active drugs.

5.2 Treatment of MAC

Transmission of the mycobacteria included in the MAC is varied, but mainly through birds and water (Marras et al., 2005). Infection has been related to recreational hot-tubs and can cause a hypersensitivity pneumonitis like syndrome in exposed patients (Embril et al., 1997; Rickman et al., 2002; Hanak et al., 2006).

Mycobacteria included in the MAC are resistant to first-line antituberculous drugs – rifampicin, isoniazid and streptomycin - except for ethambutol, and are usually susceptible to amikacin and macrolides, in particular clarithromycin.

Initial treatment includes ethambutol, clarithromycin or azithromycin and a third drug according to susceptibility test results. Duration of treatment is from 6 to 9 months for small lesions and up to 12-24 months in case of dissemination. Combination of ethambutol, a macrolide and rifampicin has been used successfully due to their synergism and good tolerance (Field & Cowie, 2003). Some authors recommend maintenance of the macrolide 12 more months once patients convert to negative, thus reducing the number of relapses (ATS, 1997). The importance of macrolides relies on the intracellular penetrance of both, the antibiotic and the bacteria. First recommendations included clarithromycin (Field & Cowie, 2003) and then azithromycin (Griffith et al., 2001), but always in combination and not in monotherapy as initial drugs.

M. avium is the most common cause of immune reconstitution inflammatory syndrome caused by NTM (Field & Cowie, 2006). IFN-γ is a macrophage activator in response to mycobacteria. Patients with disseminated MAC infection, with relapses or poor prognosis, respond favorably to inhaled IFN-γ (Holland et al., 1994; Hallstrand et al., 2004).

In exceptional cases, when infection is localized and with persistent lung affection, surgery has been applied. Post-operative morbidity and complications that include hemorrhages, bronchopleural fistula and empyema are possible.

5.3 Treatment of *M. abscessus* and other RGM

This group of mycobacteria is ubiquitous and can survive in adverse conditions. They can grow in any culture media used in bacteriology in less than 7 days, with the risk of not being evaluated or being considered as contaminants. Although it includes various species, the most relevant and virulent in CF patients is *M. abscessus*. This mycobacterium can cause skin infection, lung disease or even disseminate. Its treatment is difficult due to its multiresistance, not only to the classic, already mentioned antituberculous drugs, including ethambutol, but also to ampicillin, amoxicillin-clavulanate, cefoxitin, ciprofloxacin, erythromycin, sulfamethoxazole and tobramycin. It is universally susceptible to amikacin, and a recommended treatment is the combination of amikacin, clarithromycin and imipenem for 6 to 9 months (Yang et al., 2003). There can be initial improvement, but relapses are very frequent, in which case, therapy should be extended and/or a drug should be changed according to susceptibility testing. Other alternative therapeutic agents include the new oxazolidinone, linezolid, that is active against RGM (Wallace et al., 2001) with good therapeutic results (Morales et al, 2007). An open line includes the new quinolones gatifloxacin and moxifloxacin.

In the presence of big lung abscesses, a very rare presentation, surgical drainage might be necessary and can potentially lead to extrapulmonary seeding of the infecting mycobacteria and be an added risk if lung transplantation is needed.

Recommended suppressive therapy includes oral clarithromycin and aerosolized amikacin (Cullen et al., 2000; Colin AA, 2000). Monotherapy must always be avoided, since the most common cause of macrolide resistance is the use of clarithromycin as single drug in patients with CF and disseminated cutaneous infection (Wallace et al., 1996).

6. Prophylaxis

Given the extensive and varied presence of NTM in the environment and their variable susceptibility to antibiotics, the inevitable environmental exposure of CF patients and the lack of person-to-person transmission, primary chemoprophylaxis is not indicated. The only situation in which clarithromycin or azithromycin would be recommended is in HIV positive patients over 6 years of age and with a CD4 count of less than $50/\mu L$, with risk of MAC infection (American Academy of Pediatrics, 2006).

Clinical and radiological monitoring is important, including intensive and selective search for NTM, in pulmonary samples from suspected foci, especially in young adults with impaired lung disease, *Aspergillus* spp. and steroid treatment.

On the other hand, it is important to take into consideration the life style of the patient, with a watchful attitude towards surrounding environment, being aware that it constitutes an unavoidable but reducible risk. Recently, a practical and excellent guideline in this regard has been published (Avery et al., 2009)

7. Peri-transplant considerations

7.1 Pre-transplant

As has been discussed, NTM infections must be kept in mind in the differential diagnosis of any lung disease in CF patients, especially when approaching an indication of LTx. Identification and *in vitro* susceptibility of the mycobacteria are required to ensure proper treatment and to achieve complete recovery before transplantation.

In particular, so difficult is the treatment of *M. abscessus* infection, that it has been considered a strong relative contraindication to LTx (Orens et al., 2006). Recently, Gilljama et al., reported their experience in three double LTx CF patients with ongoing therapy, and a fourth with recent treatment for *M. abscessus* lung infection. The first three developed skin infection and abscesses. Recovery was finally accomplished and pulmonary function was re-established after a prolonged 7 years long follow-up. With this, they conclude that LTx is feasible but may involve severe complications.

7.2 Post-Transplant

Infection and graft rejection in organ recipients are the two main causes of morbidity and mortality. Transplant may lead to the reactivation of a previously undetected infection, to its dissemination or to its initial onset. NTM have emerged as important pathogens in these patients, especially in LTx, causing pulmonary and extrapulmonary infections (Malouf & Glanville, 1999). These bacteria have also been identified as a potential cause of graft dysfunction and mortality by themselves or together with other opportunistic pathogens, which is a very common situation. In particular, infection by *M. abscessus* may be fatal

(Sanguinetti et al., 2001; Fairhurst et al., 2002) or resolve even when disseminated (Morales et al, 2007)

7.3 Donor

Even though we have not found any documented case of NTM infection in the organ donor, mycobacteriosis would be hypothetically a relative contraindication for transplantation. Systematic search of NTM in the bronchoaspirate of donors must be done to introduce treatment as soon as possible.

8. Final considerations

- Life expectancy and quality of life have improved in CF patients and their treatments have turned/become more aggressive.
- NTM cause frequent pulmonary infection especially related to advancing age and lung function deterioration. *M. abscessus* and MAC are the most frequently isolated NTM.
- Early clinical suspicion is important. The routine or selective mycobacterial search according to known risk factors is an important decision. No comparative studies indicate which option is the most effective.
- NTM must be decontaminated, cultured and typified thoroughly, since species identification is crucial for treatment and other clinical considerations.
- When a NTM is isolated from a sputum sample, both clinician and microbiologist will determine whether it should be considered a contaminant, colonization or infective agent, with the consequent attitude.
- It is important to perform correctly the *in vitro* susceptibility tests and to try new antibiotics against NTM.
- Ensure treatment compliance, since it will prevent the emergence of antibiotic resistance, infection relapse and poor outcome.
- Since there are no primary chemoprophylaxis recommendations, patients should be oriented to a healthy life style.
- If the moment for the lung transplant arrives, all the previously mentioned considerations should be taken very seriously, since the probability for infection and dissemination are greater due to the immunosuppressive therapy.
- These processes pose significant social and health burdens (school absenteeism, work and family limitations, doctor visits, hospitalization, diagnostic testing and treatment) with the resulting economic impact.

Future should rely on early suspicion and adequate search for NTM, the use of modern microbiological techniques applied directly on the sample, safer and more active antibiotics, research of mycobacterial virulence factors and the determinants for persistence of infection.

9. References

AdéKambi, T., Colson, P., & Drancourt M. 2003. *rpoB*-based identification of nonpigmented and late-pigmenting rapidly growing mycobacteria. *J Clin Microbiol*, Vol 41, No 12,(December,2003),pp. 5699-5708.

Adékambi, T., Reynaud -Gaubert, M., Greub, G., Gevaudan, MJ., La Scola, B., Raoult, D., & and Drancourt, M. 2004. Amoebal coculture of *Mycobacterium massiliense* sp. nov. from the sputum of a patient of hemoptoic pneumonia. *J Clin Microbiol*, Vol 42, No 12, (December, 2004), pp. 5493-5501.

Adékambi, T., Berger, P., Raoult, D., & Drancourt, M. 2006. *rpo*B gene sequence based characterization of emerging non-tuberculous mycobacteria with description of *Mycobacterium bolletii* sp. nov., *Mycobacterium phocaicum* sp. nov. and *Mycobacterium aubagnense* sp. nov. *Int J Syst Evol Microbiol* Vol 56, Pt 1, (January, 2006), pp. 133-143.

American Academy of Pediatrics. 2006. Micobacterias no tuberculosas, enfermedades. In: Pickening LK., Baker, CJ., Long SS. And McMillan JA. Eds. *Red book:Enfermedades infecciosas en Pediatría.* 27ª ed.Editorial Médica Panamericana, Madrid, Spain, 2007, pp.757-763. ISBN 978-950-06-0548-9

American Thoracic Society. Diagnosis and treatment of disease caused by nontuberculous mycobacteria. *Am J Respir Crit Care Med*, Vol 156, No 2, Pt2, (August, 1997), pp. S1-S25.

Avery, RK., Michaels, MG., & AST Infectious Diseases Community of Practice. 2009. Strategies for safe-living following solid organ transplantation. *Am J Transplant*, Vol 9, No 4 Suppl, (December 2009), pp. S252-S257.

Boxerbaum, B. 1980. Isolation of rapidly growing mycobacteria in patients with cystic fibrosis. *J Pediatr*, Vol 96, No 4, (April,1980), pp. 689-691.

Brown-Elliot, BA, Griffith, DE., & Wallace RJ Jr. 2002. Newly described or emerging human species of non tuberculous mycobacteria. *Infect Dis Clin North Am*, Vol 16, No 1 (Mars, 2002), pp. 187-220.

Burns, JL., Emerson, J., Stapp, JR., Yim, DL., Krzewinski, J., Louden, L., Ramsey, BW., & Clausen, CR. 1998. Microbiology of sputum from patients at cystic fibrosis centers in the United States. *Clin Infect Dis*, Vol 27, No 1 (July,1998), pp. 158-163.

Burns, JL.,& Saiman L. 1999. *Burkholderia cepacia* infections in cystic fibrosis. *Pediatr Infect Dis*, Vol 18, No 2, (February, 1999), pp. 155-156.

Butler WR & Guthertz, LS. 2001. Mycolic acid analysis by high-performance liquid chromatography for identification of Mycobacterium species. *Clin Microbiol Rev*, Vol 14, No 4,(October, 2001), pp. 704-726.

Colin, AA. 2000. Erradication of *Mycobacterium abscessus* in a chronically infected patient with cystic fibrosis. *Pediatr Pulmonol*, Vol 30, No 3, (September,2000),pp.267-268.

Cousins, D., Francis, B., & Dawson, D. 1996. Multiplex PCR provides a low-cost alternative to DNA probe methods for rapid identification of *Mycobacterium avium* and *Mycobacterium intracellulare*, Vol 34, No 9, (September, 1996), pp. 2331-2333.

Cullen, AR., Cannon CL., Mark EJ., & Colin, AA. 2000. *Mycobacterium abscessus* infection in CF. *Am J Respir Crit Care*, Vol 161, No 2, Pt 1, (February,2000),pp. 641-645.

Daley, CL. & Griffith, DE. 2002. Pulmonary disease caused by rapidy growing mycobacteria. *Clin Chest Med*, Vol 23, No 3, (September, 2002), pp. 623-632.

Davis, PB., Drumm, M., & Konstan, MW. 1996. Cystic Fibrosis. *Am J Respir Crit Care Med*, Vol 154, No 5 (November,1996), pp. 1229-1256.

Embril, J., Warren, P., Yakrus, M., Stark, R., Corne, S., Forrest, D., & Hershfield, E. 1997. Pulmonary illness associated with exposure to *Mycobacterium-avium* complex in hot tub water: hypersensitivity pneumonitis or infection?. *Chest*, Vol 111, No 3, (Mars, 1997), pp. 813-816.

Erasmus, JJ., McAdams, HP.,Farrell MA., & Patz, EFJr. 1999. Pulmonary nontuberculous mycobacterial infection: radiologic manifestations. Radiographics, Vol 19, No 6, (November-December,1999), pp. 1487-1505.

Esther, CR Jr., Esserman DA, Gilligan P, Kerr A, & Noone PG. 2010. Chronic *Mycobacterium abscessus* infection and lung function decline in cystic fibrosis. *J Cyst Fibros*, Vol 9, No 2, (March, 2010),pp.117-123.

Fairhurst, RM., Kubak, BM., Shpiner, RB., Levine, MS., Pegues, DA., & Ardehali, A. 2002. *Mycobacterium abscessus* empyema in a lung transplant recipient. *J Heart Lung Transplant*, Vol 21, No 3, (Mars, 2002),pp. 391-394.

Fauroux, B., Delaisi, B., Clement A., Saizou, C., Moissenett, D., Truffot-Pernot, C., Tournier, G., & Vu, T. 1997. Mycobacterial lung disease in cystic fibrosis : a prospective study. *Pediatr Infect Dis*, Vol 16, No 4, (April,1997),pp. 354-358.

Field, SK., & Cowie, RL. 2003. Treatment of *Mycobacterium avium*-intracellulare complex lung disease with a macrolide, ethambutol, and clofazimine. *Chest*, Vol 124, No 4,(October, 2003),pp. 1482-1486.

Field, SK., & Cowie RL. 2006. Lung disease due to the more common nontuberculous mycobacteria. *Chest*, Vol 129, No 6, (June, 2006),pp.1653-1672.

FitzSimmons, SC. 1993. The changing epidemiology of cystic fibrosis. *J Pediatr*, Vol 122, No 1, (January,1993), pp. 1-9.

Gilljama, M., Schersténb, H., Silverbornb, M., Jönssonc, B., & Hollsingd, AE. 2010. Lung transplantation in patients with cystic fibrosis and *Mycobacterium abscessus* infection. *J Cyst Fibros*, Vol 9, No 4, (July, 2010),pp.272-276.

Goo, JM., & Im, J-G. 2002. CT of tuberculosis and nontuberculous mycobacterial infections. *Radiol Clin North Am*, Vol 40, No 1,(January, 2002),pp. 73-87.

Griffith, DE., Girard, WM., & Wallace RJ Jr. 1993. Clinical features of pulmonary disease caused by rapidly growing mycobacteria. An analysis of 154 patients. *Am Rev Respir Dis*, Vol 147, No 5, (May,1993),pp. 1271-1278.

Griffith, DE. 2003. Emergence of nontuberculous mycobacteria as pathogens in cystic fibrosis. *Am J Respir Crit Care Med*, Vol 167, No 6, (Mars, 2003), pp. 810-812.

Griffith, DE., Brown, BA., Girard, WM., Griffith, BE., Couch, LA., & Wallace RJ Jr. Azithromycin-containing regimens for treatment of *Mycobacterium avium* complex lung disease. *Clin Infect Dis*, Vol 32, No 11, (June, 2001), pp. 1547-1553.

Griffith, DE., Aksamit, T.,Brown-Elliot, BA., Catanzaro, A., Daley, C., Gordin, F., Holland, SM., Horsburgh, R., Huitt, G., Iademarco, MF., Iseman, M., Olivier, K., Ruoss, S., von Reyn, CF., Wallace, RJ Jr., & Winthrop, K; ATS mycobacterial diseases subcommitte; American Thoracic Society; Infectious Disease Society of America. 2007. An official ATS/IDSA statement:diagnosis, treatment and prevention on non tuberculous mycobacterial diseases. *Am J Respir Crit Care Med*, Vol 175, No 4, (February, 2007),pp. 367-416.

Hallstrand, TS., Ochs HD., Zhu Q, & Liles, WC. 2004. Inhaled IFN- gamma for persistent nontuberculous mycobacterial pulmonary disease due to functional IFN-gamma deficiency. *Eur Respir J*, Vol 24, No 3,(September, 2004),pp.367-370.

Hanak, V., Kalra, S., Aksamit TR., Hartman, TE., Tazelaar HD., & Ryu, JH. 2006. Hot tub lung: presenting features and clinical course of 21 patients. *Respir Med*, Vol 100, No 4,(April, 2006), pp.610-615.

Hayes, D Jr. 2005. *Mycobacterium abscessus* and other nontuberculous mycobacteria: evolving respiratory pathogens in cystic fibrosis: a case report and review. *South Med J*, Vol 98, No 6, (June, 2005),pp. 657-661.

Hjelte, L., Petrini, B., Kaellenenius, G., & Strandvik, B. 1990. Perspective study of mycobacterial infections in patients with cystic fibrosis. *Thorax*, Vol 45, No 5, (May, 1990), pp. 397-400.

Holland, SM., Eisenstein, EM., Kuhns, DB., Turner, ML., Fleisher, TA., Strober, W., & Gallin, JL.1994. Treatment of refractary disseminated infection with interferon gamma: A preliminary report. *N Eng Jmed*, Vol 330, No 19, (May, 1994), pp. 1348-1355.

Huang, JH., Kao, PN., Adi, V., & Ruoss, SJ. 1999. *Mycobacterium avium-intracellulare* pulmonary infection in HIV-negative patients without preexisting lung disease: diagnostic and management limitations. *Chest*, Vol 115, No 4, (April,1999), pp. 1033-1040.

Jönsson, BE., Gilljam, M., Lindblad, A., Ridell, M., Wold, AE., & Welinder-Olsson, C. 2007. Molecular biology of *Mycobacterium abscessus* with focus on cystic fibrosis. *J Clin Microbiol*, Vol 45, No 5, (May, 2007), pp. 1497-1504.

Kent, PT., & Kubica, GP. 1983. Public health mycobacteriology: a guide for the level III laboratory. Atlanta. Centers for Disease Control.

Kim, HY, Yun, YJ., Park, CG., Lee, DH., Cho, YK., Park, BJ., Joo, SI., Kim, EC., Hur, YJ, Kim, BJ., & KooK, YH. 2007. Outbreak of *Mycobacterium massiliense* infection associated with intramuscular injections.*J Clin microbiol*, Vol 45, No 9, (September, 2007), pp.3127-3130.

Leite, CQ., da Silva Rocha, A., de Andrade Leite, SR., Ferreira, RM., Suffys, PN, de Souza Fonseca, L., & Saad, MH. 2005. A comparison of mycolic acid analysis for nontuberculous mycobacteria identification by thin-layer chromatography and molecular methods. *Microbiol Immunol*, Vol 49, No 7,(2005), pp.571-578.

Levy, I., Grisaru-Soen, G., Lerner-Geva, L., Kerem, E., Blau, H., Bentur, L., Aviram, M., Rivlin, J., Picard, E., Lavy, A., Yahav, Y., & Rahav, G. 2008. Multicenter cross-sectional study of nontuberculous mycobacterial infections among cystic fibrosis patientes, Israel. *Emerg Infect Dis*, Vol 14, No 3, (Mars, 2008), pp. 378-374.

Lynch,DA., Simone, PM., Fox, MA, Bucher, BL., & Heinig, MJ.1995. CT features of pulmonary *Mycobacterium avium* complex infection. *J Comput Assist Tomogr*, Vol 19, No 3, (May-June, 1995), pp.353-360.

Malouf, MA., & Glanville, AR. 1999. The spectrum of mycobacterial infection after lung transplantation. Am J Respir Crit Care Med, Vol 160, No 5 Pt 1, (November, 1999), pp. 1611-1616.

Marras, TK., Wallace, RJ Jr., Koth, LL, Stulbarg, MS., Cowl, CT., & Daley, CL.2005. Hypersensitivity pneumonitis reaction to *Mycobacterium avium* in household water. *Chest*, Vol 127, No 2, (February, 2005), pp. 664-671.

Maycher, B., O´Connor, R., & Long, R. 2000. Computed tomographic abnormalities in Mycobacterium avium complex lung disease include the mosaic pattern of reduced lung attenuation. *Can Assoc Radiol J*, Vol 51, No 2, (April,2000), pp. 93-102.

Metchock, BG., Nolte FS., & Wallace, RJ Jr. 1999. Mycobacterium. In: Murray PR, Baron EJ, Pfaller MA, Tenover FC, Yolken RH, editors. Manual of clinical microbiology. Washington, DC: ASM Press, 1999, pp., 399-437.

Morales, P., Ros JA, Blanes, M., Pérez-Enguix, D., Saiz, V., & Santos. M. 2007. Successful recovery after disseminated infection due to *Mycobacterium abscessus* in a lung transplant patient: subcutaneous nodule as first manifestation- a case report. *Transplant Proc*, Vol 39, No 7, (September, 2007), pp. 2413-2415.

Morales,P., Santos, M., Hadjilidis, D., & Aris, RM. Mycobacterial infections in cardiothoracic transplantation. pp. 161-173. In ISHLT. Monograph Series: Diagnosis and Management of Infectious diseases in Cardiothoracic Transplantation and mechanical ciculatory support. Mooney, ML., Hannan, MM., Husain, S, Kirklin, JK. (Eds). 2011. Elsevier Ed. Philadelphia,P.A. ISSN-1930-2134.

Mussaffi, H., Rivlin, J., Shalit, I., Ephros, M., & Blau, H. 2005. Nontuberculous mycobacteria in cystic fibrosis associated with allergic bronchopulmonary aspergillosis and steroid therapy. *Eur Respir J*, Vol 25, No 2, (February, 2005),pp. 324-328.

Oliver, A., Maiz, L., Cantón, R., Escobar, H., Baquero, E., & Gómez-Mampaso, E. 2001. Nontuberculous mycobacteria in patients with cystic fibrosis. *CID*, Vol 32, No 9, (May, 2001), pp. 1298-1303.

Olivier, KN., Yankaskas, JR., & Knowles, MR. 1996. Nontuberculous mycobacterial pulmonary disease in cystic fibrosis. *Semin Respir Infect*, Vol 11, No 4, (December ,1996), pp. 272-284.

Olivier, KN., Weber, DJ., Wallace, RJ Jr., Faiz, AR., Lee JH., Zhang, Y., Brown-Elliot, BA., Handler, A., Wilson, RW., Schechter, MS., Edwards, LJ., Chakraborti, S., & Knowles, R., for the Nontuberculous Mycobacteria in Cistic Fibrosis Study Group. 2003. Nontuberculous Mycobacteria. I: Multicenter prevalence study in Cystic Fibrosis. *Am J Respir Crit Care Med*, Vol 167, No 6, (Mars , 2003), pp. 828-834.

Orens, JB., Estenne, M., Arcasoy,S., Conte, JV., Corris, P., Egan, JJ., Egan, T., Keshavjee, S., Knoop, C., Kotloff, R., Martinez, FJ., Nathan, S., Palmer, S., Patterson, A., Singer, L., Snell, G., Studer, S., Vachiery, JL., Glanville, AR.; Pulmonary Scientific Council of the International Society for Heart and Lung Transplantation. 2006. International guidelines for the selection of lung transplant candidates: 2006 Update – A consensus report from the pulmonary scientific council of the international society for heart and lung transplantation. J Heart Lung Transplant Vol 25, No 7, (July, 2006), pp. 745–755.

Parker, BC., Ford, MA., Gruft H., & Falkinham JO III. 1983. Epidemiology of infection by nontuberculous mycobacteria.IV.Preferential aerosolization of *Mycobacterium intracellulare* from natural water. *Am Rev Respir Dis,* Vol 128, No 4 (October, 1983),pp.652-656.

Pottumarthy, S., Wells, VC., & Morris, AJ. 2000. A comparison of seven tests for serological diagnosis of tuberculosis. *J Clin Microbiol,* Vol 38, No 6,(June,2000), pp. 2227-2231.

Pierre-Audigier, C., Ferroni, A., Sermet-Gaudelus, I., Le Bourgeois, M., Offredo, C., Vu-Thien, H., Fauroux, B., Mariani, P., Munck, A., Bingen, E., Guillemot, D., Quesne, G., Vincent, V., Berche, P., & Gaillard, JL. 2005. Age-related prevalence and distribution of nontuberculous mycobacterial species among patients with cystic fibrosis. *J Clin Microbiol,* Vol 43, No 7, (July, 2005), pp. 3467-3470.

Primm, TP., Lucero, CA., & Falkinham, JO III. 2004. Health impacts of environmental mycobacteria. *Clin Microbiol Rev,* Vol 17, No 1 (January, 2004), pp. 98-106.

Prince, DS., Peterson, DD., Steiner, RM., Gottlieb, JE, Scott, R., Israel HL, Figueroa WG., & Fish, JE. 1989. Infection with *Mycobacterium avium* complex in patients without predisposing conditions. *N Eng J Med,* Vol 321,No 13, (September,1989), pp. 863-868.

Ramsey BW. 1996. Management of pulmonary disease in patients with cystic fibrosis. *N Eng J Med,* Vol 335, No 3 (July,1996), pp. 179-188.

Rickman, OB., Ryu, JH., Fidler, ME., & Kalra, S. 2002. Hypersensitivity pneumonitis associated with *Mycobacterium avium* complex and hot tube use. *Mayo Clin Proc,* Vol 77, No 11, (November, 2002), pp.1233-1237.

Rodman, DM., Polis, JM., Heltshe, SL, Sontag MK, Chacon C, Rodman RV, Brayshaw SJ, Huitt GA, Iseman MD, Saavedra MT, Taussig LM, Wagener JS, Accurso FJ, Nick JA. 2005. Late diagnosis defines a unique population of long-term survivors of cystic fibrosis. *Am J Respir Crit Care Med,* Vol 171, No 6, (Mars, 2005), pp. 621-626.

Roux, AL., Catherinot, E., Ripoll, F., Soismier, N., Macheras, E., Ravilly, S, Bellis, G., Vibet, MA., Le Roux E, Lemonnier, L., Gutierrez, C., Vincent, V., Fauroux, B., Rottman, M., Guillemot, D, Gaillard, JL, & Herrman JL., for the OMA Group. 2009. Multicenter study of prevalence of nontuberculous *Mycobacteria* in patients with cystic fibrosis in France. *J Clin Microbiol,* Vol 47,No 12, (December, 2009),pp. 4124-4128.

Runyon, EH. 1959. Anonymous mycobacteria in pulmonary disease. *Med Clin North Am,* Vol 43, No 1, (January, 1959), pp. 273-290.

Sanguinetti, M., Ardito F., Fiscarelli E., La Sorda, M., D'Argenio, P., Ricciotti, G., & Fadda, G. 2001. Fatal pulmonary infection due to multidrug-resistant *Mycobacterium abscessus* in a patient with cystic fibrosis. *J Clin Microbiol,* Vol 39, No 2,(February,2001),pp. 816-819.

Sermet-Gaudelus, I., Le Bourgeois, M., Pierre-Audigier, C., Offredo, C., Guillemot, D., Halley, S., Akoua-Koffi, C., Vincent, V, Sivadon-Tardy, V., Ferroni, A., Berche, P-, Scheinmann, P., Lenoir, G., & Gaillard, JL. 2003. *Mycobacterium abscessus* and children with cystic fibrosis. *Emerg Infect Dis,* Vol 9, No 12, (December, 2003),pp.1587-1591.

Schölvink, E., Wilkinson, KA., Whelan, AO., Martineau, AR., Levin, M., & Wlkinson, RJ. 2004. Gamma interferon-based immunodiagnosis of tuberculosis: comparison between whole-blood and enzyme-linked immunospot methods. *J Clin Microbiol*, Vol 42, No 2, (February, 2004),pp.829-831.

Taylor, JL., & Palmer, SM. 2006. *Mycobacterium abscessus* chest wall and pulmonary infection in a cystic fibrosis lung transplant recipient. *J Heart Lung* Transplant, Vol 25, No 8, (August, 2006), pp. 985-988.

Viana-Niero, C., Lima, KV., Lopes, ML, Rabello, MC., Marsola, IR., Brilhanthe, VC., Durham, AM., & Leao, SC. 2008. Molecular characterization of *Mycobacterium massiliense* and *Mycobacterium bolletii* in isolated collected from outbreaks of infections after laparoscopic surgeries cosmetic procedures. *J Clin Microbiol*, Vol 46, No 3, (Mars,2008),pp.850-855.

Wallace, RJ Jr., Brown, BA., Griffith, DE., Girard, WM., & Murphy, DT. 1996. Clarithromycin regimens for pulmonary *Mycobacterium avium* complex. The first 50 patients. *Am J Respir Crit Care Med*, Vol 153, No 6 Pt 1, (June,1996),pp.1762-1772.

Wallace, RJ Jr., Brown, BA., & Griffith DE. 1998. Nosocomial outbreaks/pseudo-outbreaks caused by nontuberculous mycobacteria. *Annu Rev Microbiol*, Vol, 52, pp. 453-490.

Wallace, RJ Jr., Brown-Elliott, BA., Ward, SC., Crist, CJ., Mann, LB., & Wilson, RW. 2001. Activities of linezolid against rapidly growing mycobacteria. *Antimicrob Agents Chemother*, Vol 45, No 3, (Mars, 2001), pp. 764-767.

Wayne, PA.: National Committee for Clinical Laboratory Standards. 2000. Susceptibility testing of mycobacteria, Nocardia, and other aerobic actinomycetes. 2nd ed. Tentative standard M24-T2.

Welsh, MJ. 1990. Abnormal regulation of ion channels in cystic fibrosis epithelia. *FASEB J*, Vol 4, No 10,(July, 1990), pp. 2718-2725.

Whittier, S., Olivier, K., Gilligan, P., Knowles, M., & Della-Latta, P. 1997. Proficiency testing of clinical microbiology laboratories using modified decontamination procedures for detection of nontuberculous mycobacteria in sputum samples from CF patients. *J Clin Microbiol*, Vol 35, No 10,(October,1997), pp. 2706-2708.

Williams, MM., Yakrus, MA., Arduino, MJ,, Cooksey RC., Crane CB., Banerjee, SN., Hilborn, ED., & Donlan, RM. 2009. Structural analysis of biofilm formation by rapidly and slowly growing nontuberculous mycobacteria. *Appl Environ Microbiol*, Vol 75, No 7, (April, 2009), pp. 2091-2098.

Woods, GL. 2000. Susceptibility testing for mycobacteria. 2000. *Clin Infect Di*s, Vol 31, No 5, (November, 2000), pp.1209-1215.

Yang, SC., Hisueh, PR., Lai, HC., Teng, LJ., Huang, LM., Chen, JM., Wang, SK., Shie, DC., Ho, SW., & Luh, KT. 2003. High prevalence of antimicrobial resistance in rapidly growing mycobacteria in Taiwan. *Antimicrobial Agent Chemother*, Vol 47, No 6, (June,2003),pp 1958-1962.

Zelazny AM, Root JM, Shea YR, Colombo RE, Shamputa IC, Stock F, Conlan S, McNulty S, Brown-Elliott BA, Wallace RJ Jr, Olivier KN, Holland SM, Sampaio EP. 2009. Cohort study of molecular identification and typing of *Mycobacterium abscessus*, *Mycobacterium massiliense*, and *Mycobacterium bolletii*. *J Clin Microbiol*, Vol 47, No 7, (July, 2009), pp. 1985-1995.

Zhang, Y., Rajagopalan, M., Brown, BA., & Wallace, RJ Jr. 1997. Randomly amplified polymorphic DNA PCR for comparison of *Mcobacterium abscessus* strains from nosocomial outbreaks. *J Clin Microbiol*, Vol 35, No 12, (December,1997),pp. 3132-3139.

8

Pseudomonas aeruginosa Biofilm Formation in the CF Lung and Its Implications for Therapy

Gregory G. Anderson
Indiana University Purdue University Indianapolis
USA

1. Introduction

Numerous microorganisms colonize or are associated with the airways of individuals with Cystic Fibrosis (CF). Impairment of the mucociliary clearance in CF lungs leads to a greater number of microbes present for the simple fact that they are not physically removed (Gibson, Burns et al. 2003; Boucher 2004). Microbes thrive in the large mucus plugs in CF airways, probably due to optimal growth temperatures and the abundance of nutrients. Additionally, CF patients display defective antimicrobial peptide activity in their lungs, which can further enhance microbial colonization (Gibson, Burns et al. 2003; Boucher 2004). As a result of these abnormalities, CF lungs are extraordinarily susceptible to infection with a number of bacteria, fungi, and viruses, including *Pseudomonas aeruginosa*, *Staphylococcus aureus*, *Burkholderia cepacia* complex, *Stenotrophomonas maltophilia*, *Haemophilus influenzae*, *Aspergillus fumigatus*, *Candida albicans*, Respiratory Syncytial virus, and Influenza Virus (Govan and Deretic 1996; Lyczak, Cannon et al. 2002; Saiman and Siegel 2004; Lipuma 2010). The relative abundance and rate of isolation of these various microorganisms varies over time. For instance, early in life, *S. aureus* is the most often isolated microbe, but by adolescence to young adulthood, *P. aeruginosa* becomes the predominate microorganism isolated from the airways (Gibson, Burns et al. 2003; Pressler, Bohmova et al. 2011).

P. aeruginosa is a Gram-negative bacterium that causes opportunistic infections. With a large number of genes involved in metabolism of many different substrates, as well as numerous regulatory genes, this bacterium has the genetic flexibility to colonize a wide range of different habitats (Stover, Pham et al. 2000; Yoon and Hassett 2004; Gomez and Prince 2007). Though typically considered an obligate aerobe, *P. aeruginosa* had been shown to undergo anaerobic respiration, in particular by denitrification processes utilizing nitrate, nitrite, or nitric oxide as terminal electron acceptors (Davies, Lloyd et al. 1989; Yoon and Hassett 2004). Furthermore, *P. aeruginosa* produces an arsenal of virulence factors, including pili, flagella, exopolysaccharides, proteases, elastase, lipases, iron chelators (pyoverdine and pyochelin), and a number of different toxins, including pyocyanin, hydrogen cyanide, exotoxin A, and the Type III Secretion System (T3SS) toxins ExoS, ExoT, ExoU, and ExoY (Lyczak, Cannon et al. 2000; Ran, Hassett et al. 2003; Shaver and Hauser 2004; Sadikot, Blackwell et al. 2005; Yahr and Wolfgang 2006; Gomez and Prince 2007). Utilizing these pathogenic tools, *P. aeruginosa* can infect a wide range of hosts, including animals (Rahme, Stevens et al. 1995), plants (Rahme, Stevens et al. 1995), insects (Miyata, Casey et al. 2003), nematodes (Gallagher and Manoil 2001), and fungi (Hogan and Kolter 2002). In humans, in addition to CF lung infections, *P. aeruginosa* can cause acute pneumonia (especially in the context of ventilator-associated pneumonia), burn wound infections, ulcerative keratitis, otitis media, otitis externa, bacteremia, urinary tract infections, and meningitis (Lyczak, Cannon et al. 2000; Sadikot, Blackwell et al. 2005; Moore and Flaws 2011).

The unique pathogenic characteristics of *P. aeruginosa* also promote efficient infection in the CF lung. Studies suggest that 20%-25% of CF infants have had a positive *P. aeruginosa* culture in the United States, and infection rates steadily increase with increasing age, such that 80% of adults 25 years old and older are chronically infected with *P. aeruginosa* (Gibson, Burns et al. 2003; Stuart, Lin et al. 2010; Woodward, Brown et al. 2010). Initially, individuals with CF experience intermittent infection, wherein transient colonization is followed by *P. aeruginosa*-free periods (Hoiby, Frederiksen et al. 2005; Stuart, Lin et al. 2010). Clinically, intermittent infection has been defined as either 1) "at least 1 isolate of [*P. aeruginosa*] with normal [*P. aeruginosa*] antibody levels," or 2) "[*P. aeruginosa*] cultures were positive in 50% or less of the 12 months" (Stuart, Lin et al. 2010). Other definitions are possible. These initial, intermittent strains are thought to originate from the environment, but there have also been cases of epidemic strains, demonstrating the potential for direct or indirect person-to-person spread (Salunkhe, Smart et al. 2005; Lipuma 2010; Mowat, Paterson et al. 2011; Saiman 2011). Following the intermittent colonization period, *P. aeruginosa* eventually establishes chronic infection (Gibson, Burns et al. 2003; Pressler, Bohmova et al. 2011). One of the hallmark characteristics of chronic *P. aeruginosa* infection in the CF lung is a switch in the colony morphology of *P. aeruginosa* isolates from a non-mucoid to a mucoid phenotype (Gibson, Burns et al. 2003; Yoon and Hassett 2004). It has been estimated that this conversion to mucoidy takes approximately 1.8 years to occur (Stuart, Lin et al. 2010). Because of mucoidy and other changes (as described below), the bacteria in the chronic state survive the intense immune reaction that occurs in the CF lung as well as the high-dose antibiotic treatment given to CF patients to kill infecting microbes (Lyczak, Cannon et al. 2002; Gomez and Prince 2007). Because of their location within the mucus airway plugs, these mucoid bacteria are further protected from immune clearance (Worlitzsch, Tarran et al. 2002; Bjarnsholt, Jensen et al. 2009). Thus, once the chronic infection is established, *P. aeruginosa* persists for the life of the individual. This chronic colonization is the cause of much of the morbidity and mortality associated with CF (Gibson, Burns et al. 2003).

Chronic *P. aeruginosa* infection also contributes significantly to the economic burden associated with treatment and care for individuals with CF. Recent studies have calculated an average of $48,098 (US) in overall medical costs per CF patient per year in the United States, with similar estimates for some European countries (Ouyang, Grosse et al. 2009). Thus, with approximately 30,000 CF individuals in the United States (Gibson, Burns et al. 2003), CF accounts for over $1.4 billion (US) in medical expenditures in the United States alone. This calculation is a gross underestimate because it omits increased costs for transplantation, malnutrition, CF-associated diabetes, and other complications (Ouyang, Grosse et al. 2009). Additional analysis has estimated that the costs of treatment with the anti-Pseudomonal antibiotic tobramycin can reach $22,481 per person per year in the United States, which is nearly half of the aforementioned per person total expenditures ($48,098) (Woodward, Brown et al. 2010). It is evident, then, that development of more effective anti-Pseudomonal therapies might lead to decreased *P. aeruginosa* infection rates and decreased economic burden. Development of new drugs will come through a better understanding of the mechanisms used by *P. aeruginosa* to establish chronic infection.

2. Transition to the chronic infection phenotype

2.1 Biofilm formation

It is generally well accepted that the chronic nature of *P. aeruginosa* in the CF lung results from the association of the bacteria into organized structures called biofilms (Gibson, Burns et al. 2003; Gomez and Prince 2007). Biofilms are communities of microorganisms bound to a surface, or to each other. During biofilm formation, bacteria undergo phenotypic, and often genotypic, changes that lead to self-aggregation and transition to a lifestyle distinct from their free-swimming (planktonic) counterparts (Costerton, Lewandowski et al. 1995). Numerous infectious states involve a biofilm component, including *P. aeruginosa* infection in the CF lung, infectious kidney stones, bacterial endocarditis, otitis media, chronic prostatitis, urinary tract infections, periodontitis, and medical device-related infections (Costerton 2001; Donlan and Costerton 2002; Parsek and Singh 2003). Often, these biofilm infections are chronic and/or recurrent.

While the characteristics of biofilms vary depending upon microbial species and growth conditions, there are several general properties that can be used to describe and define biofilms (Figure 1). Focusing specifically on *P. aeruginosa*, biofilm formation is initiated as planktonic bacteria bind to a surface via their polar flagella (O'Toole and Kolter 1998; Sauer, Camper et al. 2002), although pili have also been shown to mediate attachment to cells and other surfaces (Woods, Straus et al. 1980; Chiang and Burrows 2003). At this point, the bacterium can spin in place as the flagellum continues to rotate (Sauer, Camper et al. 2002; Hinsa, Espinosa-Urgel et al. 2003; Caiazza and O'Toole 2004). However, this initial attachment is reversible because polarly-bound bacteria can detach and swim away from the site of initial attachment (Sauer, Camper et al. 2002; Hinsa, Espinosa-Urgel et al. 2003; Caiazza and O'Toole 2004; Monds, Newell et al. 2007). This initial reversible attachment stage has been referred to as a "sampling" of the surface before full commitment to biofilm formation has been made (Caiazza and O'Toole 2004). Full commitment to the biofilm mode of growth is signaled as the initially-bound *P. aeruginosa* rods lay down on the surface along their long axis (Sauer, Camper et al. 2002; Caiazza and O'Toole 2004). The bacteria become irreversibly bound at this point and remain on the surface (Stoodley, Sauer et al. 2002)(Figure 1: Inset). Next, through type IV pilus-mediated twitching motility, the individual bacteria begin to associate into structures called microcolonies (O'Toole, Kaplan et al. 2000; Sauer, Camper et al. 2002). Through the efforts of specific signaling molecules called quorum sensing signals (described below), and the resultant change in gene expression, these microcolonies mature into large structures, which can reach a thickness of 100 μM, depending upon the growth conditions (Sauer, Camper et al. 2002). During the maturation process, the constituent bacteria begin to excrete polysaccharides, such that the bacteria in the mature biofilm are encased in a matrix of exopolysaccharides that they produced (Costerton, Lewandowski et al. 1995; Ryder, Byrd et al. 2007). DNA and protein have also been shown to be components of *P. aeruginosa* biofilms (Parsek and Singh 2003; Bjarnsholt, Tolker-Nielsen et al. 2010). Finally, as the biofilm ages, a sub-population of the bacteria break away from the biofilm bulk, revert to the planktonic state (become motile), and disperse from the biofilm (O'Toole, Kaplan et al. 2000; Sauer, Camper et al. 2002; Kirov, Webb et al. 2007; Harmsen, Yang et al. 2010). Dispersion events appear to be influenced by the production of virulent bacteriophage from dormant prophage (Rice, Tan et al. 2009). While very few studies investigating *P. aeruginosa* biofilm formation on living tissue have been performed, it is thought that these steps are conserved during infection (Hoffmann, Rasmussen et al. 2005; Anderson, Moreau-Marquis et al. 2008; Moreau-Marquis, Bomberger et al. 2008; Woodworth, Tamashiro et al. 2008; Moreau-Marquis, Redelman et al. 2010)(Figure 1).

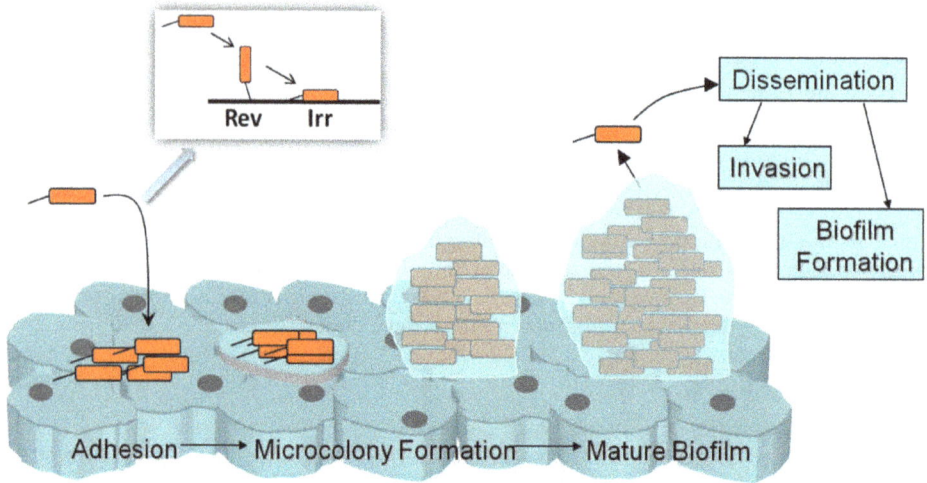

Fig. 1. Proposed biofilm formation cascade on living tissue. It is thought that many of the steps involved in bacterial biofilm formation on non-living surfaces also occur as bacteria form biofilms on human cells. Inset: Initially *P. aeruginosa* bind reversibly (Rev) by their flagellum. Irreversible binding (Irr) begins when the bacteria lay down on the surface along their long axis. See text for details.

2.2 Quorum sensing

As mentioned above, the production of quorum sensing (QS) molecules greatly influences biofilm maturation. QS is a method of self-recognition and cell density-dependent gene regulation (Cooley, Chhabra et al. 2008; Galloway, Hodgkinson et al. 2011). As a population of bacteria grows, small molecules (the QS signal) are produced and secreted. Once the density of the population is sufficiently high, the QS signal binds to an intracellular receptor that activates (or represses) a sub-set of genes (Galloway, Hodgkinson et al. 2011). Recognition of the QS signal is a stochastic process and the probability of a QS molecule binding to a receptor is low until the culture reaches a threshold density (Galloway, Hodgkinson et al. 2011). Hence, QS molecules allow bacteria to "sense the quorum", or the relative density of the population, and in this manner, they can coordinate their behaviors (Cooley, Chhabra et al. 2008). Because of the high bacterial density achieved in biofilms, QS plays a large role in regulating gene expression during biofilm development (Bjarnsholt, Tolker-Nielsen et al. 2010). *P. aeruginosa* contains 3 overlapping QS systems: Las, Rhl, and PQS (Wagner, Bushnell et al. 2003; Harmsen, Yang et al. 2010; Heeb, Fletcher et al. 2011). These systems regulate expression of virulence factors, exopolysaccharides, and other factors important for biofilm formation (Sauer, Camper et al. 2002; Wagner, Bushnell et al. 2003; Bjarnsholt, Tolker-Nielsen et al. 2010; Heeb, Fletcher et al. 2011). It has been found that QS systems are activated during biofilm maturation, and that mutation of QS genes leads to aberrations in overall biofilm architecture and sensitivity of the biofilm to stresses (Sauer, Camper et al. 2002; Bjarnsholt, Tolker-Nielsen et al. 2010; Harmsen, Yang et al. 2010; Heeb, Fletcher et al. 2011). As detailed below, much research is being devoted to the development of QS inhibitors for the disruption of biofilms.

2.3 The acute/chronic infection regulatory switch

There are numerous phenotypic changes that occur as planktonic *P. aeruginosa* transitions to the biofilm state, including a general decrease in expression of toxins and other tissue damaging virulence factors important for acute infections (Furukawa, Kuchma et al. 2006; Gooderham and Hancock 2009; Bjarnsholt, Tolker-Nielsen et al. 2010; Diaz, King et al. 2011). This suggests that *P. aeruginosa* displays 2 different infection phenotypes: an acute infection phenotype characterized by production of toxins, and a chronic infection phenotype characterized by biofilm formation and secretion of exopolysaccharides. In fact, recent evidence has revealed an inverse regulation of biofilm formation and virulence attributes associated with acute infections (Goodman, Kulasekara et al. 2004; Furukawa, Kuchma et al. 2006; Harmsen, Yang et al. 2010). For instance, expression of the AlgU alternative sigma factor leads to decreased expression of T3SS and increased production of the biofilm exopolysaccharide alginate (Wu, Badrane et al. 2004; Diaz, King et al. 2011). Similarly, the SadARS (also known as RocARS) three component regulatory system positively regulates biofilm maturation but inhibits the transcription of genes encoding components of the T3SS (Kuchma, Connolly et al. 2005; Kulasekara, Ventre et al. 2005). The LadS and GacS sensor proteins also enhance biofilm formation and exopolysaccharide production, but repress T3SS (Ventre, Goodman et al. 2006; Gooderham and Hancock 2009; Harmsen, Yang et al. 2010; Diaz, King et al. 2011). These sensors activate GacA, which, in addition to modulation of T3SS and exopolysaccharide production, can alter levels of pyocyanin, hydrogen cyanide, elastase, and lipase (Burrowes, Baysse et al. 2006; Gooderham and Hancock 2009). On the other hand, the regulatory protein RetS (also known as RtsM) inhibits the actions of GacA, and expression of RetS negatively influences exopolysaccharide production and biofilm formation but positively regulates T3SS gene expression and production of the toxins ToxA and LipA (Goodman, Kulasekara et al. 2004; Laskowski, Osborn et al. 2004). This alternate regulation of genes involved in acute toxicity and genes involved in biofilm formation suggests that during an infection, local environmental conditions might influence the infection phenotype of *P. aeruginosa*, producing an acute, toxic infection or a chronic, biofilm infection. Indeed, taking the human lung as an example, *P. aeruginosa* infection can lead to either acute pneumonia or, in the case of the CF lung, chronic colonization (Chastre and Fagon 2002; Furukawa, Kuchma et al. 2006). Depending upon the activity levels of the various acute and chronic regulators, a variety of intermediate bacterial phenotypes could occur on the acute to chronic spectrum. Investigation into this Acute/Chronic regulatory switch, and how it impacts human infections, is ongoing.

2.4 Evidence for biofilm formation in the CF lung

Numerous lines of evidence have confirmed that *P. aeruginosa* persists in CF lungs as biofilms. Perhaps most importantly, microscopic examinations of sputum samples and lung tissue sections have revealed the presence of microcolonies and large biofilm-like structures in the airways (Lam, Chan et al. 1980; Singh, Schaefer et al. 2000; Worlitzsch, Tarran et al. 2002; Bjarnsholt, Jensen et al. 2009; Hoiby, Ciofu et al. 2010; Hoiby, Ciofu et al. 2011). These biofilms can grow to larger than 100 μM in diameter (Worlitzsch, Tarran et al. 2002), and the bacteria within these biofilms have been identified as *P. aeruginosa* by fluorescent *in situ* hybridization (FISH) (Bjarnsholt, Jensen et al. 2009). Studies have suggested that in those individuals without sufficient antimicrobial therapy, these biofilms exist throughout the lungs, whereas in those patients that have had aggressive antibiotic therapy, biofilms are confined to the conductive zone and are absent from the lower airways (Bjarnsholt, Jensen et al. 2009).

As further confirmation of biofilm formation in the CF lung, *P. aeruginosa* QS signaling molecules have been identified and characterized in CF patient sputum samples (Singh, Schaefer et al. 2000). Importantly, the ratios and relative proportion of the different QS molecules was similar to that of *P. aeruginosa* biofilms grown on abiotic surfaces. These data suggest that the bacteria within CF airways receive signals that induce them toward a chronic biofilm infection phenotype.

Indeed, *P. aeruginosa* isolates from CF airways display a number of characteristics indicative of biofilm formation. The conversion to mucoidy seen with chronically-infecting strains results from an overproduction of the biofilm exopolysaccharide alginate (Gibson, Burns et al. 2003; Ramsey and Wozniak 2005). Initially, steep hypoxic gradients in the mucus plugs of the CF airways stimulate the production of alginate (Worlitzsch, Tarran et al. 2002; Yoon and Hassett 2004). Over time, mutations in the gene *mucA*, encoding the membrane-localized anti-sigma factor MucA, result in constitutive expression of the alginate biosynthesis genes, through activation of the alternative sigma factor AlgU (Ohman and Chakrabarty 1981; Hughes and Mathee 1998; Hentzer, Teitzel et al. 2001; Ramsey and Wozniak 2005; Hoiby, Ciofu et al. 2010). It is thought that the constant oxidative stress encountered in the CF lung environment induces these mutations (Yoon and Hassett 2004; Hoiby, Ciofu et al. 2010).

CF lung isolates also accumulate mutations in T3SS genes (Dacheux, Attree et al. 2001; Jain, Ramirez et al. 2004; Smith, Buckley et al. 2006). Studies have shown an increasing number of T3SS defective isolates with increasing length of *P. aeruginosa* colonization (Jain, Ramirez et al. 2004). However, T3SS-competent bacteria have also been isolated from the lungs of CF patients (Dacheux, Toussaint et al. 2000; Jain, Ramirez et al. 2004; Jain, Bar-Meir et al. 2008), and it is possible that hyperactivation of AlgU might inhibit T3SS in these strains (Wu, Badrane et al. 2004; Diaz, King et al. 2011). Thus, both mutation and regulation appear to inhibit T3SS production in the CF lung during chronic infection, and this decrease in T3SS further supports the hypothesis that *P. aeruginosa* forms biofilms in the CF lung.

Intriguingly, many other mutations appear in genes involved in acute toxicity, including genes for lipopolysaccharide (LPS) biosynthesis, twitching motility, regulation of exotoxin A, pyoverdine synthesis, and QS factors (Smith, Buckley et al. 2006). A particular subset of chronic CF isolates, called small-colony variants (SCVs) due to their small colony morphology on agar plates, contains mutations in intracellular signaling proteins that lead to altered expression of polysaccharides, flagella, and type VI secretion (Starkey, Hickman et al. 2009). Thus, chronic CF *P. aeruginosa* isolates generally display a decrease in acute virulence. It is interesting to note that several studies have shown decreased virulence of chronic *P. aeruginosa* strains in mouse models of acute infection (Smith, Buckley et al. 2006; Bragonzi, Paroni et al. 2009). This adapted virulence of SCVs and other chronic CF isolates is thought to promote bacterial survival in the CF lung environment. T3SS toxins and other secreted factors are highly immunogenic, and mutation might protect the infecting bacteria from immune clearance. Furthermore, decreased bacterial toxicity would potentially inhibit the destruction of the biofilm habitat.

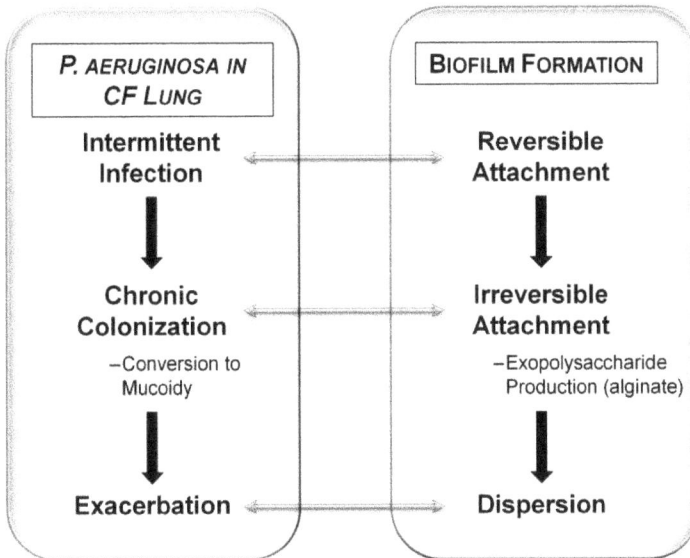

Fig. 2. Similarities between *P. aeruginosa* colonization of the CF lung and *in vitro P. aeruginosa* biofilm formation. The transition from reversible to irreversible attachment is mirrored in the transition from intermittent to chronic colonization. Similarly, just as bacteria in mature biofilms secrete exopolysaccharides, the conversion to mucoidy observed with CF isolates signals the overproduction of the exopolysaccharide alginate. Finally, it is possible that bacteria present during an exacerbation could represent bacteria that have dispersed from the biofilm and reverted to the planktonic phenotype expressing acute virulence factors.

Taken together, the presence of biofilm-like microcolonies and QS molecules, the increase in alginate production, and the decrease in T3SS and other acute infection phenotype factors strongly indicate that *P. aeruginosa* persists in the CF lung as biofilms. When comparing the biofilm formation cascade to the history of *P. aeruginosa* in an individual with CF, several intriguing parallels become apparent (Figure 2). Thus, the progression of intermittent infection, followed by chronic infection and conversion to mucoidy, is analogous to reversible binding, followed by irreversible binding and maturation of the *in vitro* biofilms, albeit chronic infection occurs on a much longer time scale than biofilms grown in the laboratory.

3. Consequences of biofilm formation in the CF lung

The formation of *P. aeruginosa* biofilms promotes chronic infection in the CF airways. As discussed in the following sections, several unique properties of biofilms contribute to this bacterial persistence, including antibiotic resistance, resistance to the activities of the immune system, and the high-frequency generation of bacterial mutants. Additionally, it has been found that *P. aeruginosa* contact with airway fluid leads to reduced flagella production (Wolfgang, Jyot et al. 2004), which potentially limits spread of the microorganism. Indeed, bacterial colonizers of the CF lung generally remain localized to the airways, and systemic spread rarely occurs (Govan and Deretic 1996). The biofilms that result from the growth and accumulation of infecting bacteria confer several survival advantages.

3.1 Antibiotic resistance

Biofilm bacteria are more resistant to many stresses than their planktonic counterparts (Costerton, Stewart et al. 1999; Stewart and Costerton 2001; Donlan and Costerton 2002; Dunne 2002; Patel 2005). In fact, biofilm bacteria can display up to 1,000 fold greater antibiotic resistance than planktonic bacteria (Mah and O'Toole 2001). This increased antibiotic resistance is due to several factors, including reduced antibiotic diffusion through the biofilm exopolysaccharide matrix, reduced growth rates of biofilm bacteria, the development of dormant persister cells, and the production of specific antibiotic-resistance factors (Donlan and Costerton 2002; Mah, Pitts et al. 2003; Lewis 2005; del Pozo and Patel 2007; Anderson 2008). All of these factors appear to influence the antibiotic-resistant nature of *P. aeruginosa* biofilms. In particular, alginate has been shown to retard the movement of cationic antimicrobial peptides, quaternary ammonium compounds, and aminoglycosides (including tobramycin) through *P. aeruginosa* biofilms (Nichols, Dorrington et al. 1988; Campanac, Pineau et al. 2002; Chan, Burrows et al. 2005). Additionally, *P. aeruginosa* produces biofilm-specific antimicrobial inhibitors (Mah, Pitts et al. 2003). Antibiotic treatment of *P. aeruginosa* biofilms also stimulates increased production of resistance factors, such as β-lactamases and antibiotic efflux pumps (Whiteley, Bangera et al. 2001; Bagge, Schuster et al. 2004). Further compounding the problem of biofilm antibiotic resistance, chronic *P. aeruginosa* CF isolates can accumulate mutations in antibiotic resistance genes, resulting in increased expression and activity of the resistance factors. These mutations confer increased survival in the presence of particular antibiotics (Smith, Buckley et al. 2006). The combination of these activities enables *P. aeruginosa* biofilms to survive the intense, often daily, antibiotic treatment regime taken by individuals with CF.

3.2 Immune resistance

P. aeruginosa biofilms also persist despite the high level inflammatory reaction that occurs in the CF lung (Gibson, Burns et al. 2003; Boucher 2004). The biofilm matrix acts as a shield preventing opsonophagocytosis of biofilm bacteria (Worlitzsch, Tarran et al. 2002; Gibson, Burns et al. 2003; Parsek and Singh 2003). In sputum and lung samples, neutrophils have been seen surrounding *P. aeruginosa* biofilms, but they have rarely been observed within the biofilms (Bjarnsholt, Jensen et al. 2009; Hoiby, Ciofu et al. 2010). *P. aeruginosa* can also counteract the effects of harmful chemical species produced by immune cells. Alginate has been shown to protect biofilm bacteria from reactive oxygen species (Cochran, Suh et al. 2000; Battan, Barnes et al. 2004; Gomez and Prince 2007; Hoiby, Ciofu et al. 2010), and denitrification pathways expressed in *P. aeruginosa* can metabolize reactive nitrogen intermediates, such as nitric oxide (Davies, Lloyd et al. 1989; Yoon and Hassett 2004). Thus, neutrophils appear to be recruited to CF lung biofilms, but the bacteria are protected from attack. Of greatest concern, lysis of spent neutrophils has been shown to add to biofilm viscosity and volume due to the release of DNA and protein (Walker, Tomlin et al. 2005; Parks, Young et al. 2009).

Chronic biofilm growth might also inhibit immune recognition of *P. aeruginosa*. Reduced production of flagella, T3SS, and acute phase virulence factors in biofilms can lead to reduced antibody detection of these antigens (Adamo, Sokol et al. 2004; Jain, Ramirez et al. 2004; Wolfgang, Jyot et al. 2004; Smith, Buckley et al. 2006; Starkey, Hickman et al. 2009). Furthermore, some chronic *P. aeruginosa* isolates display a modified LPS, which can further contribute to immune evasion (Ernst, Yi et al. 1999).

3.3 The insurance hypothesis

Biofilm formation can also result in genetic diversity. In addition to mutations in virulence factors and antibiotic resistance factors, a host of other *P. aeruginosa* genes are mutated within biofilms (Boles, Thoendel et al. 2004; Smith, Buckley et al. 2006; Starkey, Hickman et al. 2009). It is thought that the constant stress encountered in the CF lung environment leads to DNA damage, and hence mutations. Several studies have found mutations in DNA mismatch repair genes in chronic CF *P. aeruginosa* isolates, which enhances the mutation rate (Smith, Buckley et al. 2006; Doring, Parameswaran et al. 2011). It has been suggested that this genetic diversification with *P. aeruginosa* biofilms supports the "Insurance Hypothesis", which states that diversity within a population provides protection for the community as a whole against a wide range of adverse or changing conditions (Boles, Thoendel et al. 2004). In other words, in the CF lung, mutation of individual *P. aeruginosa* cells within a biofilm will give rise to subpopulations with resistance to a wide range of different stresses and the ability to grow in a variety of different environments. In fact, it has been shown that genetic diversity within *P. aeruginosa* biofilms confers protection from oxidative stress (Boles, Thoendel et al. 2004). In this manner, genotypic changes, along with antibiotic resistance and immune evasion, promote *P. aeruginosa* survival and chronic infection in the CF lung.

3.4 Seed for recurring exacerbations?

Considering the presence of a large persistent population of *P. aeruginosa* in the lungs of individuals with CF, it is possible that biofilms serve as a reservoir of bacterial pathogens that emerge during a pulmonary exacerbation (VanDevanter and Van Dalfsen 2005). Indeed, during an exacerbation, lung function decreases while the symptoms of bacterial infection increase (VanDevanter, O'Riordan et al. 2010). Clinically, exacerbations have been defined as a sudden worsening of symptoms requiring physician intervention and the need for altered antibiotic treatment (Rogers, Hoffman et al. 2011), although some clinicians and researchers argue for more objective criteria (Bilton, Canny et al. 2011). This definition implies that bacterial activity is a large part of an exacerbation. However, the role of bacteria during an exacerbation remains a mystery. Some studies have shown that bacterial densities increase during an exacerbation (Mowat, Paterson et al. 2011), while others report similar bacterial levels before and during an exacerbation (Stressmann, Rogers et al. 2011). It has also been suggested that a virulent sub-population of bacteria emerge during an exacerbation, thus leading to symptoms of acute infection (Jaffar-Bandjee, Lazdunski et al. 1995; Stressmann, Rogers et al. 2011). In support of this hypothesis, researchers have found increased levels of *P. aeruginosa* exoenzyme S, exotoxin A, elastase, and alkaline protease in sputum samples during exacerbations (Grimwood, Semple et al. 1993; Jaffar-Bandjee, Lazdunski et al. 1995).

Moreover, it has been shown that high-dose antibiotic intervention for exacerbations decreases bacterial density and results in improved pulmonary symptoms, indication that bacterial activity plays a large role in initiation and progression of an exacerbation (Jaffar-Bandjee, Lazdunski et al. 1995; VanDevanter, O'Riordan et al. 2010; Tunney, Klem et al. 2011). Thus, during an exacerbation, it is possible that some fraction of the biofilm bacteria disperses from the biofilm and reverts to the acute planktonic phenotype, which will cause more tissue damage and lead to greater immune stimulation (Figure 2).

4. Treatment of *P. aeruginosa* infections of the CF lung: Triumphs and challenges

Treatment of *P. aeruginosa* lung infections remains challenging. The best course of action might be prevention of infection through aggressive infection control procedures. These procedures are meant to prevent person-to-person transmission as well as transmission from contaminated surfaces. It has been found that sputum-encased *P. aeruginosa* can survive on inanimate surfaces for up to 8 days (Saiman and Siegel 2004). Thus, thorough cleaning and sterilization of clinical rooms, apparatuses, and home respirators is recommended (Saiman and Siegel 2004; Saiman 2011). Furthermore, healthcare workers should practice good hand and respiratory hygiene (Saiman and Siegel 2004; Hoiby, Ciofu et al. 2011; Saiman 2011). Isolation and separation of individuals infected with particular pathogens, such as *P. aeruginosa* and multi-drug resistant bacteria, has also been suggested to reduce patient-to-patient spread. Many clinics also encourage re-gowning and re-gloving with each new patient contact. However, despite the best infection control protocols, most CF individuals still acquire *P. aeruginosa*, either from environmental sources or from other CF patients. As discussed below, there are a number of antimicrobial therapies implemented to control lung infection with *P. aeruginosa*.

4.1 Antibiotic treatments

Numerous antibiotics have been used to treat CF lung infection with *P. aeruginosa*, although the aminoglycoside antibiotic tobramycin has most often been used and has been studied the most (Gibson, Burns et al. 2003; Ryan, Singh et al. 2011). In order to achieve high concentration in the airways, tobramycin and other antibiotics are often inhaled in a nebulized form (Ryan, Singh et al. 2011). Studies have investigated the efficacy of a number of inhaled antibiotics, including tobramycin, colistin, gentamicin, ceftazidime, cephaloridine, aztreonam lysine, taurolidine, and a gentamicin/carbenicillin combination (Ryan, Singh et al. 2011). The use of inhaled antibiotics, can lead to increased lung function and decreased exacerbation frequency over placebo (Ryan, Singh et al. 2011). During stable periods, inhaled antibiotics such as tobramycin or colistin can be given as chronic suppressive therapies to maintain low bacterial levels within the airways (Hoiby, Ciofu et al. 2011). An economics study estimated that increased usage of inhaled tobramycin would lead to increased cost for medication but decreased physician and hospital visits. This would have a net decrease in healthcare costs (Woodward, Brown et al. 2010). It has also been suggested that this maintenance therapy be supplemented with 2-week courses of intravenous (IV) antibiotic combinations every 3 months for added anti-Pseudomonal pressure (Hoiby, Ciofu et al. 2011). In addition to antimicrobial therapies, other medications such as DNase and hypertonic saline are widely used to increase airway clearance (Fuchs, Borowitz et al. 1994; Donaldson, Bennett et al. 2006; Elkins, Robinson et al. 2006; Parks, Young et al. 2009).

However, despite suppressive therapies, pulmonary exacerbations still occur. The types of antibiotics, dosing, and treatment schedules for exacerbation therapy vary greatly country-to-country and site-to-site. Synergy and a reduction in antibiotic resistance have been shown with thrice daily IV infusions of an aminoglycoside antibiotic and a β-lactam antibiotic (Bals, Hubert et al. 2011; Plummer and Wildman 2011). A recent study has found that twice daily treatments of tobramycin and ceftazidime are just as effective as thrice daily infusions, and this reduced treatment regimen can be safer and more convenient than a three times a day schedule. Studies have demonstrated that the bacterial response to antibiotic treatment is completed within 14 days (Adeboyeku, Jones et al. 2011), although in some cases, patients respond better to shorter or longer treatments (VanDevanter, O'Riordan et al. 2010; Plummer and Wildman 2011). Many more antibiotic treatment regimens are used in clinics and hospitals, and optimization of therapy for an individual exacerbation event often relies on symptoms and pulmonary function testing. Home-based IV antibiotic therapy of exacerbation has also been explored as an alternative to inpatient treatment. At-home therapy, while requiring specialized training for family members and friends, can reduce costs to families and hospitals, reduce incidence of hospital-acquired infections, improve disease manifestations, and can be more convenient for the affected individual (Balaguer and Gonzalez de Dios 2008).

4.2 Early colonization eradication

The period of intermittent infection, before the establishment of chronic *P. aeruginosa* biofilms, presents a unique opportunity for therapeutic intervention. Many studies have shown the efficacy of early aggressive antibiotic therapy to eradicate *P. aeruginosa* during this early colonization period. In the Copenhagen Model, which has been in place for over 20 years in the Copenhagen CF center, infected CF patients are given inhaled colistin and IV ciprofloxacin for 3 months (Hoiby, Frederiksen et al. 2005; Hansen, Pressler et al. 2008). 80% of patients treated with this regimen were free of chronic *P. aeruginosa* infection for up to 15 years, and the bacterial isolates recovered exhibited little resistance to colistin and ciprofloxacin (Hansen, Pressler et al. 2008). In a different study of other European CF centers, treatment with inhaled colistin and IV ciprofloxacin for 3 months was found to be 81% effective (Taccetti, Campana et al. 2005). In this study, treated patients were completely free from *P. aeruginosa* infection for an average of 18 months, and 73% of subsequent *P. aeruginosa* infections were found to involve a genotypically distinct strain, suggesting that the original isolate had been eradicated (Taccetti, Campana et al. 2005). This treatment was also associated with reduced overall treatment costs and little development of antibiotic resistance (Taccetti, Campana et al. 2005).

There are numerous variations on eradication therapies, and many studies evaluating the efficacy of these treatments (Stuart, Lin et al. 2010; Hayes, Feola et al. 2011). In an effort to develop standardized treatment guidelines for early eradication therapies, there have been 2 large, multicenter studies: the Early Inhaled Tobramycin for Eradication (ELITE) study in Europe, and the Early *Pseudomonas* Infection Control (EPIC) program in the United States. The

EPIC program, the results of which have yet to be published, is comparing standard culture-based therapy with twice daily inhaled tobramycin (300 mg) for 28 days every yearly quarter (Stuart, Lin et al. 2010; Hayes, Feola et al. 2011). The tobramycin-treatment group is further split into groups that additionally receive 14 days of either oral ciprofloxacin or oral placebo. The ELITE study treated participants for 28 days with twice daily inhaled tobramycin (300mg/5mL), and found that 93% of those treated were *P. aeruginosa*-free after 1 month (Ratjen, Munck et al. 2010). 66% of participants were free of *P. aeruginosa* infection for 2 years (Ratjen, Munck et al. 2010). Similar results were obtained with individuals treated for 56 days.

The early promise of eradication therapy studies demonstrates that these treatments will likely enhance overall patient health and reduce healthcare costs related to *P. aeruginosa* infection. Indeed, such early eradication protocols have dramatically increased the age at which chronic *P. aeruginosa* infection is established (Hoiby, Frederiksen et al. 2005; Hansen, Pressler et al. 2008). Furthermore, eradication can be achieved regardless of the age of the patient, provided there has been no evidence of prior *P. aeruginosa* infection (Hayes, Feola et al. 2011). However, even with constant monitoring and treatment, intermittent *P. aeruginosa* infection will eventually give way to chronic biofilm formation. It is well established that once chronic infection is initiated, eradication of *P. aeruginosa* from the CF lung is essentially impossible (Hoiby, Frederiksen et al. 2005; Hansen, Pressler et al. 2008).

4.3 Antibiotic resistance

Perhaps not surprisingly, treatment of CF lung infections with large doses of antibiotics leads to high levels of antibiotic resistance. Resistance of a CF lung isolate to a particular antibiotic is generally associated with treatment with that antibiotic (Emerson, McNamara et al. 2010). Greater resistance leads to longer therapies, which consequently induces more resistance (Plummer and Wildman 2011). The formation of *P. aeruginosa* biofilms plays a large role in the emergence of antibiotic resistance. In addition to the general resistance of biofilms and other stresses (Costerton, Stewart et al. 1999; Stewart and Costerton 2001; Donlan and Costerton 2002; Dunne 2002; Patel 2005), the high mutation rate and generation of diversity that occurs in *P. aeruginosa* biofilms results in variant strains that display increased resistance to antibiotics, through mutation of antibiotic targets and increased production and activity of multidrug efflux pumps (Smith, Buckley et al. 2006; Bals, Hubert et al. 2011; Mowat, Paterson et al. 2011). Moreover, the SCVs that develop in biofilms, and appear with increasing prevalence in CF patient sputum samples over time, are more innately resistant to a multitude of antibiotics (Starkey, Hickman et al. 2009; Bals, Hubert et al. 2011). The appearance of multidrug-resistant *P. aeruginosa* clones, which are associated with more severe lung disease and declining lung function (Plummer and Wildman 2011), has lead to an antibiotic dilemma. Novel antimicrobial strategies must be developed to combat these multidrug-resistant *P. aeruginosa* infections in the CF lung.

5. Hope for the future: Novel therapies and model systems

Recent investigations into anti-Pseudomonal treatments, with an eye toward inhibiting *P. aeruginosa* biofilm formation, have led to new drugs and novel implementation strategies of existing antimicrobials (Table 1). Likewise, advances in CF lung infection model systems are leading to new insights into the nature of chronic *P. aeruginosa* infection in the CF lung.

Strategy	References
Anti-biofilm Testing	
MBEC testing of current antibiotics	(Ceri, Olson et al. 1999; Keays, Ferris et al. 2009; Moskowitz, Emerson et al. 2011)
Quorum Sensing Inhibitors	
Furanones	(Steinberg, Schneider et al. 1997; Hentzer, Riedel et al. 2002)
Garlic extract	(Rasmussen and Givskov 2006; Harmsen, Yang et al. 2010)
Patulin	(Rasmussen, Skindersoe et al. 2005)
Penicillin acid	(Rasmussen, Skindersoe et al. 2005)
cis-2 decanoic acid	(Bjarnsholt, Tolker-Nielsen et al. 2010)
Salicylic acid	(Bjarnsholt, Tolker-Nielsen et al. 2010)
4-NPO	(Rasmussen and Givskov 2006; Bjarnsholt, Tolker-Nielsen et al. 2010)
Solenopsin A	(Bjarnsholt, Tolker-Nielsen et al. 2010)
Azithromycin	(Skindersoe, Alhede et al. 2008; Bjarnsholt, Tolker-Nielsen et al. 2010)
Clarithromycin	(Wozniak and Keyser 2004)
Ceftazidime	(Skindersoe, Alhede et al. 2008)
Ciprofloxacin	(Skindersoe, Alhede et al. 2008)
Inhaled Antibiotics	
Aztreonam lysine	(McCoy, Quittner et al. 2008; Retsch-Bogart, Burns et al. 2008; Parkins and Elborn 2010)
Levofloxacin	(Anderson 2010; Bals, Hubert et al. 2011)
Fosfomycin/Tobramycin	(Anderson 2010)
Tobramycin, inhalable powder	(Bals, Hubert et al. 2011)
Ciprofloxacin, inhalable powder	(Anderson 2010; Bals, Hubert et al. 2011)
Liposomally-encased Antibiotics	
Amikacin	(Anderson 2010; Bals, Hubert et al. 2011)
Tobramycin	(Bals, Hubert et al. 2011)
Polymyxin B	(Bals, Hubert et al. 2011)
New Antibiotics	
Tigecycline	(Parkins and Elborn 2010)
Doripenem	(Parkins and Elborn 2010)
Ceftibiprole	(Parkins and Elborn 2010)
Tomopenem	(Parkins and Elborn 2010)
CXA-101	(Parkins and Elborn 2010; Bals, Hubert et al. 2011)
NXL104/Ceftazidime	(Parkins and Elborn 2010)
ACHN-490	(Parkins and Elborn 2010)
CB182,804	(Parkins and Elborn 2010)
BLI-489/Pipericillin	(Parkins and Elborn 2010)
Disruption of Iron Metabolism	
Gallium	(Kaneko, Thoendel et al. 2007)
Desferasirox	(Moreau-Marquis, O'Toole et al. 2009)
Desferoxamine	(Moreau-Marquis, O'Toole et al. 2009)
Virulence Factor Modulation	
T3SS Inhibitors	(Aiello, Williams et al. 2010)
Vaccination	(Doring and Pier 2008)

Table 1. Novel and Emerging Therapies for *P. aeruginosa* Infection of CF Lungs

5.1 Novel therapies

5.1.1 Anti-biofilm strategies

Because biofilm formation plays an integral role in the persistence and antibiotic resistance of *P. aeruginosa* in the CF lung, many researchers have begun searching out ways to specifically destroy biofilms. The most obvious place to start in the development of anti-biofilm therapies is testing the efficacy of our current antibiotics against *P. aeruginosa* biofilms (Moskowitz, Emerson et al. 2011)(Table 1). In one retrospective analysis, the reported planktonic antibiotic susceptibilities of *P. aeruginosa* CF isolates were compared to the antibiotic susceptibilities of these strains grown as biofilms (Keays, Ferris et al. 2009). Those patients that were treated with antibiotics that could kill biofilm-state bacteria experienced lower treatment failure, decreased exacerbation risk, and decreased hospital stays (Keays, Ferris et al. 2009). Other studies have also shown that treatment tailored to biofilm susceptibility patterns can be effective (Moskowitz, Emerson et al. 2011). The recent development of the Minimum Biofilm Eradication Concentration (MBEC) Assay (also known as the Calgary Biofilm Device, distributed through Innovotech, Edmonton, CA), has permitted high throughput analysis of biofilm formation and biofilm susceptibilities of *P. aeruginosa* and other CF pathogens (Ceri, Olson et al. 1999; Tomlin, Malott et al. 2005; Davies, Harrison et al. 2007; Alfa and Howie 2009). Anti-biofilm therapies developed using the MBEC or other biofilm assays can thus be of great clinical benefit.

Another promising avenue of anti-biofilm research is the identification of molecules that interrupt QS signaling (Geske, Wezeman et al. 2005; Rasmussen and Givskov 2006; Galloway, Hodgkinson et al. 2011)(Table 1). By interfering with inter-bacterial communication and gene regulation, these compounds can lead to the dispersion of biofilm bacteria as well as alter virulence factor production. Generally, QS inhibitors fall into one of three categories: 1) those that block production of the QS signaling molecule, 2) those that degrade the QS molecule, and 3) those that prevent bacterial recognition of the QS signal (Rasmussen and Givskov 2006). Many large screens of natural compounds have been completed or are taking place to identify novel QS inhibitors, and several active compounds have emerged from these studies. For instance, halogenated furanones from the alga *Delisea pulchra* and synthetic furanones have been shown to block *P. aeruginosa* QS and biofilm formation, and they lead to increased *P. aeruginosa* killing when used in combination with traditional antibiotics (Steinberg, Schneider et al. 1997; Hentzer, Riedel et al. 2002; Bjarnsholt, Tolker-Nielsen et al. 2010). Likewise, garlic extract, patulin and penicillic acid from *Penicillium* species, *cis*-2-decanoic acid from *P. aeruginosa*, salicylic acid, 4-nitro-pyridine-N-oxide (4-NPO), and solenopsin A from fire ant venom have all demonstrated inhibition of *P. aeruginosa* QS, and some have shown direct biofilm disruption activity (Rasmussen, Skindersoe et al. 2005; Rasmussen and Givskov 2006; Bjarnsholt, Tolker-Nielsen et al. 2010; Harmsen, Yang et al. 2010). Some of these QS inhibitors, such as garlic extract, patulin, 4-NPO, and furanones, have also displayed a therapeutic effect in models of *P. aeruginosa* infection (Rasmussen and Givskov 2006). Importantly, it is thought that resistance to QS inhibitors will not develop because these compounds do not directly affect bacterial growth, and thus exert little selective pressure (Bjarnsholt, Tolker-Nielsen et al. 2010).

Intriguingly, it has been found that some traditional antibiotics can affect biofilm formation and virulence factor production through QS inhibition or other mechanisms. For instance, azithromycin, ceftazidime, and ciprofloxacin were all shown to affect *P. aeruginosa* QS and virulence factor production (Skindersoe, Alhede et al. 2008; Bjarnsholt, Tolker-Nielsen et al. 2010). Sub-inhibitory concentrations of clarithromycin can also alter biofilm morphology (Wozniak and Keyser 2004). Thus, treatment with these antibiotics has yielded unexpected consequences for *P. aeruginosa* infection.

5.1.2 Newer antimicrobial strategies

Development of traditional antibiotics, and novel delivery methods for antibiotics, has also yielded some successes (Table 1). Several new antibiotics have recently hit the markets in various countries, including tigecycline, doripenem, and the 5th generation cephalosporin ceftibiprole (Parkins and Elborn 2010). Many more antibiotics with potential efficacy against Gram-negative CF pathogens are in development, such as tomopenem, CXA-101, NXL104/ceftazidime, ACHN-490, CB182,804, and BLI-489/pipericillin (Parkins and Elborn 2010; Bals, Hubert et al. 2011). However, because many of these compounds are derivatives of existing antibiotics, resistance and toxicity might hinder further research on these novel therapies (Parkins and Elborn 2010).

On the other hand, the development of inhaled versions of existing antibiotics has been shown to improve delivery times and concentrate the antibiotic at the site of infection (Anderson 2010; Bals, Hubert et al. 2011; Ryan, Singh et al. 2011). Nebulized tobramycin has been used for years as an effective anti-Pseudomonal therapy, and many other inhaled antibiotic formulation have been studied (Ryan, Singh et al. 2011). Recently, Aztreonam Lysine for Inhalation has been approved in many countries for treatment of chronic CF lung infections, and studies have shown that use of this drug can improve quality of life and pulmonary function of CF patients, while decreasing *P. aeruginosa* burden and lower exacerbation severity (McCoy, Quittner et al. 2008; Retsch-Bogart, Burns et al. 2008; Anderson 2010; Parkins and Elborn 2010; Bals, Hubert et al. 2011). Work continues on other inhaled antibiotics, including aerosolized levofloxacin, fosfomycin/tobramycin, and inhalable dry powers of tobramycin and ciprofloxacin (Anderson 2010; Bals, Hubert et al. 2011). Inhalation of liposomally-encased antibiotics shows great promise for therapy of biofilm infections, as liposome delivery is thought to increase the penetration of biofilms (Smith 2005; Bals, Hubert et al. 2011). Patients treated with liposomally-encased amikacin showed improved lung function and reduction in sputum *P. aeruginosa* levels (Anderson 2010; Bals, Hubert et al. 2011). Similarly, liposomal encasement of tobramycin and polymyxin B might hold great promise as alternative treatments for chronic CF infections (Bals, Hubert et al. 2011).

Looking toward the future, there is great interest in identifying and developing novel chemical agents that disrupt bacterial metabolism, adhesins, virulence factor production, efflux pump activity, and bacterial intracellular signaling (Parkins and Elborn 2010; Bals, Hubert et al. 2011)(Table 1). Indeed, treatment with iron chelators (desferasirox and desferoxamine) or gallium, which is a non-reducible mimic for iron, can interfere with *P. aeruginosa* metabolism, resulting in biofilm disruption and protection against *P. aeruginosa* infection in animal models (Kaneko, Thoendel et al. 2007; DeLeon, Balldin et al. 2009; Moreau-Marquis, O'Toole et al. 2009). Inhibitors of *P. aeruginosa* T3SS have also been found

(Aiello, Williams et al. 2010). Further screening of chemical compound libraries will likely reveal many additional molecules with anti-Pseudomonal activity.

5.1.3 Vaccination

Vaccines against *P. aeruginosa* have also been proposed as a potential therapy for preventing chronic CF infections (Table 1). Researchers have explored vaccines against *P. aeruginosa* LPS, alginate, flagella, outer membrane proteins, pili, T3SS components, DNA, and killed whole bacteria (Doring and Pier 2008). Many of these vaccines have been tested in clinical trials, with moderate efficacy. It is thought that clearance and prevention of *P. aeruginosa* infection by aggressive early eradication programs masks the true effectiveness of these vaccines, and none of them have reached the market (Doring and Pier 2008). Passive immunotherapy with monoclonal antibodies or pooled immune serum has also been investigated for anti-Pseudomonal therapy (Doring and Pier 2008).

5.2 Novel model systems

5.2.1 Animal models

Researchers have tried for decades to develop an animal CF model that can maintain a chronic *P. aeruginosa* infection. Mice with various *CFTR* alleles and/or overexpression of βENaC have been tested as infection models, but *P. aeruginosa* is generally cleared from the lungs of these animals (Grubb and Boucher 1999; Mall, Grubb et al. 2004; Wilke, Buijs-Offerman et al. 2011; Zhou, Duerr et al. 2011). Mice and humans have very different lung physiologies, which most likely account for the inability to establish chronic infection in "CF" mice (Wilke, Buijs-Offerman et al. 2011). The recently developed pig and ferret CF animal models have been reported to develop spontaneous bacterial infections, and it is possible that chronic *P. aeruginosa* infection could be reproduced in these animals (Fisher, Zhang et al. 2011). However, these CF animals generally require surgery to correct the meconium ileus that develops in the young (Fisher, Zhang et al. 2011). Thus, the cost of these model systems is high.

5.2.2 Artificial sputum

In order to model the CF lung environment *in vitro*, several groups have created artificial sputum media. These media replicate the experimentally-determined composition of CF sputum samples, and they can support similar *P. aeruginosa* growth rates, gene expression patterns, nutritional preferences, and QS patterns as found in CF sputum (Sriramulu, Lunsdorf et al. 2005; Palmer, Aye et al. 2007). These media have also been useful for investigations of *P. aeruginosa* biofilm formation (Sriramulu, Lunsdorf et al. 2005; Garbe, Wesche et al. 2010). These models could lead to a better understanding of metabolic flux in *P. aeruginosa* biofilms in the context of CF lung infection.

5.2.3 Biofilms co-cultured with airway cells

Recently, several investigators have developed *P. aeruginosa* biofilms on cultured airway cells *in vitro* (Figure 3). These co-culture biofilm models were developed to more closely mimic the CF lung environment and potential signals that the bacteria receive from mammalian cells during infection. In one model, *P. aeruginosa* bind to a monolayer or air-liquid interface differentiated layer of immortalized CF-derived (*CFTR* ΔF508 homozygous) bronchial epithelial cells (Moreau-Marquis, Bomberger et al. 2008; Moreau-Marquis, Redelman et al. 2010). Fresh culture medium then flows across the system and large bacterial aggregates form on the epithelial cells.   The aggregates appear morphologically similar to biofilms formed on abiotic surfaces (Moreau-Marquis, Bomberger et al. 2008; Moreau-Marquis, Redelman et al. 2010). Furthermore, formation of these co-culture biofilms requires factors necessary for abiotic biofilm formation, and bacteria within co-culture biofilms display a pattern of gene expression consistent with that found in abiotic biofilms. In a different study, similar co-culture biofilms were formed by static incubation of *P. aeruginosa* and CF airway cells in the presence of arginine (Anderson, Moreau-Marquis et al. 2008; Moreau-Marquis, Redelman et al. 2010). Importantly, in both systems, the antibiotic resistance of the co-culture biofilms was greatly increased compared to both planktonic bacteria and abiotic biofilms (Anderson, Moreau-Marquis et al. 2008; Moreau-Marquis, Bomberger et al. 2008; Moreau-Marquis, O'Toole et al. 2009). It was also discovered that the co-culture biofilms displayed a different genetic response to tobramycin treatment than biofilms formed on plastic (Anderson, Moreau-Marquis et al. 2008). These data suggest that the surface upon which a biofilm forms can affect the properties of that biofilm, and they also offer clues into the high antibiotic resistance of *P. aeruginosa* biofilms that form in the CF lung. *P. aeruginosa* biofilms have also been shown to form on cultured mouse nasal septal epithelial cells (Woodworth, Tamashiro et al. 2008).

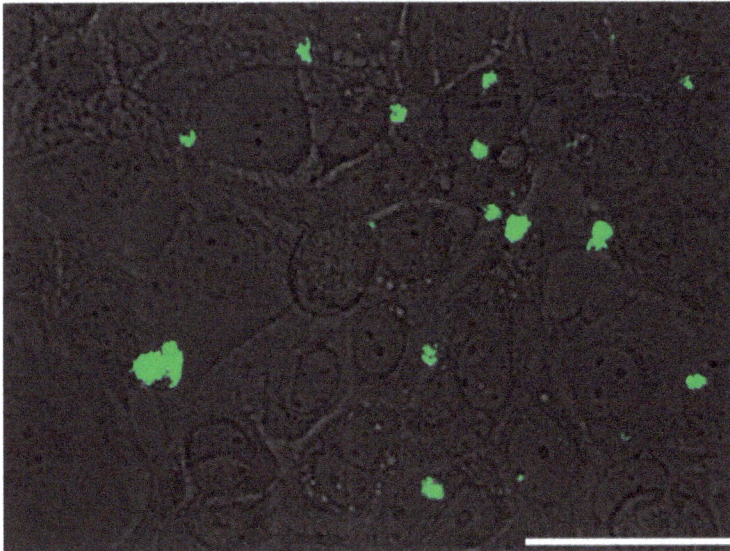

Fig. 3. *P. aeruginosa* biofilm microcolonies on cultured human CF-derived airway cells. Immortalized human bronchial epithelial cells, originally isolated from an individual with CF, were inoculated with *P. aeruginosa* constitutively expressing green fluorescent protein. Biofilm microcolonies (green) are attached to the surface of the cells. Bar = 50μm.

6. Conclusion

There have been a number of great advances in recent years in anti-Pseudomonal therapy of CF lung infections. In particular, early eradication treatments appear to show much promise in delaying the onset of chronic *P. aeruginosa* biofilm formation. The increasing arsenal against *P. aeruginosa*, including inhaled aztreonam and liposomal amikacin, will likely prove a benefit for *P. aeruginosa* treatment. Eradication of chronic *P. aeruginosa* may be possible, but it will take creative thinking. It is clear that new anti-biofilm treatments need to be discovered and implemented. The development of clinically-relevant models will further aid this process by providing appropriate systems for testing novel molecules. With renewed focus on the biofilm nature of the infection, much progress can be made toward eliminating chronic *P. aeruginosa* from the CF lung.

7. Acknowledgements

Many thanks are given to C. Redelman, C. McCaslin, and M. Howenstine for helpful comments and technical support. This work was supported by RSFG from IUPUI and PRF from Purdue University to GGA.

8. References

Adamo, R., S. Sokol, G. Soong, M. I. Gomez and A. Prince (2004). Pseudomonas aeruginosa flagella activate airway epithelial cells through asialoGM1 and toll-like receptor 2 as well as toll-like receptor 5. *Am J Respir Cell Mol Biol* 30(5): 627-34.

Adeboyeku, D., A. L. Jones and M. E. Hodson (2011). Twice vs three-times daily antibiotics in the treatment of pulmonary exacerbations of cystic fibrosis. *J Cyst Fibros* 10(1): 25-30.

Aiello, D., J. D. Williams, H. Majgier-Baranowska, I. Patel, N. P. Peet, J. Huang, S. Lory, T. L. Bowlin and D. T. Moir (2010). Discovery and characterization of inhibitors of Pseudomonas aeruginosa type III secretion. *Antimicrob Agents Chemother* 54(5): 1988-99.

Alfa, M. J. and R. Howie (2009). Modeling microbial survival in buildup biofilm for complex medical devices. *BMC Infect Dis* 9: 56.

Anderson, G. G., S. Moreau-Marquis, B. A. Stanton and G. A. O'Toole (2008). In vitro analysis of tobramycin-treated Pseudomonas aeruginosa biofilms on cystic fibrosis-derived airway epithelial cells. *Infect Immun* 76(4): 1423-33.

Anderson, G. G., O'Toole. G. A. (2008). Innate and Induced Resistance Mechanisms of Bacterial Biofilms. *Bacterial Biofilms*. T. Romeo. Berlin, Springer-Verlag. 322: 85-105.

Anderson, P. (2010). Emerging therapies in cystic fibrosis. *Ther Adv Respir Dis* 4(3): 177-85.

Bagge, N., M. Schuster, M. Hentzer, O. Ciofu, M. Givskov, E. P. Greenberg and N. Hoiby (2004). Pseudomonas aeruginosa biofilms exposed to imipenem exhibit changes in global gene expression and beta-lactamase and alginate production. *Antimicrob Agents Chemother* 48(4): 1175-87.

Balaguer, A. and J. Gonzalez de Dios (2008). Home intravenous antibiotics for cystic fibrosis. *Cochrane Database Syst Rev*(3): CD001917.

Bals, R., D. Hubert and B. Tummler (2011). Antibiotic treatment of CF lung disease: from bench to bedside. *J Cyst Fibros* 10 Suppl 2: S146-51.

Battan, P. C., A. I. Barnes and I. Albesa (2004). Resistance to oxidative stress caused by ceftazidime and piperacillin in a biofilm of Pseudomonas. *Luminescence* 19(5): 265-70.

Bilton, D., G. Canny, S. Conway, S. Dumcius, L. Hjelte, M. Proesmans, B. Tummler, V. Vavrova and K. De Boeck (2011). Pulmonary exacerbation: towards a definition for use in clinical trials. Report from the EuroCareCF Working Group on outcome parameters in clinical trials. *J Cyst Fibros* 10 Suppl 2: S79-81.

Bjarnsholt, T., P. O. Jensen, M. J. Fiandaca, J. Pedersen, C. R. Hansen, C. B. Andersen, T. Pressler, M. Givskov and N. Hoiby (2009). Pseudomonas aeruginosa biofilms in the respiratory tract of cystic fibrosis patients. *Pediatr Pulmonol* 44(6): 547-58.

Bjarnsholt, T., T. Tolker-Nielsen, N. Hoiby and M. Givskov (2010). Interference of Pseudomonas aeruginosa signalling and biofilm formation for infection control. *Expert Rev Mol Med* 12: e11.

Boles, B. R., M. Thoendel and P. K. Singh (2004). Self-generated diversity produces "insurance effects" in biofilm communities. *Proc Natl Acad Sci U S A* 101(47): 16630-5.

Boucher, R. C. (2004). New concepts of the pathogenesis of cystic fibrosis lung disease. *Eur Respir J* 23(1): 146-58.

Bragonzi, A., M. Paroni, A. Nonis, N. Cramer, S. Montanari, J. Rejman, C. Di Serio, G. Doring and B. Tummler (2009). Pseudomonas aeruginosa microevolution during cystic fibrosis lung infection establishes clones with adapted virulence. *Am J Respir Crit Care Med* 180(2): 138-45.

Burrowes, E., C. Baysse, C. Adams and F. O'Gara (2006). Influence of the regulatory protein RsmA on cellular functions in Pseudomonas aeruginosa PAO1, as revealed by transcriptome analysis. *Microbiology* 152(Pt 2): 405-18.

Caiazza, N. C. and G. A. O'Toole (2004). SadB is required for the transition from reversible to irreversible attachment during biofilm formation by Pseudomonas aeruginosa PA14. *J Bacteriol* 186(14): 4476-85.

Campanac, C., L. Pineau, A. Payard, G. Baziard-Mouysset and C. Roques (2002). Interactions between biocide cationic agents and bacterial biofilms. *Antimicrob Agents Chemother* 46(5): 1469-74.

Ceri, H., M. E. Olson, C. Stremick, R. R. Read, D. Morck and A. Buret (1999). The Calgary Biofilm Device: new technology for rapid determination of antibiotic susceptibilities of bacterial biofilms. *J Clin Microbiol* 37(6): 1771-6.

Chan, C., L. L. Burrows and C. M. Deber (2005). Alginate as an auxiliary bacterial membrane: binding of membrane-active peptides by polysaccharides. *J Pept Res* 65(3): 343-51.

Chastre, J. and J. Y. Fagon (2002). Ventilator-associated pneumonia. *Am J Respir Crit Care Med* 165(7): 867-903.

Chiang, P. and L. L. Burrows (2003). Biofilm formation by hyperpiliated mutants of Pseudomonas aeruginosa. *J Bacteriol* 185(7): 2374-8.

Cochran, W. L., S. J. Suh, G. A. McFeters and P. S. Stewart (2000). Role of RpoS and AlgT in Pseudomonas aeruginosa biofilm resistance to hydrogen peroxide and monochloramine. *J Appl Microbiol* 88(3): 546-53.

Cooley, M., S. R. Chhabra and P. Williams (2008). N-Acylhomoserine lactone-mediated quorum sensing: a twist in the tail and a blow for host immunity. *Chem Biol* 15(11): 1141-7.

Costerton, J. W. (2001). Cystic fibrosis pathogenesis and the role of biofilms in persistent infection. *Trends Microbiol* 9(2): 50-2.

Costerton, J. W., Z. Lewandowski, D. E. Caldwell, D. R. Korber and H. M. Lappin-Scott (1995). Microbial biofilms. *Annu Rev Microbiol* 49: 711-45.

Costerton, J. W., P. S. Stewart and E. P. Greenberg (1999). Bacterial biofilms: a common cause of persistent infections. *Science* 284(5418): 1318-22.

Dacheux, D., I. Attree and B. Toussaint (2001). Expression of ExsA in trans confers type III secretion system-dependent cytotoxicity on noncytotoxic Pseudomonas aeruginosa cystic fibrosis isolates. *Infect Immun* 69(1): 538-42.

Dacheux, D., B. Toussaint, M. Richard, G. Brochier, J. Croize and I. Attree (2000). Pseudomonas aeruginosa cystic fibrosis isolates induce rapid, type III secretion-dependent, but ExoU-independent, oncosis of macrophages and polymorphonuclear neutrophils. *Infect Immun* 68(5): 2916-24.

Davies, J. A., J. J. Harrison, L. L. Marques, G. R. Foglia, C. A. Stremick, D. G. Storey, R. J. Turner, M. E. Olson and H. Ceri (2007). The GacS sensor kinase controls phenotypic reversion of small colony variants isolated from biofilms of Pseudomonas aeruginosa PA14. *FEMS Microbiol Ecol* 59(1): 32-46.

Davies, K. J., D. Lloyd and L. Boddy (1989). The effect of oxygen on denitrification in Paracoccus denitrificans and Pseudomonas aeruginosa. *J Gen Microbiol* 135(9): 2445-51.

del Pozo, J. L. and R. Patel (2007). The challenge of treating biofilm-associated bacterial infections. *Clin Pharmacol Ther* 82(2): 204-9.

DeLeon, K., F. Balldin, C. Watters, A. Hamood, J. Griswold, S. Sreedharan and K. P. Rumbaugh (2009). Gallium maltolate treatment eradicates Pseudomonas aeruginosa infection in thermally injured mice. *Antimicrob Agents Chemother* 53(4): 1331-7.

Diaz, M. R., J. M. King and T. L. Yahr (2011). Intrinsic and extrinsic regulation of type III secretion gene expression in Pseudomonas aeruginosa. *Frontiers in Microbiology* 2.

Donaldson, S. H., W. D. Bennett, K. L. Zeman, M. R. Knowles, R. Tarran and R. C. Boucher (2006). Mucus clearance and lung function in cystic fibrosis with hypertonic saline. *N Engl J Med* 354(3): 241-50.

Donlan, R. M. and J. W. Costerton (2002). Biofilms: survival mechanisms of clinically relevant microorganisms. *Clin Microbiol Rev* 15(2): 167-93.

Doring, G., I. G. Parameswaran and T. F. Murphy (2011). Differential adaptation of microbial pathogens to airways of patients with cystic fibrosis and chronic obstructive pulmonary disease. *FEMS Microbiol Rev* 35(1): 124-46.

Doring, G. and G. B. Pier (2008). Vaccines and immunotherapy against Pseudomonas aeruginosa. *Vaccine* 26(8): 1011-24.

Dunne, W. M., Jr. (2002). Bacterial adhesion: seen any good biofilms lately? *Clin Microbiol Rev* 15(2): 155-66.

Elkins, M. R., M. Robinson, B. R. Rose, C. Harbour, C. P. Moriarty, G. B. Marks, E. G. Belousova, W. Xuan and P. T. Bye (2006). A controlled trial of long-term inhaled hypertonic saline in patients with cystic fibrosis. *N Engl J Med* 354(3): 229-40.

Emerson, J., S. McNamara, A. M. Buccat, K. Worrell and J. L. Burns (2010). Changes in cystic fibrosis sputum microbiology in the United States between 1995 and 2008. *Pediatr Pulmonol* 45(4): 363-70.

Ernst, R. K., E. C. Yi, L. Guo, K. B. Lim, J. L. Burns, M. Hackett and S. I. Miller (1999). Specific lipopolysaccharide found in cystic fibrosis airway Pseudomonas aeruginosa. *Science* 286(5444): 1561-5.

Fisher, J. T., Y. Zhang and J. F. Engelhardt (2011). Comparative biology of cystic fibrosis animal models. *Methods Mol Biol* 742: 311-34.

Fuchs, H. J., D. S. Borowitz, D. H. Christiansen, E. M. Morris, M. L. Nash, B. W. Ramsey, B. J. Rosenstein, A. L. Smith and M. E. Wohl (1994). Effect of aerosolized recombinant human DNase on exacerbations of respiratory symptoms and on pulmonary function in patients with cystic fibrosis. The Pulmozyme Study Group. *N Engl J Med* 331(10): 637-42.

Furukawa, S., S. L. Kuchma and G. A. O'Toole (2006). Keeping their options open: acute versus persistent infections. *J Bacteriol* 188(4): 1211-7.

Gallagher, L. A. and C. Manoil (2001). Pseudomonas aeruginosa PAO1 kills Caenorhabditis elegans by cyanide poisoning. *J Bacteriol* 183(21): 6207-14.

Galloway, W. R., J. T. Hodgkinson, S. D. Bowden, M. Welch and D. R. Spring (2011). Quorum sensing in Gram-negative bacteria: small-molecule modulation of AHL and AI-2 quorum sensing pathways. *Chem Rev* 111(1): 28-67.

Garbe, J., A. Wesche, B. Bunk, M. Kazmierczak, K. Selezska, C. Rohde, J. Sikorski, M. Rohde, D. Jahn and M. Schobert (2010). Characterization of JG024, a pseudomonas aeruginosa PB1-like broad host range phage under simulated infection conditions. *BMC Microbiol* 10: 301.

Geske, G. D., R. J. Wezeman, A. P. Siegel and H. E. Blackwell (2005). Small molecule inhibitors of bacterial quorum sensing and biofilm formation. *J Am Chem Soc* 127(37): 12762-3.

Gibson, R. L., J. L. Burns and B. W. Ramsey (2003). Pathophysiology and management of pulmonary infections in cystic fibrosis. *Am J Respir Crit Care Med* 168(8): 918-51.

Gomez, M. I. and A. Prince (2007). Opportunistic infections in lung disease: Pseudomonas infections in cystic fibrosis. *Curr Opin Pharmacol* 7(3): 244-51.

Gooderham, W. J. and R. E. Hancock (2009). Regulation of virulence and antibiotic resistance by two-component regulatory systems in Pseudomonas aeruginosa. *FEMS Microbiol Rev* 33(2): 279-94.

Goodman, A. L., B. Kulasekara, A. Rietsch, D. Boyd, R. S. Smith and S. Lory (2004). A signaling network reciprocally regulates genes associated with acute infection and chronic persistence in Pseudomonas aeruginosa. *Dev Cell* 7(5): 745-54.

Govan, J. R. and V. Deretic (1996). Microbial pathogenesis in cystic fibrosis: mucoid Pseudomonas aeruginosa and Burkholderia cepacia. *Microbiol Rev* 60(3): 539-74.

Grimwood, K., R. A. Semple, H. R. Rabin, P. A. Sokol and D. E. Woods (1993). Elevated exoenzyme expression by Pseudomonas aeruginosa is correlated with exacerbations of lung disease in cystic fibrosis. *Pediatr Pulmonol* 15(3): 135-9.

Grubb, B. R. and R. C. Boucher (1999). Pathophysiology of gene-targeted mouse models for cystic fibrosis. *Physiol Rev* 79(1 Suppl): S193-214.

Hansen, C. R., T. Pressler and N. Hoiby (2008). Early aggressive eradication therapy for intermittent Pseudomonas aeruginosa airway colonization in cystic fibrosis patients: 15 years experience. *J Cyst Fibros* 7(6): 523-30.

Harmsen, M., L. Yang, S. J. Pamp and T. Tolker-Nielsen (2010). An update on Pseudomonas aeruginosa biofilm formation, tolerance, and dispersal. *FEMS Immunol Med Microbiol* 59(3): 253-68.

Hayes, D., Jr., D. J. Feola, B. S. Murphy, R. J. Kuhn and G. A. Davis (2011). Eradication of Pseudomonas aeruginosa in an adult patient with cystic fibrosis. *Am J Health Syst Pharm* 68(4): 319-22.

Heeb, S., M. P. Fletcher, S. R. Chhabra, S. P. Diggle, P. Williams and M. Camara (2011). Quinolones: from antibiotics to autoinducers. *FEMS Microbiol Rev* 35(2): 247-74.

Hentzer, M., K. Riedel, T. B. Rasmussen, A. Heydorn, J. B. Andersen, M. R. Parsek, S. A. Rice, L. Eberl, S. Molin, N. Hoiby, S. Kjelleberg and M. Givskov (2002). Inhibition of quorum sensing in Pseudomonas aeruginosa biofilm bacteria by a halogenated furanone compound. *Microbiology* 148(Pt 1): 87-102.

Hentzer, M., G. M. Teitzel, G. J. Balzer, A. Heydorn, S. Molin, M. Givskov and M. R. Parsek (2001). Alginate overproduction affects Pseudomonas aeruginosa biofilm structure and function. *J Bacteriol* 183(18): 5395-401.

Hinsa, S. M., M. Espinosa-Urgel, J. L. Ramos and G. A. O'Toole (2003). Transition from reversible to irreversible attachment during biofilm formation by Pseudomonas fluorescens WCS365 requires an ABC transporter and a large secreted protein. *Mol Microbiol* 49(4): 905-18.

Hoffmann, N., T. B. Rasmussen, P. O. Jensen, C. Stub, M. Hentzer, S. Molin, O. Ciofu, M. Givskov, H. K. Johansen and N. Hoiby (2005). Novel mouse model of chronic Pseudomonas aeruginosa lung infection mimicking cystic fibrosis. *Infect Immun* 73(4): 2504-14.

Hogan, D. A. and R. Kolter (2002). Pseudomonas-Candida interactions: an ecological role for virulence factors. *Science* 296(5576): 2229-32.

Hoiby, N., O. Ciofu and T. Bjarnsholt (2010). Pseudomonas aeruginosa biofilms in cystic fibrosis. *Future Microbiol* 5(11): 1663-74.

Hoiby, N., O. Ciofu, H. K. Johansen, Z. J. Song, C. Moser, P. O. Jensen, S. Molin, M. Givskov, T. Tolker-Nielsen and T. Bjarnsholt (2011). The clinical impact of bacterial biofilms. *Int J Oral Sci* 3(2): 55-65.

Hoiby, N., B. Frederiksen and T. Pressler (2005). Eradication of early Pseudomonas aeruginosa infection. *J Cyst Fibros* 4 Suppl 2: 49-54.

Hughes, K. T. and K. Mathee (1998). The anti-sigma factors. *Annu Rev Microbiol* 52: 231-86.

Jaffar-Bandjee, M. C., A. Lazdunski, M. Bally, J. Carrere, J. P. Chazalette and C. Galabert (1995). Production of elastase, exotoxin A, and alkaline protease in sputa during pulmonary exacerbation of cystic fibrosis in patients chronically infected by Pseudomonas aeruginosa. *J Clin Microbiol* 33(4): 924-9.

Jain, M., M. Bar-Meir, S. McColley, J. Cullina, E. Potter, C. Powers, M. Prickett, R. Seshadri, B. Jovanovic, A. Petrocheilou, J. D. King and A. R. Hauser (2008). Evolution of Pseudomonas aeruginosa type III secretion in cystic fibrosis: a paradigm of chronic infection. *Transl Res* 152(6): 257-64.

Jain, M., D. Ramirez, R. Seshadri, J. F. Cullina, C. A. Powers, G. S. Schulert, M. Bar-Meir, C. L. Sullivan, S. A. McColley and A. R. Hauser (2004). Type III secretion phenotypes of Pseudomonas aeruginosa strains change during infection of individuals with cystic fibrosis. *J Clin Microbiol* 42(11): 5229-37.

Kaneko, Y., M. Thoendel, O. Olakanmi, B. E. Britigan and P. K. Singh (2007). The transition metal gallium disrupts Pseudomonas aeruginosa iron metabolism and has antimicrobial and antibiofilm activity. *J Clin Invest* 117(4): 877-88.

Keays, T., W. Ferris, K. L. Vandemheen, F. Chan, S. W. Yeung, T. F. Mah, K. Ramotar, R. Saginur and S. D. Aaron (2009). A retrospective analysis of biofilm antibiotic susceptibility testing: a better predictor of clinical response in cystic fibrosis exacerbations. *J Cyst Fibros* 8(2): 122-7.

Kirov, S. M., J. S. Webb, Y. O'May C, D. W. Reid, J. K. Woo, S. A. Rice and S. Kjelleberg (2007). Biofilm differentiation and dispersal in mucoid Pseudomonas aeruginosa isolates from patients with cystic fibrosis. *Microbiology* 153(Pt 10): 3264-74.

Kuchma, S. L., J. P. Connolly and G. A. O'Toole (2005). A three-component regulatory system regulates biofilm maturation and type III secretion in Pseudomonas aeruginosa. *J Bacteriol* 187(4): 1441-54.

Kulasekara, H. D., I. Ventre, B. R. Kulasekara, A. Lazdunski, A. Filloux and S. Lory (2005). A novel two-component system controls the expression of Pseudomonas aeruginosa fimbrial cup genes. *Mol Microbiol* 55(2): 368-80.

Lam, J., R. Chan, K. Lam and J. W. Costerton (1980). Production of mucoid microcolonies by Pseudomonas aeruginosa within infected lungs in cystic fibrosis. *Infect Immun* 28(2): 546-56.

Laskowski, M. A., E. Osborn and B. I. Kazmierczak (2004). A novel sensor kinase-response regulator hybrid regulates type III secretion and is required for virulence in Pseudomonas aeruginosa. *Mol Microbiol* 54(4): 1090-103.

Lewis, K. (2005). Persister cells and the riddle of biofilm survival. *Biochemistry (Mosc)* 70(2): 267-74.

Lipuma, J. J. (2010). The changing microbial epidemiology in cystic fibrosis. *Clin Microbiol Rev* 23(2): 299-323.

Lyczak, J. B., C. L. Cannon and G. B. Pier (2000). Establishment of Pseudomonas aeruginosa infection: lessons from a versatile opportunist. *Microbes Infect* 2(9): 1051-60.

Lyczak, J. B., C. L. Cannon and G. B. Pier (2002). Lung infections associated with cystic fibrosis. *Clin Microbiol Rev* 15(2): 194-222.

Mah, T. F. and G. A. O'Toole (2001). Mechanisms of biofilm resistance to antimicrobial agents. *Trends Microbiol* 9(1): 34-9.

Mah, T. F., B. Pitts, B. Pellock, G. C. Walker, P. S. Stewart and G. A. O'Toole (2003). A genetic basis for Pseudomonas aeruginosa biofilm antibiotic resistance. *Nature* 426(6964): 306-10.

Mall, M., B. R. Grubb, J. R. Harkema, W. K. O'Neal and R. C. Boucher (2004). Increased airway epithelial Na+ absorption produces cystic fibrosis-like lung disease in mice. *Nat Med* 10(5): 487-93.

McCoy, K. S., A. L. Quittner, C. M. Oermann, R. L. Gibson, G. Z. Retsch-Bogart and A. B. Montgomery (2008). Inhaled aztreonam lysine for chronic airway Pseudomonas aeruginosa in cystic fibrosis. *Am J Respir Crit Care Med* 178(9): 921-8.

Miyata, S., M. Casey, D. W. Frank, F. M. Ausubel and E. Drenkard (2003). Use of the Galleria mellonella caterpillar as a model host to study the role of the type III secretion system in Pseudomonas aeruginosa pathogenesis. *Infect Immun* 71(5): 2404-13.

Monds, R. D., P. D. Newell, R. H. Gross and G. A. O'Toole (2007). Phosphate-dependent modulation of c-di-GMP levels regulates Pseudomonas fluorescens Pf0-1 biofilm formation by controlling secretion of the adhesin LapA. *Mol Microbiol* 63(3): 656-79.

Moore, N. M. and M. L. Flaws (2011). Epidemiology and pathogenesis of Pseudomonas aeruginosa infections. *Clin Lab Sci* 24(1): 43-6.

Moreau-Marquis, S., J. M. Bomberger, G. G. Anderson, A. Swiatecka-Urban, S. Ye, G. A. O'Toole and B. A. Stanton (2008). The {Delta}F508-CFTR mutation results in increased biofilm formation by Pseudomonas aeruginosa by increasing iron availability. *Am J Physiol Lung Cell Mol Physiol* 295(1): L25-37.

Moreau-Marquis, S., G. A. O'Toole and B. A. Stanton (2009). Tobramycin and FDA-approved iron chelators eliminate Pseudomonas aeruginosa biofilms on cystic fibrosis cells. *Am J Respir Cell Mol Biol* 41(3): 305-13.

Moreau-Marquis, S., C. V. Redelman, B. A. Stanton and G. G. Anderson (2010). Co-culture Models of Pseudomonas aeruginosa Biofilms Grown on Live Human Airway Cells. *J Vis Exp*(44): e2186.

Moskowitz, S. M., J. C. Emerson, S. McNamara, R. D. Shell, D. M. Orenstein, D. Rosenbluth, M. F. Katz, R. Ahrens, D. Hornick, P. M. Joseph, R. L. Gibson, M. L. Aitken, W. W. Benton and J. L. Burns (2011). Randomized trial of biofilm testing to select antibiotics for cystic fibrosis airway infection. *Pediatr Pulmonol* 46(2): 184-92.

Mowat, E., S. Paterson, J. L. Fothergill, E. A. Wright, M. J. Ledson, M. J. Walshaw, M. A. Brockhurst and C. Winstanley (2011). Pseudomonas aeruginosa Population Diversity and Turnover in Cystic Fibrosis Chronic Infections. *Am J Respir Crit Care Med* 183(12): 1674-9.

Nichols, W. W., S. M. Dorrington, M. P. Slack and H. L. Walmsley (1988). Inhibition of tobramycin diffusion by binding to alginate. *Antimicrob Agents Chemother* 32(4): 518-23.

O'Toole, G., H. B. Kaplan and R. Kolter (2000). Biofilm formation as microbial development. *Annu Rev Microbiol* 54: 49-79.

O'Toole, G. A. and R. Kolter (1998). Flagellar and twitching motility are necessary for Pseudomonas aeruginosa biofilm development. *Mol Microbiol* 30(2): 295-304.

Ohman, D. E. and A. M. Chakrabarty (1981). Genetic mapping of chromosomal determinants for the production of the exopolysaccharide alginate in a Pseudomonas aeruginosa cystic fibrosis isolate. *Infect Immun* 33(1): 142-8.

Ouyang, L., S. D. Grosse, D. D. Amendah and M. S. Schechter (2009). Healthcare expenditures for privately insured people with cystic fibrosis. *Pediatr Pulmonol* 44(10): 989-96.

Palmer, K. L., L. M. Aye and M. Whiteley (2007). Nutritional cues control Pseudomonas aeruginosa multicellular behavior in cystic fibrosis sputum. *J Bacteriol* 189(22): 8079-87.

Parkins, M. D. and J. S. Elborn (2010). Aztreonam lysine: a novel inhalational antibiotic for cystic fibrosis. *Expert Rev Respir Med* 4(4): 435-44.

Parkins, M. D. and J. S. Elborn (2010). Newer antibacterial agents and their potential role in cystic fibrosis pulmonary exacerbation management. *J Antimicrob Chemother* 65(9): 1853-61.

Parks, Q. M., R. L. Young, K. R. Poch, K. C. Malcolm, M. L. Vasil and J. A. Nick (2009). Neutrophil enhancement of Pseudomonas aeruginosa biofilm development: human F-actin and DNA as targets for therapy. *J Med Microbiol* 58(Pt 4): 492-502.

Parsek, M. R. and P. K. Singh (2003). Bacterial biofilms: an emerging link to disease pathogenesis. *Annu Rev Microbiol* 57: 677-701.

Patel, R. (2005). Biofilms and antimicrobial resistance. *Clin Orthop Relat Res* 437: 41-7.

Plummer, A. and M. Wildman (2011). Duration of intravenous antibiotic therapy in people with cystic fibrosis. *Cochrane Database Syst Rev*(1): CD006682.

Pressler, T., C. Bohmova, S. Conway, S. Dumcius, L. Hjelte, N. Hoiby, H. Kollberg, B. Tummler and V. Vavrova (2011). Chronic Pseudomonas aeruginosa infection definition: EuroCareCF Working Group report. *J Cyst Fibros* 10 Suppl 2: S75-8.

Rahme, L. G., E. J. Stevens, S. F. Wolfort, J. Shao, R. G. Tompkins and F. M. Ausubel (1995). Common virulence factors for bacterial pathogenicity in plants and animals. *Science* 268(5219): 1899-902.

Ramsey, D. M. and D. J. Wozniak (2005). Understanding the control of Pseudomonas aeruginosa alginate synthesis and the prospects for management of chronic infections in cystic fibrosis. *Mol Microbiol* 56(2): 309-22.

Ran, H., D. J. Hassett and G. W. Lau (2003). Human targets of Pseudomonas aeruginosa pyocyanin. *Proc Natl Acad Sci U S A* 100(24): 14315-20.

Rasmussen, T. B. and M. Givskov (2006). Quorum-sensing inhibitors as anti-pathogenic drugs. *Int J Med Microbiol* 296(2-3): 149-61.

Rasmussen, T. B., M. E. Skindersoe, T. Bjarnsholt, R. K. Phipps, K. B. Christensen, P. O. Jensen, J. B. Andersen, B. Koch, T. O. Larsen, M. Hentzer, L. Eberl, N. Hoiby and M. Givskov (2005). Identity and effects of quorum-sensing inhibitors produced by Penicillium species. *Microbiology* 151(Pt 5): 1325-40.

Ratjen, F., A. Munck, P. Kho and G. Angyalosi (2010). Treatment of early Pseudomonas aeruginosa infection in patients with cystic fibrosis: the ELITE trial. *Thorax* 65(4): 286-91.

Retsch-Bogart, G. Z., J. L. Burns, K. L. Otto, T. G. Liou, K. McCoy, C. Oermann and R. L. Gibson (2008). A phase 2 study of aztreonam lysine for inhalation to treat patients with cystic fibrosis and Pseudomonas aeruginosa infection. *Pediatr Pulmonol* 43(1): 47-58.

Rice, S. A., C. H. Tan, P. J. Mikkelsen, V. Kung, J. Woo, M. Tay, A. Hauser, D. McDougald, J. S. Webb and S. Kjelleberg (2009). The biofilm life cycle and virulence of Pseudomonas aeruginosa are dependent on a filamentous prophage. *ISME J* 3(3): 271-82.

Rogers, G. B., L. R. Hoffman, M. W. Johnson, N. Mayer-Hamblett, J. Schwarze, M. P. Carroll and K. D. Bruce (2011). Using bacterial biomarkers to identify early indicators of cystic fibrosis pulmonary exacerbation onset. *Expert Rev Mol Diagn* 11(2): 197-206.

Ryan, G., M. Singh and K. Dwan (2011). Inhaled antibiotics for long-term therapy in cystic fibrosis. *Cochrane Database Syst Rev*(3): CD001021.

Ryder, C., M. Byrd and D. J. Wozniak (2007). Role of polysaccharides in Pseudomonas aeruginosa biofilm development. *Curr Opin Microbiol* 10(6): 644-8.

Sadikot, R. T., T. S. Blackwell, J. W. Christman and A. S. Prince (2005). Pathogen-host interactions in Pseudomonas aeruginosa pneumonia. *Am J Respir Crit Care Med* 171(11): 1209-23.

Saiman, L. (2011). Infection prevention and control in cystic fibrosis. *Curr Opin Infect Dis* 24(4): 390-5.

Saiman, L. and J. Siegel (2004). Infection control in cystic fibrosis. *Clin Microbiol Rev* 17(1): 57-71.

Salunkhe, P., C. H. Smart, J. A. Morgan, S. Panagea, M. J. Walshaw, C. A. Hart, R. Geffers, B. Tummler and C. Winstanley (2005). A cystic fibrosis epidemic strain of Pseudomonas aeruginosa displays enhanced virulence and antimicrobial resistance. *J Bacteriol* 187(14): 4908-20.

Sauer, K., A. K. Camper, G. D. Ehrlich, J. W. Costerton and D. G. Davies (2002). Pseudomonas aeruginosa displays multiple phenotypes during development as a biofilm. *J Bacteriol* 184(4): 1140-54.

Shaver, C. M. and A. R. Hauser (2004). Relative contributions of Pseudomonas aeruginosa ExoU, ExoS, and ExoT to virulence in the lung. *Infect Immun* 72(12): 6969-77.

Singh, P. K., A. L. Schaefer, M. R. Parsek, T. O. Moninger, M. J. Welsh and E. P. Greenberg (2000). Quorum-sensing signals indicate that cystic fibrosis lungs are infected with bacterial biofilms. *Nature* 407(6805): 762-4.

Skindersoe, M. E., M. Alhede, R. Phipps, L. Yang, P. O. Jensen, T. B. Rasmussen, T. Bjarnsholt, T. Tolker-Nielsen, N. Hoiby and M. Givskov (2008). Effects of antibiotics on quorum sensing in Pseudomonas aeruginosa. *Antimicrob Agents Chemother* 52(10): 3648-63.

Smith, A. W. (2005). Biofilms and antibiotic therapy: is there a role for combating bacterial resistance by the use of novel drug delivery systems? *Adv Drug Deliv Rev* 57(10): 1539-50.

Smith, E. E., D. G. Buckley, Z. Wu, C. Saenphimmachak, L. R. Hoffman, D. A. D'Argenio, S. I. Miller, B. W. Ramsey, D. P. Speert, S. M. Moskowitz, J. L. Burns, R. Kaul and M. V. Olson (2006). Genetic adaptation by Pseudomonas aeruginosa to the airways of cystic fibrosis patients. *Proc Natl Acad Sci U S A* 103(22): 8487-92.

Sriramulu, D. D., H. Lunsdorf, J. S. Lam and U. Romling (2005). Microcolony formation: a novel biofilm model of Pseudomonas aeruginosa for the cystic fibrosis lung. *J Med Microbiol* 54(Pt 7): 667-76.

Starkey, M., J. H. Hickman, L. Ma, N. Zhang, S. De Long, A. Hinz, S. Palacios, C. Manoil, M. J. Kirisits, T. D. Starner, D. J. Wozniak, C. S. Harwood and M. R. Parsek (2009). Pseudomonas aeruginosa rugose small-colony variants have adaptations that likely promote persistence in the cystic fibrosis lung. *J Bacteriol* 191(11): 3492-503.

Steinberg, P. D., R. Schneider and S. Kjelleberg (1997). Chemical defenses of seaweeds against microbial colonization. *Biodegradation* 8(3): 211-220.

Stewart, P. S. and J. W. Costerton (2001). Antibiotic resistance of bacteria in biofilms. *Lancet* 358(9276): 135-8.

Stoodley, P., K. Sauer, D. G. Davies and J. W. Costerton (2002). Biofilms as complex differentiated communities. *Annu Rev Microbiol* 56: 187-209.

Stover, C. K., X. Q. Pham, A. L. Erwin, S. D. Mizoguchi, P. Warrener, M. J. Hickey, F. S. Brinkman, W. O. Hufnagle, D. J. Kowalik, M. Lagrou, R. L. Garber, L. Goltry, E. Tolentino, S. Westbrock-Wadman, Y. Yuan, L. L. Brody, S. N. Coulter, K. R. Folger, A. Kas, K. Larbig, R. Lim, K. Smith, D. Spencer, G. K. Wong, Z. Wu, I. T. Paulsen, J. Reizer, M. H. Saier, R. E. Hancock, S. Lory and M. V. Olson (2000). Complete genome sequence of Pseudomonas aeruginosa PA01, an opportunistic pathogen. *Nature* 406(6799): 959-64.

Stressmann, F. A., G. B. Rogers, P. Marsh, A. K. Lilley, T. W. Daniels, M. P. Carroll, L. R. Hoffman, G. Jones, C. E. Allen, N. Patel, B. Forbes, A. Tuck and K. D. Bruce (2011). Does bacterial density in cystic fibrosis sputum increase prior to pulmonary exacerbation? *J Cyst Fibros.*

Stuart, B., J. H. Lin and P. J. Mogayzel, Jr. (2010). Early eradication of Pseudomonas aeruginosa in patients with cystic fibrosis. *Paediatr Respir Rev* 11(3): 177-84.

Taccetti, G., S. Campana, F. Festini, M. Mascherini and G. Doring (2005). Early eradication therapy against Pseudomonas aeruginosa in cystic fibrosis patients. *Eur Respir J* 26(3): 458-61.

Tomlin, K. L., R. J. Malott, G. Ramage, D. G. Storey, P. A. Sokol and H. Ceri (2005). Quorum-sensing mutations affect attachment and stability of Burkholderia cenocepacia biofilms. *Appl Environ Microbiol* 71(9): 5208-18.

Tunney, M. M., E. R. Klem, A. A. Fodor, D. F. Gilpin, T. F. Moriarty, S. J. McGrath, M. S. Muhlebach, R. C. Boucher, C. Cardwell, G. Doering, J. S. Elborn and M. C. Wolfgang (2011). Use of culture and molecular analysis to determine the effect of antibiotic treatment on microbial community diversity and abundance during exacerbation in patients with cystic fibrosis. *Thorax* 66(7): 579-84.

VanDevanter, D. R., M. A. O'Riordan, J. L. Blumer and M. W. Konstan (2010). Assessing time to pulmonary function benefit following antibiotic treatment of acute cystic fibrosis exacerbations. *Respir Res* 11: 137.

VanDevanter, D. R. and J. M. Van Dalfsen (2005). How much do Pseudomonas biofilms contribute to symptoms of pulmonary exacerbation in cystic fibrosis? *Pediatr Pulmonol* 39(6): 504-6.

Ventre, I., A. L. Goodman, I. Vallet-Gely, P. Vasseur, C. Soscia, S. Molin, S. Bleves, A. Lazdunski, S. Lory and A. Filloux (2006). Multiple sensors control reciprocal expression of Pseudomonas aeruginosa regulatory RNA and virulence genes. *Proc Natl Acad Sci U S A* 103(1): 171-6.

Wagner, V. E., D. Bushnell, L. Passador, A. I. Brooks and B. H. Iglewski (2003). Microarray analysis of Pseudomonas aeruginosa quorum-sensing regulons: effects of growth phase and environment. *J Bacteriol* 185(7): 2080-95.

Walker, T. S., K. L. Tomlin, G. S. Worthen, K. R. Poch, J. G. Lieber, M. T. Saavedra, M. B. Fessler, K. C. Malcolm, M. L. Vasil and J. A. Nick (2005). Enhanced Pseudomonas aeruginosa biofilm development mediated by human neutrophils. *Infect Immun* 73(6): 3693-701.

Whiteley, M., M. G. Bangera, R. E. Bumgarner, M. R. Parsek, G. M. Teitzel, S. Lory and E. P. Greenberg (2001). Gene expression in Pseudomonas aeruginosa biofilms. *Nature* 413(6858): 860-4.

Wilke, M., R. M. Buijs-Offerman, J. Aarbiou, W. H. Colledge, D. N. Sheppard, L. Touqui, A. Bot, H. Jorna, H. R. de Jonge and B. J. Scholte (2011). Mouse models of cystic fibrosis: phenotypic analysis and research applications. *J Cyst Fibros* 10 Suppl 2: S152-71.

Wolfgang, M. C., J. Jyot, A. L. Goodman, R. Ramphal and S. Lory (2004). Pseudomonas aeruginosa regulates flagellin expression as part of a global response to airway fluid from cystic fibrosis patients. *Proc Natl Acad Sci U S A* 101(17): 6664-8.

Woods, D. E., D. C. Straus, W. G. Johanson, Jr., V. K. Berry and J. A. Bass (1980). Role of pili in adherence of Pseudomonas aeruginosa to mammalian buccal epithelial cells. *Infect. Immun.* 29(3): 1146-1151.

Woodward, T. C., R. Brown, P. Sacco and J. Zhang (2010). Budget impact model of tobramycin inhalation solution for treatment of Pseudomonas aeruginosa in cystic fibrosis patients. *J Med Econ* 13(3): 492-9.

Woodworth, B. A., E. Tamashiro, G. Bhargave, N. A. Cohen and J. N. Palmer (2008). An in vitro model of Pseudomonas aeruginosa biofilms on viable airway epithelial cell monolayers. *Am J Rhinol* 22(3): 235-8.

Worlitzsch, D., R. Tarran, M. Ulrich, U. Schwab, A. Cekici, K. C. Meyer, P. Birrer, G. Bellon, J. Berger, T. Weiss, K. Botzenhart, J. R. Yankaskas, S. Randell, R. C. Boucher and G. Doring (2002). Effects of reduced mucus oxygen concentration in airway Pseudomonas infections of cystic fibrosis patients. *J Clin Invest* 109(3): 317-25.

Wozniak, D. J. and R. Keyser (2004). Effects of subinhibitory concentrations of macrolide antibiotics on Pseudomonas aeruginosa. *Chest* 125(2 Suppl): 62S-69S; quiz 69S.

Wu, W., H. Badrane, S. Arora, H. V. Baker and S. Jin (2004). MucA-mediated coordination of type III secretion and alginate synthesis in Pseudomonas aeruginosa. *J Bacteriol* 186(22): 7575-85.

Yahr, T. L. and M. C. Wolfgang (2006). Transcriptional regulation of the Pseudomonas aeruginosa type III secretion system. *Mol Microbiol* 62(3): 631-40.

Yoon, S. S. and D. J. Hassett (2004). Chronic Pseudomonas aeruginosa infection in cystic fibrosis airway disease: metabolic changes that unravel novel drug targets. *Expert Rev Anti Infect Ther* 2(4): 611-23.

Zhou, Z., J. Duerr, B. Johannesson, S. C. Schubert, D. Treis, M. Harm, S. Y. Graeber, A. Dalpke, C. Schultz and M. A. Mall (2011). The ENaC-overexpressing mouse as a model of cystic fibrosis lung disease. *J Cyst Fibros* 10 Suppl 2: S172-82.

9

Outcome and Prevention of *Pseudomonas aeruginosa-Staphylococcus aureus* Interactions During Pulmonary Infections in Cystic Fibrosis

Gabriel Mitchell and François Malouin
Université de Sherbrooke
Canada

1. Introduction

Several microorganisms take advantages of the most common single gene disorder afflicting Caucasians and colonize the airways of cystic fibrosis (CF) patients. Although CF is a multi-system disorder, the associated mortality is mostly due to respiratory problems subsequent to chronic bacterial infections. CF is the result of mutations in the cystic fibrosis transmembrane conductance regulator (CFTR) which is a cAMP-regulated chloride channel and a regulator of the activity of other channels. Consequently, there is a significant dehydration of the airway mucus when CFTR is dysfunctional. However, the exact reason why CF predisposes the lungs to microbial infections is not completely understood. It is thought that the obstruction of the airways by mucus and the proinflammatory status associated with this disease may be part of the explanation (Lyczak *et al.*, 2002; Riordan, 2008).

The recalcitrance of CF pathogens to antibiotic therapies is a major problem and is responsible for most of the morbidity and the mortality associated with CF (Chmiel & Davis, 2003; Lyczak *et al.*, 2002). The ever-growing and overwhelming problems caused by antibiotic-resistant bacteria in human medicine have not spared CF patients. Antibiotic-resistant bacteria are frequently recovered from CF samples (George *et al.*, 2009; Parkins & Elborn, 2010). The evolution of drug resistance has been accelerated by the extensive use of an antibiotic arsenal which has become limited due to insufficient innovation in the development of antimicrobials (Shah, 2005; Talbot *et al.*, 2006). Indeed, the development of new classes of antibiotics has been almost abandoned for the last four decades and antibiotics that were introduced during this period usually consisted of new-generation molecules derived from existing antibiotics (Wenzel *et al.*, 2005). Furthermore, long-term infections of the CF airways not only allow pathogens to adapt and circumvent the host immune system, but also allow them time to adapt to antibiotic therapies (Goerke & Wolz, 2010; Hogardt & Heesemann, 2010). Several mechanisms that decrease the susceptibility to antimicrobials are known to be at play in the CF airways. Conventional resistance mechanisms include the upregulation of bacterial efflux pumps and mutations of antibiotic target molecules (Høiby *et al.*, 2010). In addition, the formation of persister cells (Mulcahy *et al.*, 2010) and of small-colony variants (Goerke & Wolz, 2010; Proctor *et al.*, 2006; Schneider *et al.*, 2008) as well as bacterial growth in biofilms (Høiby *et al.*, 2010; Mitchell *et al.*, 2010a,

2010b; Wagner & Iglewski, 2008) are mechanisms that are well known for their involvement in difficult-to-treat infections (Galli *et al.*, 2007; Stewart, 2002).

The formation of bacterial biofilms may explain, at least in part, the failure of many antimicrobial therapies. Biofilm-growing bacteria are highly persistent in CF because they appear to be physically protected from the host immune system and are inherently resistant to antimicrobials (Costerton *et al.*, 1999; Davies & Bilton, 2009; Høiby *et al.*, 2010; Stewart, 2002). These bacteria are thought to be as much as 1000 times more resistant to antimicrobials than their planktonic counterparts (George *et al.*, 2009). Biofilms also represent complex integrated polymicrobial communities that are strongly influenced by cell-to-cell intraspecies and interspecies communications (Costerton *et al.*, 1999; Hall-Stoodley *et al.*, 2004; Stoodley *et al.*, 2002). The different species of microbes found in polymicrobial infections such as in CF most probably respond to each other's chemical signals in order to survive and this is likely to influence the course of any particular infection (Brogden *et al.*, 2005; Ryan & Dow, 2008).

In the surge to develop new therapies against CF pathogens, multiple aspects should be considered. Indeed, several diverse phenotypic adaptations confer a selective advantage in the host environment or toward antibiotic therapies. Also to consider are the various bacterial signals used for cell-to-cell communication that are involved in the establishment and the development of an infection. These mechanisms enable pathogens from polymicrobial communities to adjust their behavior in response to other neighboring bacteria and they deserve particular attention. This chapter aims to describe some of the mechanisms used by *Pseudomonas aeruginosa* and *Staphylococcus aureus* for their mutual coexistence and persistence in the host environment, and to emphasize those that are potential targets for the development of anti-pathogenesis therapies.

2. Microbiology of CF

Colonization of the CF airways by bacteria usually occurs in infancy and results in the establishment of chronic infections which eventually lead to respiratory failure and death (Harrison, 2007; Lyczak *et al.*, 2002). Recent investigations have shown that the CF airways are colonized by complex polymicrobial communities constituted by numerous bacterial species and not only by the relatively few predominant species originally described that include *P. aeruginosa*, *S. aureus*, *Heamophilus influenzae*, bacteria from the *Burkholderia cepacia* complex and *Stenotrophomonas maltophilia* (Sibley & Surette, 2011). Notwithstanding this polymicrobial mixture, *P. aeruginosa* and *S. aureus* are still among the most prevalent and dominant bacterial species encountered in CF (Canadian Cystic Fibrosis Foundation, 2009; Cystic Fibrosis Foundation, 2009; European Cystic Fibrosis Society, 2007). It is also important to note that the prevalence of the different pathogens varies as a function of the age of patients, with *S. aureus* and *H. influenzae* being more frequent in early childhood and *P. aeruginosa* being more important as patients become older. Several other microorganisms such as *Mycobacterium* spp., pathogenic viruses, fungal pathogens (*e.g. Aspergillus fulmigatus*) and yeasts (*e.g. Candida albicans*) have also been recovered from the CF airways and may also contribute to disease (Harrison, 2007; Lyczak *et al.*, 2002; Moskowitz *et al.*, 2005). It should be kept in mind that the chronically infected CF airways represent a complex and diverse ecosystem and that the precise contribution of the different microbes to the morbidity of the disease remains undetermined, even for the less frequently encountered microorganisms (Harrison, 2007).

2.1 Pathogenesis of *P. aeruginosa* in CF

P. aeruginosa is a Gram-negative bacterium that has the ability to survive in several different natural environments. However, it is better known as an opportunistic antibiotic-resistant human pathogen often encountered in hospital settings (Bodey *et al.*, 1983). This bacterium is also known as the major cause of lung function decline and mortality in CF (Lyczak *et al.*, 2002). *P. aeruginosa* establishes infections using several virulence factors. The production of these virulence factors varies as a function of the cell density of the bacterial population and is controlled by cell-to-cell chemical communication, *i.e.* quorum-sensing or QS (R. S. Smith & Iglewski, 2003). QS systems are used by many bacteria to promote collective behaviors and depend on the action of diffusible signal molecules. QS systems are typically composed of a signal synthase that produces the signal molecule and a signal receptor that modulates the expression of target genes subsequent to the binding of the signal molecule.

QS in *P. aeruginosa* is controlled by the *las* and *rhl* N-acylhomoserine lactone (AHL) regulatory circuits and by the 2-alkyl-4-quinolone (AQ) system (Dubern & Diggle, 2008). In the *las* and *rhl* system, the *lasI* and *rhlI* gene products direct the synthesis of the homoserine lactones (HSL) 3-oxo-C12-HSL and C4-HSL, which interact with the transcription regulators LasR and RhlR, respectively, and activate target promoters. The *las* and *rhl* systems are hierarchically connected and interact together to regulate the production of several virulence determinants such as pyocyanin biosynthesis and biofilm formation (Dubern & Diggle, 2008; R. S. Smith & Iglewski, 2003). The AQ system is also interconnected with *las* and *rhl* and leads to the production of 2-heptyl-4-quinolone (HHQ) and the *Pseudomonas* quinolone signal (PQS). Both HHQ and PQS also have a role in cell-to-cell communication. However, PQS has a number of other biologically important functions (Dubern & Diggle, 2008). *P. aeruginosa* produces several other quinolone compounds, some of which, such as 4-hydroxy-2-heptylquinoline-N-oxide (HQNO), have antibiotic activity (Leisinger & Margraff, 1979; Lépine *et al.*, 2004; Machan *et al.*, 1992). It should also be kept in mind that the control of virulence factors by these systems is growth and environment dependent. This complex mixture of factors allows *P. aeruginosa* to modulate its behavior only when necessary (Williams & Camara, 2009). Interestingly, *P. aeruginosa* QS signals not only serve for intraspecies communications, but are also known to affect other microorganisms and the host (Williams & Camara, 2009). The association between the environment, *P. aeruginosa* QS systems and virulence is schematized in Fig. 1.

Substantial adaptive and genetic changes occur in the genome of *P. aeruginosa* during chronic infections of the CF airways (Foweraker *et al.*, 2005; E. E. Smith *et al.*, 2006; Sriramulu *et al.*, 2005). These changes cause bacteria to diversify and to exhibit characteristics differing from isolates found in the environment outside the body. The adaptation of *P. aeruginosa* during persistent infection of CF lungs can often lead to antimicrobial resistance, alginate overproduction and improved metabolic fitness. Overall, *P. aeruginosa* seems able to adopt a less aggressive profile by repressing its virulence factors and its immunostimulatory products, by growing in biofilms and by metabolically adapting to the microaerobic environment created by airway mucus plugs (Hogardt & Heesemann, 2010). Of these characteristics it appears that the formation of drug-resistant biofilms is strongly associated with the persistence of this bacterium in the CF airways (Høiby *et al.*, 2010; Wagner &

Iglewski, 2008). Also, non-mucoid strains that colonize CF patients can, with time, switch to the mucoid phenotype, show resistance to various antibiotics and become more difficult to eradicate from the airways (George *et al.*, 2009). Other phenotypic variants associated with chronic infections and antibiotic tolerance have also been recovered from the CF airways such as persister cells (Mulcahy *et al.*, 2010) and small-colony variants (Häußler *et al.*, 1999; Schneider *et al.*, 2008). The hypermutability of *P. aeruginosa* CF strains is thought to accelerate the development of antibiotic resistances and the adaptation required for long-term persistence in the host (Maciá *et al.*, 2005).

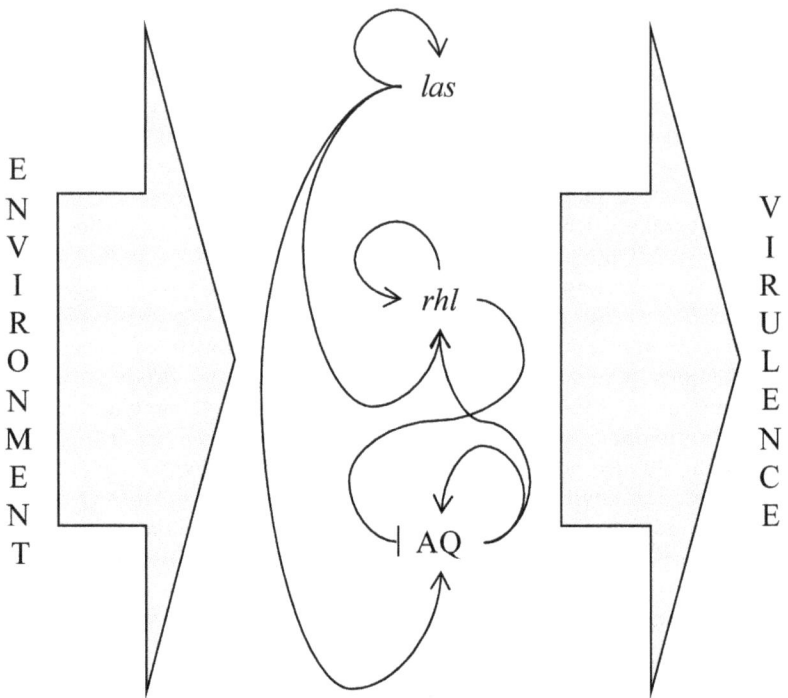

Fig. 1. The virulence of *P. aeruginosa* is controlled by interconnected quorum-sensing (QS) systems that integrate environmental cues and influence virulence gene expression. The two N-acylhomoserine lactone systems *las* and *rhl* and the 2-alkyl-4-quinolone (AQ) system are hierarchically interconnected. The *las* system is usually activated first. These QS systems regulate the production of several virulence factors as a function of growth and in response to the environment not only to influence *P. aeruginosa* behavior but also other bacteria of the microbial community as well as host-pathogen interactions.

2.2 Pathogenesis of *S. aureus* in CF

S. aureus can live as a human commensal but also can be an opportunistic Gram-positive pathogen associated with significant mortality in hospitals (Talbot *et al.*, 2006). This bacterium demonstrates an impressive versatility being able to infect several hosts, organs and body sites and cause both life-threatening and chronic infections (Archer, 1998; Goerke & Wolz, 2010). The treatment of *S. aureus* is seriously impeded by antibiotic resistance that has spread among staphylococci and is now being considered as a serious threat to the general population (Witte *et al.*, 2008).

The presence of numerous virulence genes in the genome of *S. aureus* is thought to explain the ability of this bacterium to cause a broad spectrum of diseases (Archer, 1998). The genes involved in pathogenesis are tightly controlled by complex regulatory networks that allow the bacteria to express its virulence factors as a function of the bacterial population density and of its environment (Novick, 2003). One of the most characterized regulatory systems influencing the virulence of *S. aureus* is *agr*, the quorum-sensing accessory gene regulator, that upregulates the production of several extracellular proteins while downregulating many cell-surface proteins (Novick & Geisinger, 2008). Other regulatory networks that govern the expression of accessory genes in *S. aureus* include several two-component regulatory systems and transcription factors such as the alternative sigma factor SigB (Bronner *et al.*, 2004; Novick, 2003). The activity of particular virulence regulators is thought to allow the expression of different sets of factors likely to be required at specific steps during infection or needed for different types of infections.

The contribution of *S. aureus* to the progression of disease in CF is less obvious than that of *P. aeruginosa*. Although the presence of this bacterium in the lower respiratory tract is considered as representative of a pathologic situation, there are still questions concerning the impact of *S. aureus* on the progression of the disease (Lyczak *et al.*, 2002). However, recent data indicate that while the prevalence of *P. aeruginosa* has declined among CF patients over the past few years, the incidence of methicillin-suceptible and methicillin-resistant *S. aureus* (MSSA and MRSA, respectively) has increased in the USA (Razvi *et al.*, 2009). Importantly, detection of persistent MRSA in the respiratory tract of CF patients has been associated with a decrease in survival and with a more rapid decline in lung function (Dasenbrook *et al.*, 2008; Dasenbrook *et al.*, 2010). Furthermore, MRSA bacteria often present a phenotype of mutiresistance to antibiotics (Chambers & Deleo, 2009; Pruneau *et al.*, 2011) and are proficient in biofilm production (Molina *et al.*, 2008).

Notwithstanding these findings, *S. aureus* often persists in the CF lungs for many months or even years and is the cause of recurrent and relapsing infections despite antibiotic treatments (Goerke & Wolz, 2010; B. C. Kahl, 2010). Long-term adaptation of *S. aureus* to the CF environment may occur through mutations (such as those causing the small-colony variant [SCV] phenotype) or through regulatory mechanisms that are still not well understood and that may result in the repression of the *agr* system and establishment of biofilms (Goerke & Wolz, 2010).

SCVs of *S. aureus* are often isolated from chronic infections such as those of the CF airways (Kahl *et al.*, 1998; Moisan *et al.*, 2006; Proctor *et al.*, 2006). The SCV phenotype is frequently caused by either mutations in genes required for electron transport (*e.g.* genes involved in the biosynthesis of hemin or menadione) or by mutations in genes enabling thymidine biosynthesis. Almost all the phenotypic characteristics of SCVs such as the slow growth (*i.e.*, the formation of pin-point colonies when grown on solid media), the altered susceptibility to aminoglycoside antibiotics and the decreased production of exotoxins can be explained by their dysfunctional electron transport (Proctor *et al.*, 2006). Several studies have reported that SCVs are less virulent than prototypical strains *in vivo* yet they can persist as well as the normal strains (Proctor *et al.*, 2006). Our group and others have demonstrated that SCVs are relatively more persistent than their normal counterparts under antibiotic pressure (Bates *et al.*, 2003; Brouillette *et al.*, 2004). A recent study supports the theory that bacterial switching between wild-type and SCV phenotypes is required to sustain chronic infections (Tuchscherr *et al.*, 2011).

The hypothesis that SCVs play a role in the development of chronic infections is well supported by *in vitro* experiments demonstrating that these variants have an increased ability to adhere to host tissue components (Mitchell *et al.*, 2008; Vaudaux *et al.*, 2002), to form biofilms (Mitchell *et al.*, 2010a, 2010b; Singh *et al.*, 2009, 2010) and to infect and persist within non-professional phagocytes (Mitchell *et al.*, 2011b; Sendi & Proctor, 2009). These *in vitro* characteristics can be explained by the impact of the defective electron transport chain on the expression of virulence factors which seem to be mostly controlled by the activity of SigB rather than by the *agr* system in SCVs (Moisan *et al.*, 2006; Senn *et al.*, 2005). This altered activation of virulence regulators triggers a sustained expression of several genes encoding cell-surface proteins (*e.g.* the fibronectin-binding protein A *fnbA* gene) and the down-regulation of several exoprotein genes (*e.g.* the hemolysin-α *hla* gene) (Mitchell *et al.*, 2008; Moisan *et al.*, 2006). The sustained expression of *fnbA* has been associated with efficient binding of SCVs to fibronectin (Mitchell *et al.*, 2008). In turn, the formation of a fibronectin bridge between *S. aureus* fibronectin-binding proteins and the $\alpha_5\beta_1$-integrin of eukaryotic cells (Sinha *et al.*, 1999) probably explains the proficient cellular internalization of SCVs (Sendi & Proctor, 2009). Additionally, the low production of exoproteins and toxins by SCVs is likely to account for their increased persistence within host cells (Sendi & Proctor, 2009). Moreover, the increased production of biofilm by SCVs in comparison with wild-type strains may possibly be explained by the relative influence and the interconnection of the *agr* system and SigB that manipulate the maturation of protein-dependent biofilms (Lauderdale *et al.*, 2009). Furthermore, SCVs have been shown to activate the innate immune response to a lesser extent than that observed with wild-type strains (Tuchscherr *et al.*, 2010). This reduced ability of SCVs to induce an inflammatory response may also be attributable to the repression of the *agr* system (Grundmeier *et al.*, 2010) and supports the idea that the SCV phenotype confers on *S. aureus* the ability to remain hidden from the host immune system inside non-professional phagocytes. However, to date, the *in vitro* observations that suggest that the formation of biofilms and the infection of host cells by SCVs allow *S. aureus* to establish long-term infections in CF patients have not been supported by *in vivo* experiments. Further work is required, especially in CF models of pulmonary infections, in order to fully understand the role of SCVs in the pathogenesis of *S. aureus*. Some of the characteristics of the normal and SCV strains are compared in Fig. 2.

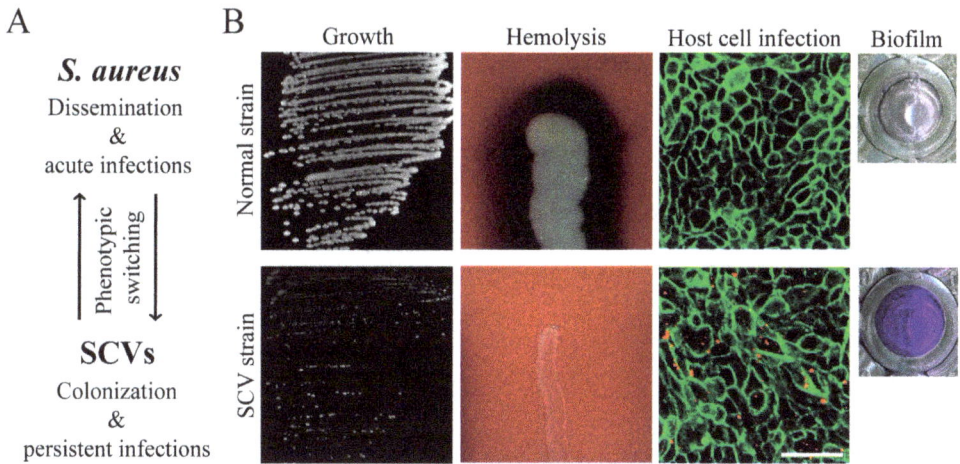

Fig. 2. The ability to switch from the normal to the small-colony variant (SCV) phenotype
may have an impact on the virulence of S. aureus. (A) S. aureus can switch from a normal to a
SCV phenotype. The normal and SCV phenotypes are associated with the dissemination of
bacteria and acute infections, and with host tissue colonization and persistent infections,
respectively. In comparison to normal strains, SCVs form pinpoint colonies, are less or non-
hemolytic on blood agar plates and have an increased ability to infect non-professional
phagocytes and to form biofilms (B). The host-cell infection pictures were prepared as
previously described (Mitchell et al., 2011a, 2011b) and show Calu-3 cells with actin colored
in green and internalized S. aureus bacteria in red. Scale bar is 50 µm. Biofilm formation was
evaluated by crystal violet staining as previously decribed (Mitchell et al., 2010a, 2010b).

3. Interspecies interactions between CF pathogens

It is now accepted that bacteria can sense signal molecules across species' boundaries and
that this signaling influences the development of microbial communities and the virulence
and persistence of pathogens during infections (Ryan & Dow, 2008). The clinical impact of
polymicrobial infections is receiving more and more recognition from the medical
community. There are indeed several examples of polymicrobial infections where at least
two different microorganisms influence the course of the disease by synergistic, additive or
antagonistic effects. Also, biofilms are thought to be of major importance for the
pathogenesis of bacteria in the context of CF lung infections (Davies & Bilton, 2009) and can
be considered as integrated and complex polymicrobial communities whose development is
controlled by interspecies communications (Stoodley et al., 2002). Accordingly, and as
previously underlined, infections of the CF airways is highly polymicrobic and there is
growing evidence that many of these microorganisms interact (Sibley & Surette, 2011) as
observed between P. aeruginosa and S. aureus (Biswas et al., 2009; Hoffman et al., 2006;
Mashburn et al., 2005; Mitchell et al., 2010b; Qazi et al., 2006; Yang et al., 2011), P. aeruginosa
and Burkholderia spp. (Bakkal et al., 2010; Chattoraj et al., 2010; Riedel et al., 2001; Weaver &
Kolter, 2004), P. aeruginosa and S. maltophilia (Ryan et al., 2008), P. aeruginosa and C. albicans
(McAlester et al., 2008), and more generally with a large proportion of the organisms found
in the CF airways (Duan et al., 2003; Sibley et al., 2008).

3.1 Interactions between *P. aeruginosa* and *S. aureus*

Given that *P. aeruginosa* and *S. aureus* are highly prevalent and commonly co-isolated from the CF airways (Harrison, 2007; Hoffman *et al.*, 2006), a great deal of effort has been directed toward the characterization of the interaction between them. Historically, synergistic interactions between these two species have been proposed and it was thought that *S. aureus* could sensitize the lungs for subsequent infections by *P. aeruginosa* (Lyczak *et al.*, 2002). However, it is now clear that antagonistic interactions also exist between these bacteria as *P. aeruginosa* has the ability to provoke lysis of *S. aureus* cells (Mashburn *et al.*, 2005; Palmer *et al.*, 2005). The structures of some *P. aeruginosa* exoproducts that are known to impact on *S. aureus* are shown in Fig. 3.

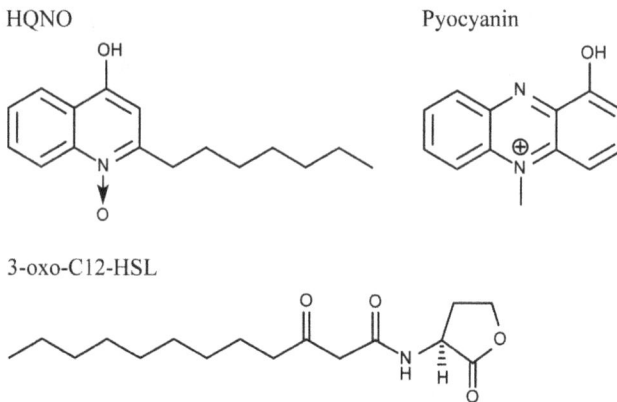

Fig. 3. Structure of *P. aeruginosa* molecules influencing *S. aureus* viability and pathogenesis.

The antistaphylococcal activities of pseudomonal HQNO (see Fig. 3) and other 4-hydroxy-2-alkylquinolines (HAQs) have been known for many years and are molecules that can generally suppress the growth of many Gram-positive bacteria (Lightbown & Jackson, 1954; Machan *et al.*, 1992). Mashburn *et al.* (2005) suggested that *P. aeruginosa* could exploit this property to lyse *S. aureus* cells in order to use the released iron for growth in low-iron environments. Interestingly, HQNO also allows some Gram-positive to grow slowly in presence of aminoglycoside antibiotics (Lightbown, 1954) and the reason for this has remained a mystery for several years. The protection provided by HQNO against the inhibitory activity of aminoglycosides was finally found to be related to the ability of this molecule to inhibit the Gram-positive electron transport chain (Hoffman *et al.*, 2006), which is required for aminoglycoside uptake (Bryan & Van Den Elzen, 1977). It was further shown that prolonged exposure of *S. aureus* to HQNO (or to *P. aeruginosa*) selects for SCVs (Hoffman *et al.*, 2006). We subsequently demonstrated that HQNO produced by *P. aeruginosa* not only stimulates the formation of *S. aureus* biofilms but also modulates the activity of virulence regulators. More particularly, while increasing the activity of SigB and the expression of *sarA*, HQNO downregulates the expression of the effector of the *agr* system (RNAIII). This modulation of regulator activities is likely to influence the expression of several virulence factors as was shown for *fnbA* and *hla* (Mitchell *et al.*, 2010b). The interaction of PQS with the cell envelope of *P. aeruginosa* is also known to trigger the release of membrane vesicles (MVs) which contain toxins, DNA, antimicrobials as well as HHQ, PQS and HQNO. It is thought that MVs are important for the trafficking of PQS within the *P. aeruginosa* population as PQS is poorly soluble in water. However, since MVs contain AQs including HQNO, they could also inhibit staphylococcal growth (Mashburn & Whiteley, 2005). Furthermore, *P. aeruginosa* produces other small-molecule respiratory inhibitors such as pyocyanin (see Fig. 3) and hydrogen cyanide which can affect the respiration of *S. aureus* (Voggu *et al.*, 2006) and potentially select for the SCV phenotype (Biswas *et al.*, 2009). Whether and how these other respiratory inhibitors influence the virulence of *S. aureus* remains to be determined. Fig. 4 shows the effect of *P. aeruginosa* on the growth of *S. aureus*, the HQNO-mediated emergence of SCVs and the stimulation of *S. aureus* biofilm production by HQNO.

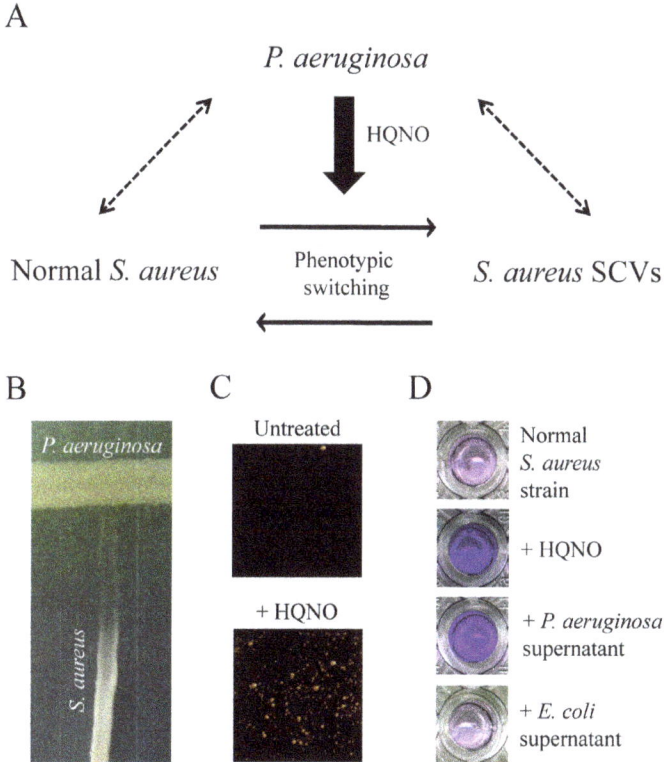

Fig. 4. *P. aeruginosa* influences the phenotypic switching of *S. aureus* and may have an impact on its virulence. (A) *P. aeruginosa* promotes the emergence of SCVs from normal *S. aureus* strains through the production of respiratory inhibitors such as HQNO and pyocyanin. Dotted arrows indicate other potential interactions between these bacterial species. (B) *P. aeruginosa* inhibits the growth of *S. aureus*. (C) HQNO stimulates the emergence of SCVs in *S. aureus*. Bacteria were treated or not with 10 µg/ml of HQNO for 18 h and plated on agar containing gentamicin at 4 µg/ml to reveal the presence of SCVs. (D) HQNO and *P. aeruginosa* culture supernatants enhance biofilm production by a normal *S. aureus* strain. *S. aureus* biofilms were produced in the presence of 10 µg/ml of HQNO or in the presence of culture supernatants from *P. aeruginosa* or *Escherichia coli* (acting as a negative control) and were revealed by crystal violet staining as previously described (Mitchell *et al.*, 2010a, 2010b).

It also appears that factors other than pseudomonal respiratory inhibitors are involved in the microbial interactions occurring between *P. aeruginosa* and *S. aureus*. Importantly, most of the antistaphylococcal activity found in *P. aeruginosa* culture supernatant is attributed to the staphylolytic endopeptidase LasA (Kessler *et al.*, 1993). Qazi *et al.* (2006) demonstrated that some long-chain 3-oxo-substituted *N*-acylhomoserine lactones (AHL) such as 3-oxo-C12-homoserine lactone (see Fig. 3) can inhibit the growth of *S. aureus* as a function of their concentrations. The 3-oxo-C12-HSL also modulates the production of *S. aureus* exotoxins and cell-surface proteins through the repression of *sarA* and *agr* by interaction with a specific and saturable receptor(s) at the cytoplasmic membrane. Furthermore, the 3-oxo-C12-HSL is capable of undergoing internal re-arrangement to form the 3-oxo-C12-tetrameric acid, which also has an inhibitory activity against Gram-positive bacteria (Kaufmann *et al.*, 2005). A recent study investigated the formation of biofilms by *P. aeruginosa-S. aureus* co-cultures using a flow chamber system and confocal microscopy (Yang *et al.*, 2011). This study demonstrated that wild-type *P. aeruginosa* facilitates *S. aureus* microcolony formation, but that *mucA* and *rpoN* mutants do not have this property and tend to outcompete *S. aureus*. A role for type IV pili in this phenomenon was proposed to occur through binding of extracellular DNA, and it was demonstrated that *P. aeruginosa* protects *S. aureus* against *Dictyostelium discoideum* phagocytosis when in co-culture biofilms.

Some studies have been carried out to substantiate the interactions between *P. aeruginosa* and *Staphylococcus epidermidis*, a bacterium closely related to *S. aureus*. It was shown that some *P. aeruginosa* extracellular products (possibly polysaccharides) provide a competitive advantage over *S. epidermidis* (Qin *et al.*, 2009). Furthermore, Pihl *et al.* (Pihl *et al.*, 2010a, 2010b) demonstrated that some *S. epidermidis* strains were better fitted than others to coexist in biofilms with *P. aeruginosa* whereas the ability of *P. aeruginosa* to inhibit *S. epidermidis* biofilms varied between clinical isolates. These authors suggested that specific *P. aeruginosa* strains might be selected during infections to counteract chronic colonization by *S. epidermidis* in order to allow the persistence and dominance of *P. aeruginosa*. Whether the genetic background of each strain also influences interspecies interactions between *S. aureus* and *P. aeruginosa* and whether the outcome of these interactions varies in each CF patient remains to be determined. Recent studies, which demontrate that *P. aeruginosa lasR* mutants are frequently found in CF, indicate that some of the abilities of this bacterium to influence the virulence of *S. aureus* may indeed be lost during CF lung infections (D'Argenio *et al.*, 2007; Hoffman *et al.*, 2009).

Other questions remain open. For example, the real impact of *S. aureus-P. aeruginosa* co-infections in CF is not known and convincing clinical data as well as co-infection in adequate experimental models are clearly missing. Whether *S. aureus* and *P. aeruginosa* have a synergistic or antagonistic effect on the progression of the disease is not known and may potentially be influenced by the nature of each clinical isolate. Furthermore, whereas the effect of *P. aeruginosa* on *S. aureus* has been studied widely, almost no investigations address the potential effect of *S. aureus* on the virulence of *P. aeruginosa*. Interestingly, Korgaonkar and Whiteley (2011) proposed a model in which *P. aeruginosa* senses surrounding bacteria by monitoring the presence of exogenous peptidoglycan and responds to it by increasing the production of the virulence factor pyocyanin.

4. New therapeutic approaches in CF

Humanity is now facing a post-antibiotic era defined by its limited capability to combat microbial infections caused by antibiotic resistant pathogens. The increased number of nosocomial and community-acquired infections caused by microorganisms resistant to at least two classes of conventional antibiotics is becoming an important public health problem. The global rise of antimicrobial resistance combined with the slow discovery and approval processes for classical antibiotics has resulted in the present urgent need for new and innovative therapeutic approaches. One of the reasons for multidrug resistance is that current antibiotics were designed around a limited number of chemical scaffolds with few major modifications since the 1980s. This has left plenty of opportunities for antibiotic resistance mechanisms to develop and spread worldwide (Shah, 2005; Talbot *et al.*, 2006). The identification of new antimicrobial targets and the development of novel therapeutic approaches may be facilitated by a better understanding of bacterial pathogenesis both at the single species and bacterial community levels. Antibiotic resistant bacteria are often recovered from CF patients but recalcitrance to antibiotic therapies is not only caused by bacterial genes that encode conventional mechanisms of antibiotic resistance. Indeed, the ever changing epidemiology of the CF airways (Razvi *et al.*, 2009) and the acquisition of bacterial phenotypes inherently resistant to antimicrobials contribute to treatment failures. Although some antibiotics have recently been approved or are close to being approved for clinical use and are promising in the context of CF (Parkins & Elborn, 2010), this section will talk about some novel therapeutic approaches that take into account the pathogenesis and the adaptation of CF pathogens in the context of polymicrobial infections. However, in order to appreciate the entirety of the efforts directed toward the cure of CF, it should be kept in mind that a number of strategies other than those using antibiotherapies are also being considered (George *et al.*, 2009).

4.1 Modulation of biofilm-forming microbial communities

The formation of biofilms by CF pathogens is thought to be a major virulence asset that promotes resistance both to antimicrobials and the host immune system (Costerton *et al.*, 1999; Davies & Bilton, 2009; Høiby *et al.*, 2010; Stewart, 2002). This fully justifies current research aimed at the development of therapeutic strategies that target biofilm formation and dispersal (Simões, 2011). Current management practices for *P. aeruginosa* infections include hygienic measures (Høiby & Pedersen, 1989), early aggressive eradication by antimicrobial therapy (Döring & Høiby, 2004), the use of nebulized DNAse (Frederiksen *et al.*, 2006) and chronic suppressive antibiotic therapy (Bjarnsholt *et al.*, 2009; Döring *et al.*, 2000). However, even if these methods are undeniably successful to a certain extent, chronic infection ultimately occurs and a gradual increase in the level of resistance is observed (Ciofu *et al.*, 1994). New therapeutic approaches specifically targeting biofilms should thus be useful in the context of CF lung infections and should decrease the occurrence or development of antibiotic resistance.

Most natural biofilms are polymicrobial (Stoodley *et al.*, 2002) and the polymicrobial nature of CF lung infections needs to be considered in novel therapeutic approaches (Sibley *et al.*, 2009; Sibley & Surette, 2011). Whereas some microbes may predispose the tissue toward the colonization by others, there may also be competition among bacterial populations and the removal of one pathogen could create an opportunity for another to expand (Harrison,

2007). On the other hand, tampering with the CF airway microbial community may lead to more effective treatment of chronic infections (Moore *et al.*, 2005). Some data even suggest that a healthy gut microflora protects against some respiratory pathogens (Alvarez *et al.*, 2001; Villena *et al.*, 2005) and that care should be taken not to deplete the gut microflora when oral or intravenous routes of antibiotic administration are used. It is also conceivable that monitoring the population dynamics of polymicrobial infections can be used to predict the efficacy of antimicrobial therapy and to optimize treatments (Rogers *et al.*, 2010). As such, the impact of antimicrobial chemotherapies on microbial communities should be assessed to detect unwanted effects. As an example, aminoglycosides, which are indicated for the management of acute exacerbations, the control of chronic infections and the eradication of recently acquired *P. aeruginosa*, have also been shown to induce bacterial biofilms in both *P. aeruginosa* (Hoffman *et al.*, 2005) and *S. aureus* (Mitchell *et al.*, 2010a).

The next sections provide examples of methods by which biofilm infections may be potentially overcome using different strategies that include targeting specific microbial phenotypes, influencing the pathogenesis of bacteria through the manipulation of cell-to-cell signaling and the enhancement of preexisting antimicrobial therapies against persistent forms of bacteria.

4.2 Targeting the persistent microbial phenotype

Bacteria often encounter unfavorable conditions during infection that limit bacterial growth and oblige the microorganisms to enter a quiescent state in order to persist within the host (Kolter *et al.*, 1993; Nataro *et al.*, 2000). Dormant bacteria are well-known for their tolerance to antibiotics normally active against rapidly dividing cells and often require prolonged periods of treatment (Coates *et al.*, 2002; Neu, 1992). The highly refractory nature of biofilms to eradication by chemotherapy is thought to be at least partly attributable to the presence of metabolically inactive cells (Fux *et al.*, 2005). The inefficacy of antibiotics against non-multiplying bacteria thus results in slow or partial death, prolonges the duration of therapy and increases the emergence of genotypic resistances. Accordingly, targeting slow-growing or non-dividing bacteria should provide substancial therapeutic benefits.

Membrane-acting agents are usually active against bacteria in all their phases of growth and are thus good candidates for the development of antimicrobials that target slow-growing and non-dividing bacteria. As an example, the novel porphyrin antibacterial agents XF-70 and XF-73 were shown to remain highly active against this type of bacteria (Ooi *et al.*, 2010). Hu *et al.* (2010) found that the small quinolone-derived compound HT61 was active against non-multiplying MSSA and MRSA by causing depolarization of the cell membrane and destruction of the cell wall. Antimicrobial peptides also interact and permeabilize the bacterial membrane and there is a good probability that they act on slow-growing bacteria that form biofilms (Batoni *et al.*, 2011). Bioactive peptides may even have additional benefits for CF therapeutic applications due to their anti-inflammatory and immunomodulating activities (Scott *et al.*, 2007; Zhang *et al.*, 2005).

The resistance of biofilms to killing by most antimicrobial agents is thought to be more specifically attributable to the presence of non-dividing persister cells (Lewis, 2007). Persisters are dormant bacteria that present a global slowdown in metabolic processes, do not divide and are tolerant to antibiotics. In other words, they have the ability to survive the effects of antibiotics without the use of drug-specific resistance mechanisms. Persisters have been described for *S. aureus* (Allison *et al.*, 2011; Singh *et al.*, 2009) and *P. aeruginosa*, with a recent study that shows the emergence of strains producing high levels of persister cells in CF patients (Mulcahy *et al.*, 2010). Currently, there are only a few therapeutic strategies that are considered for targeting persister cells. One such is the combination of conventional antibiotics with an inhibitor of an essential persister protein (Lewis, 2007). Also, repeated- or pulse-dosing of antibiotics could allow persister cells to resuscitate in order to be killed by subsequent antibiotic administration. The development of specific pro-antibiotics which could irreversibly bind to bacterial targets is also being considered (Lewis, 2007). An outstanding recent study shows that the use of specific metabolic stimuli enables the killing of persister cells with aminoglycoside antibiotics by modulating the proton-motive force required for the uptake of these drugs. The proof of concept for the latter approach has been demonstrated against biofilms and also in a model of chronic infection (Allison *et al.*, 2011).

As we have previously mentioned, SCVs are often associated with relapsing and persistent infections. In addition to the increased ability of these variants to form biofilms (Al Laham *et al.*, 2007; Häußler *et al.*, 2003; Mitchell *et al.*, 2010a, 2010b; Singh *et al.*, 2009, 2010; von Götz *et al.*, 2004), SCVs are well-known for their ability to infect and persist within non-professional phagocytes (Sendi & Proctor, 2009) and there is a limited choice of antibiotics able to act against intracellular bacteria. Nguyen *et al.* (Nguyen *et al.*, 2009a) reported a considerable decrease in the efficacy of most antibiotics against intracellular SCVs in comparison to that seen against extracellular bacteria, but, most importantly, in comparison to their efficacy against the normal-phenotype bacteria. Nevertheless, the authors noted that four antibiotics (quinupristin-dalfopristin, moxifloxacin, oritavancin and rifampicin) were more effective in killing intracellular SCVs. In addition, we recently described the first known molecule to specifically target the SCV phenotype of *S. aureus* (Mitchell *et al.*, 2011a). Tomatidine (TO) is the aglycone form of the plant secondary metabolite tomatine. The structure and the main biological activities of TO against *S. aureus* are presented in Fig. 5A. We found that TO has a bacteriostatic activity against SCVs, but not against normal strains. More importantly, we showed that TO has the ability to inhibit the replication of SCVs internalized in CF-like human airway epithelial cells (Mitchell *et al.*, 2011a). The specificity of the action of TO against SCVs was linked to the dysfunctional electron transport chain of these variants. Acordingly, HQNO sensitized normal *S. aureus* strains to TO (see Fig. 5B), which suggests that TO may be especially effective in the context where *P. aeruginosa* and *S. aureus* co-infect a CF patient. Although TO causes a marked inhibition of protein synthesis in bacteria showing a dysfunctional electron transport chain, the exact mechanism of action of TO on SCVs remains to be elucidated. Other biological activities for TO are discussed below.

4.3 Targeting virulence

Another emerging concept in the development of novel therapeutic approaches is the possibility to modulate the expression of virulence factors that are thought to be of major importance in the establishment of a particular infection. Modulators or blockers of pathogenesis are particularly interesting because it is speculated that, since they do not inhibit growth or kill bacteria, their use will not yield a strong selective pressure for resistance development. In this context, most attention has been directed toward the interference of bacterial QS and cell-to-cell signaling to inhibit virulence or biofilm

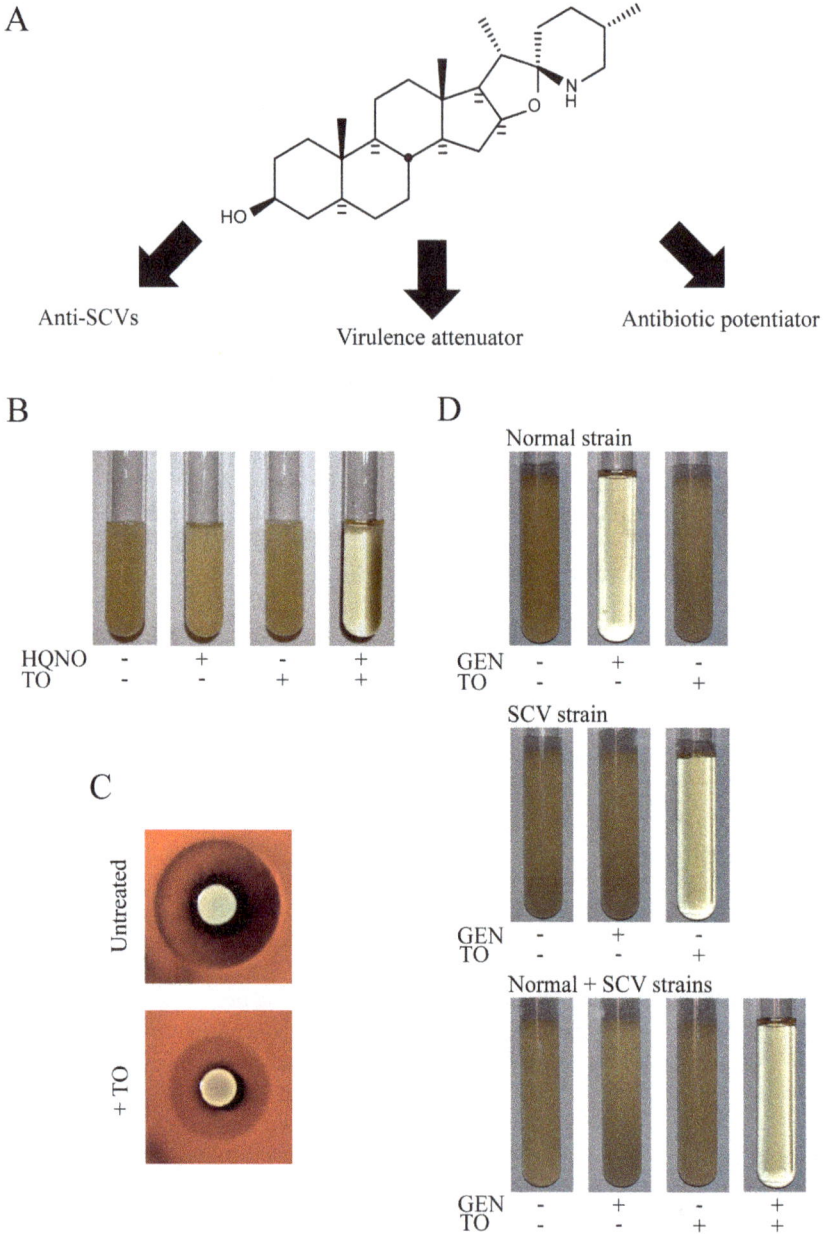

Fig. 5. Biological activities of tomatidine against *S. aureus*. (A) Tomatidine (TO) is a steroidal alkaloid molecule that inhibits both the extracellular and intracellular replication of SCVs, represses the expression of several *agr*-regulated exoproducts and potentiates the bactericidal activity of aminoglycoside antibiotics against prototypical *S. aureus*. (B) TO (8 µg/ml) inhibits the growth of a normal *S. aureus* strain in presence of HQNO (20 µg/ml).

Outcome and Prevention of Pseudomonas aeruginosa-Staphylococcus aureus Interactions
During Pulmonary Infections in Cystic Fibrosis

213

Bacteria were inoculated at 10^5-10^6 CFU/ml and incubated 24 h at 35ºC with shaking. (C) TO (8µg/ml) inhibits the hemolytic ability of a normal-growing *S. aureus* strain. (D) TO may be used in combination with aminoglycosides (*e.g.*, gentamicin [GEN]) to eradicate a population of *S. aureus* composed of normal and SCV bacteria. Bacteria were inoculated at 10^5-10^6 CFU/ml and incubated 24 h at 35ºC with shaking in presence of 4 µg/ml of GEN and/or 0.12 µg/ml of TO. The clear test tubes show no bacterial growth.

formation (Njoroge & Sperandio, 2009; Rasko & Sperandio, 2010). However, although targeting the QS systems of *P. aeruginosa* in CF infections may increase the susceptibility of biofilms to clearance by antibiotics (Hentzer *et al.*, 2003), interference with the QS *agr* system of *S. aureus* may not be a good strategy since it could increase the formation of biofilms and increase bacterial persistence (Novick & Geisinger, 2008; Otto, 2004). The discovery of compounds that attenuate or abolish the cross talk between the QS systems of different bacterial species may be more promising. It remains to be determined whether interference with interspecies communications has the potential to decrease the overall virulence or the cohesion of polymicrobial communities and more particularly of those found in CF.

Several plant products have been shown to act as "virulence attenuators" of human pathogens (González-Lamothe *et al.*, 2009). Virulence attenuators modulate the virulence or the ability of the bacterium to adapt to the host environment. This gives a competitive advantage to the host immune system. As an example, a garlic extract was shown to interfere with the QS of *P. aeruginosa*, to sensitize its biofilm to tobramycin treatments and to improve clearance of bacteria in a pulmonary mouse model (Bjarnsholt *et al.*, 2005; Rasmussen *et al.*, 2005). Ginseng extract was also shown to alter the virulence of *P. aeruginosa* by interfering with QS, destroying biofilms, promoting phagocytosis by airway phagocytes and by protecting animals from the development of chronic lung infections (Song *et al.*, 1997a, 1997b, 2010; Wu *et al.*, 2011). Some of our own transcriptional analyses of bacteria exposed to plant products have shed light on the effect of TO on the expression of virulence factors by normal *S. aureus* strains (Bouarab *et al.*, 2007). We demonstrated that TO causes a repression in the expression of many extracellular toxins and of RNAIII, the effector molecule of the *agr* system, and thus it inhibits the hemolytic activity of *S. aureus*. We further showed that TO inhibits biofilm formation by *S. aureus* SCVs, probably through the induction of bacteriostasis (Mitchell *et al.*, 2009). We suggest that the overall negative effects of TO on the virulence and the growth of both normal and SCV *S. aureus* strains could be used in the management of both acute and chronic lung infections in CF patients. Fig. 5C shows the inhibitory effect of TO on the hemolytic ability of a normal *S. aureus* strain.

Other studies have also promoted the use of virulence factor-based therapies against *S. aureus*. For example, QS autoinducing peptide variants were shown to inhibit heterologous *agr* activation and were proposed as therapeutic agents (Novick & Geisinger, 2008). Also, a blocker of the synthesis of staphyloxanthin, the golden-carotenoid pigment of *S. aureus* that promotes resistance to reactive oxygen species and host neutrophil-based killing, increased the susceptibility of *S. aureus* to killing by human blood and the innate immune clearance in a mouse infection model (Liu *et al.*, 2008). Other researchers have attempted to achieve virulence attenuation by manipulation of bacterial metabolism (Lan *et al.*, 2010; Zhu *et al.*, 2009). Another possible approach is to target the bacterial pathways for programmed cell death which have been identified in several species (Engelberg-Kulka *et al.*, 2004).

4.4 Enhancing preexisting antimicrobial therapies

The use of synergistic combinations of antimicrobial compounds is an old strategy that continues to be tantalizing especially against the polymicrobial populations found in the CF airways. Accordingly, Høiby (2011) suggests that the effectiveness of combination therapies should be tested in the context of CF lung infections. Several combinations of old antibiotics indeed showed promising synergistic effects *in vitro* and/or *in vivo* such as fosfomycin-tobramycin, tobramycin-colistin and ciprofloxacin-colistin combinations, with the ciprofloxacin-colistin combination thought to be efficient even against *P. aeruginosa* biofilms (Høiby, 2011). A large screen of double and triple antibiotic combinations was tested on biofilm-grown *B. cepacia* and *P. aeruginosa* in order to identify effective antibiotic combinations for the treatment of CF patients (Dales *et al.*, 2009). Combinations of antibiotics may also be useful in order to improve the efficiency of antimicrobial treatments against intracellular SCVs. As an example, some drug combinations that included rifampicin were most effective against intracellular *S. aureus* of both normal and SCV phenotypes. (Baltch *et al.*, 2008). Nguyen *et al.* (2009b) also showed additive or synergistic effects between oritavancin, moxifloxacin and rifampicin against intracellular SCVs.

The combination of antimicrobial agents with non-antibiotic compounds is also an attractive approach (George *et al.*, 2009). Several plant products are "antibiotic potentiators" that can act as bacterial efflux pump inhibitors, cell wall-acting agents or membrane destabilizing agents to provide synergy with conventional antibiotics (González-Lamothe *et al.*, 2009). Interestingly, we have recently demonstrated that TO potentiates the bactericidal activity of aminoglycoside antibiotics against normal *S. aureus* strains of diverse clinical origins and antibiotic susceptibility patterns (unpublished results). Although the mechanism(s) by which this effect occurs is yet unknown, TO may prove useful in combination therapy with aminoglycoside antibiotics in the treatment of CF lung infections as exemplified in Fig. 5D. According to Mohtar *et al.* (Mohtar *et al.*, 2009), a vast number of other plant products with antimicrobial activity await discovery.

5. Conclusion

Complex polymicrobial communities colonize the CF airways and interspecies interactions are likely to play a role in the course of respiratory infections. *P. aeruginosa* and *S. aureus* are prevalent pathogens often simultaneously found in CF patients and for which microbial interactions that modulate virulence are already well documented. In communities and by using intraspecies and interspecies cell-to-cell communication, these pathogens have the ability to form biofilms and to adopt persistent phenotypes such as persister cells and SCVs. These phenotypes confer non-specific resistance to antimicrobials and to the host immune system. The development of novel therapeutic approaches that take into account polymicrobial communities and the various strategies that bacteria have elaborated to adapt and persist within the CF airways should help to eradicate chronic and life-threatening infections in CF.

6. Acknowledgment

François Malouin (FM) is supported by Cystic Fibrosis Canada and by a team grant from the Fonds Québécois de la Recherche sur la Nature et les Technologies (FQRNT) with Kamal Bouarab and Éric Marsault. Gabriel Mitchell was the recipient of an Alexander-Graham-Bell

Graduate Scholarship from the Natural Sciences and Engineering Research Council of Canada and received a research scholarship from FQRNT during the course of his doctoral program. The authors would like to thank Brian Talbot for critical review of this chapter, Gilles Grondin for technical assistance as well as Alexandre Fugère, David Lalonde Séguin, Éric Brouillette, Isabelle Guay, Karine Pépin Gaudreau and Simon Boulanger for their involvement in the CF research program taking place in the FM laboratory. We thank Josée Lessard and André Cantin from the CF clinic and Eric Frost and the personnel from the clinical microbiology laboratory of the Centre Hospitalier Universitaire de Sherbrooke, and of course, we gratefully thank all CF patients for their willingness and enthusiasm in participating to this research.

7. References

Al Laham, N., Rohde, H., Sander, G., Fischer, A., Hussain, M., Heilmann, C., Mack, D., Proctor, R., Peters, G., Becker, K. & von Eiff, C. (2007). Augmented expression of polysaccharide intercellular adhesin in a defined *Staphylococcus epidermidis* mutant with the small-colony-variant phenotype. *J Bacteriol*, Vol. 189, No. 12, pp. 4494-4501.

Allison, K.R., Brynildsen, M.P. & Collins, J.J. (2011). Metabolite-enabled eradication of bacterial persisters by aminoglycosides. *Nature*, Vol. 473, No. 7346, pp. 216-220.

Alvarez, S., Herrero, C., Bru, E. & Perdigon, G. (2001). Effect of *Lactobacillus casei* and yogurt administration on prevention of *Pseudomonas aeruginosa* infection in young mice. *J Food Prot*, Vol. 64, No. 11, pp. 1768-1774.

Archer, G.L. (1998). *Staphylococcus aureus*: a well-armed pathogen. *Clin Infect Dis*, Vol. 26, No. 5, pp. 1179-1181.

Bakkal, S., Robinson, S.M., Ordonez, C.L., Waltz, D.A. & Riley, M.A. (2010). Role of bacteriocins in mediating interactions of bacterial isolates taken from cystic fibrosis patients. *Microbiology*, Vol. 156, No. Pt 7, pp. 2058-2067.

Baltch, A.L., Ritz, W.J., Bopp, L.H., Michelsen, P. & Smith, R.P. (2008). Activities of daptomycin and comparative antimicrobials, singly and in combination, against extracellular and intracellular *Staphylococcus aureus* and its stable small-colony variant in human monocyte-derived macrophages and in broth. *Antimicrob Agents Chemother*, Vol. 52, No. 5, pp. 1829-1833.

Bates, D.M., von Eiff, C., McNamara, P.J., Peters, G., Yeaman, M.R., Bayer, A.S. & Proctor, R.A. (2003). *Staphylococcus aureus menD* and *hemB* mutants are as infective as the parent strains, but the menadione biosynthetic mutant persists within the kidney. *J Infect Dis*, Vol. 187, No. 10, pp. 1654-1661.

Batoni, G., Maisetta, G., Brancatisano, F.L., Esin, S. & Campa, M. (2011). Use of antimicrobial peptides against microbial biofilms: advantages and limits. *Curr Med Chem*, Vol. 18, No. 2, pp. 256-279.

Biswas, L., Biswas, R., Schlag, M., Bertram, R. & Götz, F. (2009). Small-colony variant selection as a survival strategy for *Staphylococcus aureus* in the presence of *Pseudomonas aeruginosa*. *Appl Environ Microbiol*, Vol. 75, No. 21, pp. 6910-6912.

Bjarnsholt, T., Jensen, P.Ø., Rasmussen, T.B., Christophersen, L., Calum, H., Hentzer, M., Hougen, H.P., Rygaard, J., Moser, C., Eberl, L., Høiby, N. & Givskov, M. (2005). Garlic blocks quorum sensing and promotes rapid clearing of pulmonary *Pseudomonas aeruginosa* infections. *Microbiology*, Vol. 151, No. Pt 12, pp. 3873-3880.

Bjarnsholt, T., Jensen, P.Ø., Fiandaca, M.J., Pedersen, J., Hansen, C.R., Andersen, C.B., Pressler, T., Givskov, M. & Høiby, N. (2009). *Pseudomonas aeruginosa* biofilms in the respiratory tract of cystic fibrosis patients. *Pediatr Pulmonol*, Vol. 44, No. 6, pp. 547-558.

Bodey, G.P., Bolivar, R., Fainstein, V. & Jadeja, L. (1983). Infections caused by *Pseudomonas aeruginosa*. *Rev Infect Dis*, Vol. 5, No. 2, pp. 279-313.

Bouarab, K., Ordi, M.E., Gattuso, M., Moisan, H. & Malouin, F. (2007). Plant stress response agents affect *Staphylococcus aureus* virulence genes. abstr. C1-1483, *Proceedings of 47th Intersci. Conf. Antimicrob. Agents Chemother*, Chicago, IL.

Brogden, K.A., Guthmiller, J.M. & Taylor, C.E. (2005). Human polymicrobial infections. *Lancet*, Vol. 365, No. 9455, pp. 253-255.

Bronner, S., Monteil, H. & Prévost, G. (2004). Regulation of virulence determinants in *Staphylococcus aureus*: complexity and applications. *FEMS Microbiol Rev*, Vol. 28, No. 2, pp. 183-200.

Brouillette, E., Martinez, A., Boyll, B.J., Allen, N.E. & Malouin, F. (2004). Persistence of a *Staphylococcus aureus* small-colony variant under antibiotic pressure *in vivo*. *FEMS Immunol Med Microbiol*, Vol. 41, No. 1, pp. 35-41.

Bryan, L.E. & Van Den Elzen, H.M. (1977). Effects of membrane-energy mutations and cations on streptomycin and gentamicin accumulation by bacteria: a model for entry of streptomycin and gentamicin in susceptible and resistant bacteria. *Antimicrob Agents Chemother*, Vol. 12, No. 2, pp. 163-177.

Canadian Cystic Fibrosis Foundation (2009) *Patient data registry report*. Toronton, ON, Canada.

Chambers, H.F. & Deleo, F.R. (2009). Waves of resistance: *Staphylococcus aureus* in the antibiotic era. *Nat Rev Microbiol*, Vol. 7, No. 9, pp. 629-641.

Chattoraj, S.S., Murthy, R., Ganesan, S., Goldberg, J.B., Zhao, Y., Hershenson, M.B. & Sajjan, U.S. (2010). *Pseudomonas aeruginosa* alginate promotes *Burkholderia cenocepacia* persistence in cystic fibrosis transmembrane conductance regulator knockout mice. *Infect Immun*, Vol. 78, No. 3, pp. 984-993.

Chmiel, J.F. & Davis, P.B. (2003). State of the art: why do the lungs of patients with cystic fibrosis become infected and why can't they clear the infection? *Respir Res*, Vol. 4, pp. 8.

Ciofu, O., Giwercman, B., Pedersen, S.S. & Høiby, N. (1994). Development of antibiotic resistance in *Pseudomonas aeruginosa* during two decades of antipseudomonal treatment at the Danish CF Center. *Apmis*, Vol. 102, No. 9, pp. 674-680.

Coates, A., Hu, Y., Bax, R. & Page, C. (2002). The future challenges facing the development of new antimicrobial drugs. *Nat Rev Drug Discov*, Vol. 1, No. 11, pp. 895-910.

Costerton, J.W., Stewart, P.S. & Greenberg, E.P. (1999). Bacterial biofilms: a common cause of persistent infections. *Science*, Vol. 284, No. 5418, pp. 1318-1322.

Cystic Fibrosis Foundation (2009). Patient registry annual report, Washington, D.C.

D'Argenio, D.A., Wu, M., Hoffman, L.R., Kulasekara, H.D., Déziel, E., Smith, E.E., Nguyen, H., Ernst, R.K., Larson Freeman, T.J., Spencer, D.H., Brittnacher, M., Hayden, H.S., Selgrade, S., Klausen, M., Goodlett, D.R., Burns, J.L., Ramsey, B.W. & Miller, S.I. (2007). Growth phenotypes of *Pseudomonas aeruginosa lasR* mutants adapted to the airways of cystic fibrosis patients. *Mol Microbiol*, Vol. 64, No. 2, pp. 512-533.

Dales, L., Ferris, W., Vandemheen, K. & Aaron, S.D. (2009). Combination antibiotic susceptibility of biofilm-grown *Burkholderia cepacia* and *Pseudomonas aeruginosa* isolated from patients with pulmonary exacerbations of cystic fibrosis. *Eur J Clin Microbiol Infect Dis*, Vol. 28, No. 10, pp. 1275-1279.

Dasenbrook, E.C., Merlo, C.A., Diener-West, M., Lechtzin, N. & Boyle, M.P. (2008). Persistent methicillin-resistant *Staphylococcus aureus* and rate of FEV1 decline in cystic fibrosis. *Am J Respir Crit Care Med*, Vol. 178, No. 8, pp. 814-821.

Dasenbrook, E.C., Checkley, W., Merlo, C.A., Konstan, M.W., Lechtzin, N. & Boyle, M.P. (2010). Association between respiratory tract methicillin-resistant *Staphylococcus aureus* and survival in cystic fibrosis. *JAMA*, Vol. 303, No. 23, pp. 2386-2392.

Davies, J.C. & Bilton, D. (2009). Bugs, biofilms, and resistance in cystic fibrosis. *Respir Care*, Vol. 54, No. 5, pp. 628-640.

Döring, G., Conway, S.P., Heijerman, H.G., Hodson, M.E., Høiby, N., Smyth, A. & Touw, D.J. (2000). Antibiotic therapy against *Pseudomonas aeruginosa* in cystic fibrosis: a European consensus. *Eur Respir J*, Vol. 16, No. 4, pp. 749-767.

Döring, G. & Høiby, N. (2004). Early intervention and prevention of lung disease in cystic fibrosis: a European consensus. *J Cyst Fibros*, Vol. 3, No. 2, pp. 67-91.

Duan, K., Dammel, C., Stein, J., Rabin, H. & Surette, M.G. (2003). Modulation of *Pseudomonas aeruginosa* gene expression by host microflora through interspecies communication. *Mol Microbiol*, Vol. 50, No. 5, pp. 1477-1491.

Dubern, J.F. & Diggle, S.P. (2008). Quorum sensing by 2-alkyl-4-quinolones in *Pseudomonas aeruginosa* and other bacterial species. *Mol Biosyst*, Vol. 4, No. 9, pp. 882-888.

Engelberg-Kulka, H., Sat, B., Reches, M., Amitai, S. & Hazan, R. (2004). Bacterial programmed cell death systems as targets for antibiotics. *Trends Microbiol*, Vol. 12, No. 2, pp. 66-71.

European Cystic Fibrosis Society (2007) *Patient Registry Report*.

Foweraker, J.E., Laughton, C.R., Brown, D.F. & Bilton, D. (2005). Phenotypic variability of *Pseudomonas aeruginosa* in sputa from patients with acute infective exacerbation of cystic fibrosis and its impact on the validity of antimicrobial susceptibility testing. *J Antimicrob Chemother*, Vol. 55, No. 6, pp. 921-927.

Frederiksen, B., Pressler, T., Hansen, A., Koch, C. & Høiby, N. (2006). Effect of aerosolized rhDNase (Pulmozyme) on pulmonary colonization in patients with cystic fibrosis. *Acta Paediatr*, Vol. 95, No. 9, pp. 1070-1074.

Fux, C.A., Costerton, J.W., Stewart, P.S. & Stoodley, P. (2005). Survival strategies of infectious biofilms. *Trends Microbiol*, Vol. 13, No. 1, pp. 34-40.

Galli, J., Ardito, F., Calo, L., Mancinelli, L., Imperiali, M., Parrilla, C., Picciotti, P.M. & Fadda, G. (2007). Recurrent upper airway infections and bacterial biofilms. *J Laryngol Otol*, Vol. 121, No. 4, pp. 341-344.

George, A.M., Jones, P.M. & Middleton, P.G. (2009). Cystic fibrosis infections: treatment strategies and prospects. *FEMS Microbiol Lett*, Vol. 300, No. 2, pp. 153-164.

Goerke, C. & Wolz, C. (2009). Adaptation of *Staphylococcus aureus* to the cystic fibrosis lung. *Int J Med Microbiol*, Vol. 300, No. 8, pp. 520-525.

González-Lamothe, R., Mitchell, G., Gattuso, M., Diarra, M.S., Malouin, F. & Bouarab, K. (2009). Plant antimicrobial agents and their effects on plant and human pathogens. *Int J Mol Sci*, Vol. 10, No. 8, pp. 3400-3419.

Grundmeier, M., Tuchscherr, L., Brück, M., Viemann, D., Roth, J., Willscher, E., Becker, K., Peters, G. & Löffler, B. (2010). Staphylococcal strains vary greatly in their ability to induce an inflammatory response in endothelial cells. *J Infect Dis*, Vol. 201, No. 6, pp. 871-880.

Hall-Stoodley, L., Costerton, J.W. & Stoodley, P. (2004). Bacterial biofilms: from the natural environment to infectious diseases. *Nat Rev Microbiol*, Vol. 2, No. 2, pp. 95-108.

Harrison, F. (2007). Microbial ecology of the cystic fibrosis lung. *Microbiology*, Vol. 153, No. Pt 4, pp. 917-923.

Häußler, S., Tümmler, B., Weißbrodt, H., Rohde, M. & Steinmetz, I. (1999). Small-colony variants of *Pseudomonas aeruginosa* in cystic fibrosis. *Clin Infect Dis*, Vol. 29, No. 3, pp. 621-625.

Häußler, S., Ziegler, I., Löttel, A., von Götz, F., Rohde, M., Wehmhöhner, D., Saravanamuthu, S., Tümmler, B. & Steinmetz, I. (2003). Highly adherent small-colony variants of *Pseudomonas aeruginosa* in cystic fibrosis lung infection. *J Med Microbiol*, Vol. 52, No. Pt 4, pp. 295-301.

Hentzer, M., Wu, H., Andersen, J.B., Riedel, K., Rasmussen, T.B., Bagge, N., Kumar, N., Schembri, M.A., Song, Z., Kristoffersen, P., Manefield, M., Costerton, J.W., Molin, S., Eberl, L., Steinberg, P., Kjelleberg, S., Høiby, N. & Givskov, M. (2003). Attenuation of *Pseudomonas aeruginosa* virulence by quorum sensing inhibitors. *Embo J*, Vol. 22, No. 15, pp. 3803-3815.

Hoffman, L.R., D'Argenio, D.A., MacCoss, M.J., Zhang, Z., Jones, R.A. & Miller, S.I. (2005). Aminoglycoside antibiotics induce bacterial biofilm formation. *Nature*, Vol. 436, No. 7054, pp. 1171-1175.

Hoffman, L.R., Déziel, E., D'Argenio, D.A., Lépine, F., Emerson, J., McNamara, S., Gibson, R.L., Ramsey, B.W. & Miller, S.I. (2006). Selection for *Staphylococcus aureus* small-colony variants due to growth in the presence of *Pseudomonas aeruginosa*. *Proc Natl Acad Sci U S A*, Vol. 103, No. 52, pp. 19890-19895.

Hoffman, L.R., Kulasekara, H.D., Emerson, J., Houston, L.S., Burns, J.L., Ramsey, B.W. & Miller, S.I. (2009). *Pseudomonas aeruginosa lasR* mutants are associated with cystic fibrosis lung disease progression. *J Cyst Fibros*, Vol. 8, No. 1, pp. 66-70.

Hogardt, M. & Heesemann, J. (2010). Adaptation of *Pseudomonas aeruginosa* during persistence in the cystic fibrosis lung. *Int J Med Microbiol*, Vol. 300, No. 8, pp. 557-562.

Høiby, N. & Pedersen, S.S. (1989). Estimated risk of cross-infection with *Pseudomonas aeruginosa* in Danish cystic fibrosis patients. *Acta Paediatr Scand*, Vol. 78, No. 3, pp. 395-404.

Høiby, N., Bjarnsholt, T., Givskov, M., Molin, S. & Ciofu, O. (2010). Antibiotic resistance of bacterial biofilms. *Int J Antimicrob Agents*, Vol. 35, No. 4, pp. 322-332.

Høiby, N. (2011). Recent advances in the treatment of *Pseudomonas aeruginosa* infections in cystic fibrosis. *BMC Med*, Vol. 9, pp. 32.

Hu, Y., Shamaei-Tousi, A., Liu, Y. & Coates, A. (2010). A new approach for the discovery of antibiotics by targeting non-multiplying bacteria: a novel topical antibiotic for staphylococcal infections. *PLoS One*, Vol. 5, No. 7, pp. e11818.

Kahl, B., Herrmann, M., Everding, A.S., Koch, H.G., Becker, K., Harms, E., Proctor, R.A. & Peters, G. (1998). Persistent infection with small colony variant strains of *Staphylococcus aureus* in patients with cystic fibrosis. *J Infect Dis*, Vol. 177, No. 4, pp. 1023-1029.

Kahl, B.C. (2010). Impact of *Staphylococcus aureus* on the pathogenesis of chronic cystic fibrosis lung disease. *Int J Med Microbiol*, Vol. 300, No. 8, pp. 514-519.

Kaufmann, G.F., Sartorio, R., Lee, S.H., Rogers, C.J., Meijler, M.M., Moss, J.A., Clapham, B., Brogan, A.P., Dickerson, T.J. & Janda, K.D. (2005). Revisiting quorum sensing: Discovery of additional chemical and biological functions for 3-oxo-N-acylhomoserine lactones. *Proc Natl Acad Sci U S A*, Vol. 102, No. 2, pp. 309-314.

Kessler, E., Safrin, M., Olson, J.C. & Ohman, D.E. (1993). Secreted LasA of *Pseudomonas aeruginosa* is a staphylolytic protease. *J Biol Chem*, Vol. 268, No. 10, pp. 7503-7508.

Kolter, R., Siegele, D.A. & Tormo, A. (1993). The stationary phase of the bacterial life cycle. *Annu Rev Microbiol*, Vol. 47, pp. 855-874.

Korgaonkar, A.K. & Whiteley, M. (2011). *Pseudomonas aeruginosa* enhances production of an antimicrobial in response to N-acetylglucosamine and peptidoglycan. *J Bacteriol*, Vol. 193, No. 4, pp. 909-917.

Lan, L., Cheng, A., Dunman, P.M., Missiakas, D. & He, C. (2010). Golden pigment production and virulence gene expression are affected by metabolisms in *Staphylococcus aureus*. *J Bacteriol*, Vol. 192, No. 12, pp. 3068-3077.

Lauderdale, K.J., Boles, B.R., Cheung, A.L. & Horswill, A.R. (2009). Interconnections between Sigma B, *agr*, and proteolytic activity in *Staphylococcus aureus* biofilm maturation. *Infect Immun*, Vol. 77, No. 4, pp. 1623-1635.

Leisinger, T. & Margraff, R. (1979). Secondary metabolites of the fluorescent pseudomonads. *Microbiol Rev*, Vol. 43, No. 3, pp. 422-442.

Lépine, F., Milot, S., Déziel, E., He, J. & Rahme, L.G. (2004). Electrospray/mass spectrometric identification and analysis of 4-hydroxy-2-alkylquinolines (HAQs) produced by *Pseudomonas aeruginosa*. *J Am Soc Mass Spectrom*, Vol. 15, No. 6, pp. 862-869.

Lewis, K. (2007). Persister cells, dormancy and infectious disease. *Nat Rev Microbiol*, Vol. 5, No. 1, pp. 48-56.

Lightbown, J.W. (1954). An antagonist of streptomycin and dihydrostreptomycin produced by *Pseudomonas aeruginosa*. *J Gen Microbiol*, Vol. 11, No. 3, pp. 477-492.

Lightbown, J.W. & Jackson, F.L. (1954). Inhibition of cytochrome system of heart muscle and of *Staphylococcus aureus* by 2-heptyl-4-hydroxyquinoline-N-oxide, an antagonist of dihydrostreptomycin. *Biochem J*, Vol. 58, No. 4, pp. xlix.

Liu, C.I., Liu, G.Y., Song, Y., Yin, F., Hensler, M.E., Jeng, W.Y., Nizet, V., Wang, A.H. & Oldfield, E. (2008). A cholesterol biosynthesis inhibitor blocks *Staphylococcus aureus* virulence. *Science*, Vol. 319, No. 5868, pp. 1391-1394.

Lyczak, J.B., Cannon, C.L. & Pier, G.B. (2002). Lung infections associated with cystic fibrosis. *Clin Microbiol Rev*, Vol. 15, No. 2, pp. 194-222.

Machan, Z.A., Taylor, G.W., Pitt, T.L., Cole, P.J. & Wilson, R. (1992). 2-Heptyl-4-hydroxyquinoline N-oxide, an antistaphylococcal agent produced by *Pseudomonas aeruginosa*. *J Antimicrob Chemother*, Vol. 30, No. 5, pp. 615-623.

Maciá, M.D., Blanquer, D., Togores, B., Sauleda, J., Pérez, J.L. & Oliver, A. (2005). Hypermutation is a key factor in development of multiple-antimicrobial resistance in *Pseudomonas aeruginosa* strains causing chronic lung infections. *Antimicrob Agents Chemother*, Vol. 49, No. 8, pp. 3382-3386.

Mashburn, L.M., Jett, A.M., Akins, D.R. & Whiteley, M. (2005). *Staphylococcus aureus* serves as an iron source for *Pseudomonas aeruginosa* during *in vivo* coculture. *J Bacteriol*, Vol. 187, No. 2, pp. 554-566.

Mashburn, L.M. & Whiteley, M. (2005). Membrane vesicles traffic signals and facilitate group activities in a prokaryote. *Nature*, Vol. 437, No. 7057, pp. 422-425.

McAlester, G., O'Gara, F. & Morrissey, J.P. (2008). Signal-mediated interactions between *Pseudomonas aeruginosa* and *Candida albicans*. *J Med Microbiol*, Vol. 57, No. Pt 5, pp. 563-569.

Mitchell, G., Lamontagne, C.A., Brouillette, E., Grondin, G., Talbot, B.G., Grandbois, M. & Malouin, F. (2008). *Staphylococcus aureus* SigB activity promotes a strong fibronectin-bacterium interaction which may sustain host tissue colonization by small-colony variants isolated from cystic fibrosis patients. *Mol Microbiol*, Vol. 70, No. 6, pp. 1540-1555.

Mitchell, G., Gattuso, M., Bouarab, K. & Malouin, F. (2009). Tomatidine (TO) affects virulence regulators of prototypical *Staphylococcus aureus* (SA) and small-colony variants (SCV) of cystic fibrosis patients, abstr. C1-1341, *Proceedings of 49th Intersci. Conf. Antimicrob. Agents Chemother*, San Francisco, CA.

Mitchell, G., Brouillette, E., Séguin, D.L., Asselin, A.E., Jacob, C.L. & Malouin, F. (2010a). A role for sigma factor B in the emergence of *Staphylococcus aureus* small-colony variants and elevated biofilm production resulting from an exposure to aminoglycosides. *Microb Pathog*, Vol. 48, No. 1, pp. 18-27.

Mitchell, G., Séguin, D.L., Asselin, A.E., Déziel, E., Cantin, A.M., Frost, E.H., Michaud, S. & Malouin, F. (2010b). *Staphylococcus aureus* sigma B-dependent emergence of small-colony variants and biofilm production following exposure to *Pseudomonas aeruginosa* 4-hydroxy-2-heptylquinoline-N-oxide. *BMC Microbiol*, Vol. 10, pp. 33.

Mitchell, G., Gattuso, M., Grondin, G., Marsault, E., Bouarab, K. & Malouin, F. (2011a). Tomatidine inhibits replication of *Staphylococcus aureus* small-colony variants in cystic fibrosis airway epithelial cells. *Antimicrob Agents Chemother*, Vol. 55, No. 5, pp. 1937-1945.

Mitchell, G., Grondin, G., Bilodeau, G., Cantin, A.M. & Malouin, F. (2011b). Infection of Polarized Airway Epithelial Cells by Normal and Small-Colony Variant Strains of *Staphylococcus aureus* is Increased in Cells with Abnormal CFTR function and is influenced by NF-κB. *Infect Immun*. Vol. 79, No. 9, pp. 3541-3551.

Mohtar, M., Johari, S.A., Li, A.R., Isa, M.M., Mustafa, S., Ali, A.M. & Basri, D.F. (2009). Inhibitory and resistance-modifying potential of plant-based alkaloids against methicillin-resistant *Staphylococcus aureus* (MRSA). *Curr Microbiol*, Vol. 59, No. 2, pp. 181-186.

Moisan, H., Brouillette, E., Jacob, C.L., Langlois-Bégin, P., Michaud, S. & Malouin, F. (2006). Transcription of virulence factors in *Staphylococcus aureus* small-colony variants isolated from cystic fibrosis patients is influenced by SigB. *J Bacteriol*, Vol. 188, No. 1, pp. 64-76.

Molina, A., Del Campo, R., Máiz, L., Morosini, M.I., Lamas, A., Baquero, F. & Cantón, R. (2008). High prevalence in cystic fibrosis patients of multiresistant hospital-acquired methicillin-resistant *Staphylococcus aureus* ST228-SCC*mecI* capable of biofilm formation. *J Antimicrob Chemother*, Vol. 62, No. 5, pp. 961-967.

Moore, J.E., Shaw, A., Millar, B.C., Downey, D.G., Murphy, P.G. & Elborn, J.S. (2005). Microbial ecology of the cystic fibrosis lung: does microflora type influence microbial loading? *Br J Biomed Sci*, Vol. 62, No. 4, pp. 175-178.

Moskowitz, S.M., Gibson, R.L. & Effmann, E.L. (2005). Cystic fibrosis lung disease: genetic influences, microbial interactions, and radiological assessment. *Pediatr Radiol*, Vol. 35, No. 8, pp. 739-757.

Mulcahy, L.R., Burns, J.L., Lory, S. & Lewis, K. (2010). Emergence of *Pseudomonas aeruginosa* strains producing high levels of persister cells in patients with cystic fibrosis. *J Bacteriol*, Vol. 192, No. 23, pp. 6191-6199.

Nataro J.P., Blaser M.J. & Cunningham-Rundles S. (2000). Persistent bacterial infections: commensalism gone awry or adaptive niche?, In *Persistent Bacterial Infections*, Nataro J.P., Blaser M.J. and Cunningham-Rundles S., pp. 3-10, American Society for Microbiology Press, Washington, DC.

Neu, H.C. (1992). General therapeutic principles., In *Infectious Diseases*, Gorbach, S.L., Bartlett, J.G. and Blacklow, N.R., pp. 153-160, WB Saunders Company, Philadelphia, PA.

Nguyen, H.A., Denis, O., Vergison, A., Theunis, A., Tulkens, P.M., Struelens, M.J. & Van Bambeke, F. (2009a). Intracellular activity of antibiotics in a model of human THP-1 macrophages infected by a *Staphylococcus aureus* small-colony variant strain isolated from a cystic fibrosis patient: pharmacodynamic evaluation and comparison with isogenic normal-phenotype and revertant strains. *Antimicrob Agents Chemother*, Vol. 53, No. 4, pp. 1434-1442.

Nguyen, H.A., Denis, O., Vergison, A., Tulkens, P.M., Struelens, M.J. & Van Bambeke, F. (2009b). Intracellular activity of antibiotics in a model of human THP-1 macrophages infected by a *Staphylococcus aureus* small-colony variant strain isolated from a cystic fibrosis patient: study of antibiotic combinations. *Antimicrob Agents Chemother*, Vol. 53, No. 4, pp. 1443-1449.

Njoroge, J. & Sperandio, V. (2009). Jamming bacterial communication: new approaches for the treatment of infectious diseases. *EMBO Mol Med*, Vol. 1, No. 4, pp. 201-210.

Novick, R.P. (2003). Autoinduction and signal transduction in the regulation of staphylococcal virulence. *Mol Microbiol*, Vol. 48, No. 6, pp. 1429-1449.

Novick, R.P. & Geisinger, E. (2008). Quorum sensing in staphylococci. *Annu Rev Genet*, Vol. 42, pp. 541-564.

Ooi, N., Miller, K., Randall, C., Rhys-Williams, W., Love, W. & Chopra, I. (2010). XF-70 and XF-73, novel antibacterial agents active against slow-growing and non-dividing cultures of *Staphylococcus aureus* including biofilms. *J Antimicrob Chemother*, Vol. 65, No. 1, pp. 72-78.

Otto, M. (2004). Quorum-sensing control in Staphylococci -- a target for antimicrobial drug therapy? *FEMS Microbiol Lett*, Vol. 241, No. 2, pp. 135-141.

Palmer, K.L., Mashburn, L.M., Singh, P.K. & Whiteley, M. (2005). Cystic fibrosis sputum supports growth and cues key aspects of *Pseudomonas aeruginosa* physiology. *J Bacteriol*, Vol. 187, No. 15, pp. 5267-5277.

Parkins, M.D. & Elborn, J.S. (2010). Newer antibacterial agents and their potential role in cystic fibrosis pulmonary exacerbation management. *J Antimicrob Chemother*, Vol. 65, No. 9, pp. 1853-1861.

Pihl, M., Chávez de Paz, L.E., Schmidtchen, A., Svensäter, G. & Davies, J.R. (2010a). Effects of clinical isolates of *Pseudomonas aeruginosa* on *Staphylococcus epidermidis* biofilm formation. *FEMS Immunol Med Microbiol*, Vol. 59, No. 3, pp. 504-512.

Pihl, M., Davies, J.R., Chávez de Paz, L.E. & Svensäter, G. (2010b). Differential effects of *Pseudomonas aeruginosa* on biofilm formation by different strains of *Staphylococcus epidermidis*. *FEMS Immunol Med Microbiol*, Vol. 59, No. 3, pp. 439-446.

Proctor, R.A., von Eiff, C., Kahl, B.C., Becker, K., McNamara, P., Herrmann, M. & Peters, G. (2006). Small colony variants: a pathogenic form of bacteria that facilitates persistent and recurrent infections. *Nat Rev Microbiol*, Vol. 4, No. 4, pp. 295-305.

Pruneau, M., Mitchell, G., Moisan, H., Dumont-Blanchette, E., Jacob, C.L. & Malouin, F. (2011). Transcriptional analysis of antibiotic resistance and virulence genes in multiresistant hospital-acquired MRSA. *FEMS Immunol Med Microbiol*. Jun 10 [Epub ahead of print]

Qazi, S., Middleton, B., Muharram, S.H., Cockayne, A., Hill, P., O'Shea, P., Chhabra, S.R., Camara, M. & Williams, P. (2006). N-acylhomoserine lactones antagonize virulence gene expression and quorum sensing in *Staphylococcus aureus*. *Infect Immun*, Vol. 74, No. 2, pp. 910-919.

Qin, Z., Yang, L., Qu, D., Molin, S. & Tolker-Nielsen, T. (2009). *Pseudomonas aeruginosa* extracellular products inhibit staphylococcal growth, and disrupt established biofilms produced by *Staphylococcus epidermidis*. *Microbiology*, Vol. 155, No. Pt 7, pp. 2148-2156.

Rasko, D.A. & Sperandio, V. (2010). Anti-virulence strategies to combat bacteria-mediated disease. *Nat Rev Drug Discov*, Vol. 9, No. 2, pp. 117-128.

Rasmussen, T.B., Bjarnsholt, T., Skindersoe, M.E., Hentzer, M., Kristoffersen, P., Köte, M., Nielsen, J., Eberl, L. & Givskov, M. (2005). Screening for quorum-sensing inhibitors (QSI) by use of a novel genetic system, the QSI selector. *J Bacteriol*, Vol. 187, No. 5, pp. 1799-1814.

Razvi, S., Quittell, L., Sewall, A., Quinton, H., Marshall, B. & Saiman, L. (2009). Respiratory microbiology of patients with cystic fibrosis in the United States, 1995 to 2005. *Chest*, Vol. 136, No. 6, pp. 1554-1560.

Riedel, K., Hentzer, M., Geisenberger, O., Huber, B., Steidle, A., Wu, H., Høiby, N., Givskov, M., Molin, S. & Eberl, L. (2001). N-acylhomoserine-lactone-mediated communication between *Pseudomonas aeruginosa* and *Burkholderia cepacia* in mixed biofilms. *Microbiology*, Vol. 147, No. Pt 12, pp. 3249-3262.

Riordan, J.R. (2008). CFTR function and prospects for therapy. *Annu Rev Biochem*, Vol. 77, pp. 701-726.

Rogers, G.B., Hoffman, L.R., Whiteley, M., Daniels, T.W., Carroll, M.P. & Bruce, K.D. (2010). Revealing the dynamics of polymicrobial infections: implications for antibiotic therapy. *Trends Microbiol*, Vol. 18, No. 8, pp. 357-364.

Ryan, R.P. & Dow, J.M. (2008). Diffusible signals and interspecies communication in bacteria. *Microbiology*, Vol. 154, No. Pt 7, pp. 1845-1858.

Ryan, R.P., Fouhy, Y., Garcia, B.F., Watt, S.A., Niehaus, K., Yang, L., Tolker-Nielsen, T. & Dow, J.M. (2008). Interspecies signalling via the *Stenotrophomonas maltophilia* diffusible signal factor influences biofilm formation and polymyxin tolerance in *Pseudomonas aeruginosa*. *Mol Microbiol*, Vol. 68, No. 1, pp. 75-86.

Schneider, M., Mühlemann, K., Droz, S., Couzinet, S., Casaulta, C. & Zimmerli, S. (2008). Clinical characteristics associated with isolation of small-colony variants of *Staphylococcus aureus* and *Pseudomonas aeruginosa* from respiratory secretions of patients with cystic fibrosis. *J Clin Microbiol*, Vol. 46, No. 5, pp. 1832-1834.

Scott, M.G., Dullaghan, E., Mookherjee, N., Glavas, N., Waldbrook, M., Thompson, A., Wang, A., Lee, K., Doria, S., Hamill, P., Yu, J.J., Li, Y., Donini, O., Guarna, M.M., Finlay, B.B., North, J.R. & Hancock, R.E. (2007). An anti-infective peptide that selectively modulates the innate immune response. *Nat Biotechnol*, Vol. 25, No. 4, pp. 465-472.

Sendi, P. & Proctor, R.A. (2009). *Staphylococcus aureus* as an intracellular pathogen: the role of small colony variants. *Trends Microbiol*, Vol. 17, No. 2, pp. 54-58.

Senn, M.M., Bischoff, M., von Eiff, C. & Berger-Bächi, B. (2005). σ^B activity in a *Staphylococcus aureus hemB* mutant. *J Bacteriol*, Vol. 187, No. 21, pp. 7397-7406.

Shah, P.M. (2005). The need for new therapeutic agents: what is the pipeline? *Clin Microbiol Infect*, Vol. 11 Suppl 3, pp. 36-42.

Sibley, C.D., Duan, K., Fischer, C., Parkins, M.D., Storey, D.G., Rabin, H.R. & Surette, M.G. (2008). Discerning the complexity of community interactions using a *Drosophila* model of polymicrobial infections. *PLoS Pathog*, Vol. 4, No. 10, pp. e1000184.

Sibley, C.D., Parkins, M.D., Rabin, H.R. & Surette, M.G. (2009). The relevance of the polymicrobial nature of airway infection in the acute and chronic management of patients with cystic fibrosis. *Curr Opin Investig Drugs*, Vol. 10, No. 8, pp. 787-794.

Sibley, C.D. & Surette, M.G. (2011). The polymicrobial nature of airway infections in cystic fibrosis: Cangene Gold Medal Lecture. *Can J Microbiol*, Vol. 57, No. 2, pp. 69-77.

Simões, M. (2011). Antimicrobial strategies effective against infectious bacterial biofilms. *Curr Med Chem*, Vol. 18, No. 14, pp. 2129-2145.

Singh, R., Ray, P., Das, A. & Sharma, M. (2009). Role of persisters and small-colony variants in antibiotic resistance of planktonic and biofilm-associated *Staphylococcus aureus*: an *in vitro* study. *J Med Microbiol*, Vol. 58, No. Pt 8, pp. 1067-1073.

Singh, R., Ray, P., Das, A. & Sharma, M. (2010). Enhanced production of exopolysaccharide matrix and biofilm by a menadione-auxotrophic *Staphylococcus aureus* small-colony variant. *J Med Microbiol*, Vol. 59, No. Pt 5, pp. 521-527.

Sinha, B., Francois, P.P., Nuße, O., Foti, M., Hartford, O.M., Vaudaux, P., Foster, T.J., Lew, D.P., Herrmann, M. & Krause, K.H. (1999). Fibronectin-binding protein acts as *Staphylococcus aureus* invasin via fibronectin bridging to integrin α5β1. *Cell Microbiol*, Vol. 1, No. 2, pp. 101-117.

Smith, E.E., Buckley, D.G., Wu, Z., Saenphimmachak, C., Hoffman, L.R., D'Argenio, D.A., Miller, S.I., Ramsey, B.W., Speert, D.P., Moskowitz, S.M., Burns, J.L., Kaul, R. & Olson, M.V. (2006). Genetic adaptation by *Pseudomonas aeruginosa* to the airways of cystic fibrosis patients. *Proc Natl Acad Sci U S A*, Vol. 103, No. 22, pp. 8487-8492.

Smith, R.S. & Iglewski, B.H. (2003). *P. aeruginosa* quorum-sensing systems and virulence. *Curr Opin Microbiol*, Vol. 6, No. 1, pp. 56-60.

Song, Z., Johansen, H.K., Faber, V., Moser, C., Kharazmi, A., Rygaard, J. & Høiby, N. (1997a). Ginseng treatment reduces bacterial load and lung pathology in chronic *Pseudomonas aeruginosa* pneumonia in rats. *Antimicrob Agents Chemother*, Vol. 41, No. 5, pp. 961-964.

Song, Z., Kong, K.F., Wu, H., Maricic, N., Ramalingam, B., Priestap, H., Schneper, L., Quirke, J.M., Høiby, N. & Mathee, K. (2010). Panax ginseng has anti-infective activity against opportunistic pathogen *Pseudomonas aeruginosa* by inhibiting quorum sensing, a bacterial communication process critical for establishing infection. *Phytomedicine*, Vol. 17, No. 13, pp. 1040-1046.

Song, Z.J., Johansen, H.K., Faber, V. & Høiby, N. (1997b). Ginseng treatment enhances bacterial clearance and decreases lung pathology in athymic rats with chronic *P. aeruginosa* pneumonia. *APMIS*, Vol. 105, No. 6, pp. 438-444.

Sriramulu, D.D., Nimtz, M. & Romling, U. (2005). Proteome analysis reveals adaptation of *Pseudomonas aeruginosa* to the cystic fibrosis lung environment. *Proteomics*, Vol. 5, No. 14, pp. 3712-3721.

Stewart, P.S. (2002). Mechanisms of antibiotic resistance in bacterial biofilms. *Int J Med Microbiol*, Vol. 292, No. 2, pp. 107-113.

Stoodley, P., Sauer, K., Davies, D.G. & Costerton, J.W. (2002). Biofilms as complex differentiated communities. *Annu Rev Microbiol*, Vol. 56, pp. 187-209.

Talbot, G.H., Bradley, J., Edwards, J.E., Jr., Gilbert, D., Scheld, M. & Bartlett, J.G. (2006). Bad bugs need drugs: an update on the development pipeline from the Antimicrobial Availability Task Force of the Infectious Diseases Society of America. *Clin Infect Dis*, Vol. 42, No. 5, pp. 657-668.

Tuchscherr, L., Heitmann, V., Hussain, M., Viemann, D., Roth, J., von Eiff, C., Peters, G., Becker, K. & Löffler, B. (2010). *Staphylococcus aureus* small-colony variants are adapted phenotypes for intracellular persistence. *J Infect Dis*, Vol. 202, No. 7, pp. 1031-1040.

Tuchscherr, L., Medina, E., Hussain, M., Völker, W., Heitmann, V., Niemann, S., Holzinger, D., Roth, J., Proctor, R.A., Becker, K., Peters, G. & Löffler, B. (2011). *Staphylococcus aureus* phenotype switching: an effective bacterial strategy to escape host immune response and establish a chronic infection. *EMBO Mol Med*, Vol. 3, No. 3, pp. 129-141.

Vaudaux, P., Francois, P., Bisognano, C., Kelley, W.L., Lew, D.P., Schrenzel, J., Proctor, R.A., McNamara, P.J., Peters, G. & Von Eiff, C. (2002). Increased expression of clumping factor and fibronectin-binding proteins by *hemB* mutants of *Staphylococcus aureus* expressing small colony variant phenotypes. *Infect Immun*, Vol. 70, No. 10, pp. 5428-5437.

Villena, J., Racedo, S., Agüero, G., Bru, E., Medina, M. & Alvarez, S. (2005). *Lactobacillus casei* improves resistance to pneumococcal respiratory infection in malnourished mice. *J Nutr*, Vol. 135, No. 6, pp. 1462-1469.

Voggu, L., Schlag, S., Biswas, R., Rosenstein, R., Rausch, C. & Götz, F. (2006). Microevolution of cytochrome bd oxidase in Staphylococci and its implication in resistance to respiratory toxins released by *Pseudomonas*. *J Bacteriol*, Vol. 188, No. 23, pp. 8079-8086.

von Götz, F., Häussler, S., Jordan, D., Saravanamuthu, S.S., Wehmhöner, D., Strüßmann, A., Lauber, J., Attree, I., Buer, J., Tümmler, B. & Steinmetz, I. (2004). Expression analysis of a highly adherent and cytotoxic small colony variant of *Pseudomonas aeruginosa* isolated from a lung of a patient with cystic fibrosis. *J Bacteriol*, Vol. 186, No. 12, pp. 3837-3847.

Wagner, V.E. & Iglewski, B.H. (2008). *P. aeruginosa* Biofilms in CF Infection. *Clin Rev Allergy Immunol*, Vol. 35, No. 3, pp. 124-134.

Weaver, V.B. & Kolter, R. (2004). *Burkholderia* spp. alter *Pseudomonas aeruginosa* physiology through iron sequestration. *J Bacteriol*, Vol. 186, No. 8, pp. 2376-2384.

Wenzel, R., Bate, G. & Kirkpatrick, P. (2005). Tigecycline. *Nat Rev Drug Discov*, Vol. 4, No. 10, pp. 809-810.

Williams, P. & Camara, M. (2009). Quorum sensing and environmental adaptation in *Pseudomonas aeruginosa*: a tale of regulatory networks and multifunctional signal molecules. *Curr Opin Microbiol*, Vol. 12, No. 2, pp. 182-191.

Witte, W., Cuny, C., Klare, I., Nübel, U., Strommenger, B. & Werner, G. (2008). Emergence and spread of antibiotic-resistant Gram-positive bacterial pathogens. *Int J Med Microbiol*, Vol. 298, No. 5-6, pp. 365-377.

Wu, H., Lee, B., Yang, L., Wang, H., Givskov, M., Molin, S., Høiby, N. & Song, Z. (2011). Effects of ginseng on *Pseudomonas aeruginosa* motility and biofilm formation. *FEMS Immunol Med Microbiol*, Vol. 62, No. 1, pp. 49-56.

Yang, L., Liu, Y., Markussen, T., Høiby, N., Tolker-Nielsen, T. & Molin, S. (2011). Pattern differentiation in co-culture biofilms formed by *Staphylococcus aureus* and *Pseudomonas aeruginosa*. *FEMS Immunol Med Microbiol*.

Zhang, L., Parente, J., Harris, S.M., Woods, D.E., Hancock, R.E. & Falla, T.J. (2005). Antimicrobial peptide therapeutics for cystic fibrosis. *Antimicrob Agents Chemother*, Vol. 49, No. 7, pp. 2921-2927.

Zhu, Y., Xiong, Y.Q., Sadykov, M.R., Fey, P.D., Lei, M.G., Lee, C.Y., Bayer, A.S. & Somerville, G.A. (2009). Tricarboxylic acid cycle-dependent attenuation of *Staphylococcus aureus in vivo* virulence by selective inhibition of amino acid transport. *Infect Immun*, Vol. 77, No. 10, pp. 4256-4264.

10

Atypical Bacteria in the CF Airways: Diversity, Clinical Consequences, Emergence and Adaptation

Marchandin Hélène[1,2], Michon Anne-Laure[1,2] and Jumas-Bilak Estelle[1,3]
[1]*University Montpellier 1, Equipe Pathogènes et Environnements, UMR 5119 ECOSYM,*
[2]*University Hospital of Montpellier, Bacteriology Laboratory*
[3]*University Hospital of Montpellier, Hygiene Laboratory*
France

1. Introduction

The inventory of atypical[1] bacteria that may be found in the airways of cystic fibrosis (CF) patients besides well-known typical CF pathogens like *Staphylococcus aureus*, *Haemophilus influenzae*, *Pseudomonas aeruginosa* and *Burkholderia cepacia* complex has greatly evolved over the past decades. Progressively, species initially considered as atypical in the CF airways, mainly gram-negative bacilli including *Stenotrophomonas maltophilia*, *Achromobacter xylosoxidans* and non-tuberculous mycobacteria have received more and more attention. They are now considered as usual CF-associated bacteria although their role in the disease progression is not fully elucidated (Beringer *et al.*, 2000; Foweraker, 2009; Hauser *et al.*, 2011). At the same time, other species occasionally identified from the respiratory secretions of CF patients were in turn regarded as atypical species in CF (for a recent review, see Hauser *et al.*, 2011). This resulted from both the increasing number of metagenomic studies conducted on CF airways microbiota and a more systematic use of 16S ribosomal RNA (rRNA) gene sequencing to identify bacteria cultured from CF respiratory tract (CFRT) samples (CFRTS).

Recent findings of "new" atypical bacterial species in CF airways by both cultivation-based and cultivation-independent studies gave novel insights in microbiology of the CFRT. However, pathogenesis and clinical significance of these bacteria remain unclear, i.e. adaptation to the CF airways niche, positive or negative interaction between organisms, impact on the respiratory status of the patients. Similarly, antimicrobial susceptibility pattern is more often not investigated for atypical bacteria.

In this chapter, we propose a review of both published studies and personal findings about atypical bacterial species found in CF airways by both cultivation-based and cultivation-independent studies. Personal data came from our expertise of 16S rRNA gene-based identification of atypical bacteria cultured from CFRTS in patients attending the CF center of

---

[1]The term "atypical" will be used herein to design bacterial species rarely reported in the literature dealing with the microbiology of respiratory tract in CF patients.

the Montpellier University Hospital[2]. Most of these atypical bacteria are either environmental bacteria or belong to the human respiratory tract microbiota. In this context, examples will be mainly taken from a selected panel of bacteria in our area of expertise, including human anaerobic bacteria and environmental alphaproteobacteria: *Agrobacterium*, acetic acid bacteria, *Ochrobactrum* and *Inquilinus*.

2. CF airways, a niche for environmental opportunistic pathogens

CF airways represent a particular niche in which recent cultivation-based and cultivation-independent studies revealed several atypical microbes, which were recently reviewed by Hauser *et al.* (Hauser *et al.*, 2011). Most of these bacteria are from environmental origin and act as opportunistic pathogens. Some isolates corresponded to unknown taxa when cultivated from CFRTS and supported the description of novel species such as *Inquilinus limosus* (Coenye et al., 2002). Other isolates corresponded to species isolated for the first time in man such as the acetic acid bacteria of the genus *Gluconobacter* previously recovered from environmental and food sources only (Alauzet *et al.*, 2010). We previously reported eight other species detected in CF airways samples but so far described in food or environmental samples only: *Acetobacter fabarum*, *Advenella kashmirensis*, *Aquamicrobium lusatiense*, *Chryseobacterium bovis*, *Phyllobacterium myrsinacearum*, *Pseudomonas brenneri*, *Shinella yambaruensis* and *Sphingomonas pseudosanguinis* (Jumas-Bilak *et al.*, 2011). This diversity suggested that the microbiota of the CF airways niche was far to be fully described. Finally, other isolates were identified as environmental bacteria also known to cause opportunistic infections in immunocompromised patients, for example members of the genera *Agrobacterium* or *Ochrobactrum* (Menuet *et al.*, 2008).

2.1 Atypical bacteria identified by molecular means in our center

The following paragraphs and Table 1 present a summary about the atypical bacterial species cultivated from the respiratory tract of CF patients and identified by 16S rRNA gene sequencing in our center.

Methods performed for bacterial DNA extraction, 16S rRNA gene amplification and sequencing and sequence analysis were described elsewhere; particularly a threshold of 98.7% was considered for species identification (Stackebrandt & Ebers, 2006; Teyssier *et al.*, 2003). A total of 23 atypical taxa were identified in 30 CFRTS from 25 patients. Three patients were colonized by 2 to 3 of these atypical species recovered either in a sample or in two distantly sampled specimens. Fourteen species had never been reported in man before being identified in CF patients, 6 were previously isolated in human clinical samples but were not previously reported in CF patients and 3 species were only isolated in CF patients. Among the taxa not previously isolated in man, four have been found in cultivation-independent studies of human biological samples, *Cupriavidus metallidurans* in skin microbiota (Grice *et al.*, 2009), *Cupriavidus respiraculi* in small intestine microbiota (Franck *et al.*, 2007), *P. myrsinacearum* in vaginal microbiota (Hyman *et al.*, 2005) and *S. pseudosanguinis* in diabetic wound microbiota (Grice *et al.*, 2010). Species subjected to detailed paragraphs were not included in Table 1. They were chosen to complete available recent reviews and/or to give information from personal data.

---

[2]Caring for more than 200 children and adults each year - 95 adults and 110 children in 2009, the CF center of the Montpellier University Hospital is a large regional French CF center.

Bacterial species (Patient designation)	Non-human isolation	Isolation in non-CF patients	Isolation from CF RTS	Selected reference
Advenella kashmirensis (1)	Temperate orchard soil	NPR	NPR	Ghosh *et al.*, 2005
Aquamicrobium lusatiense (2)	Activated sludge	NPR	NPR	Fritsche *et al.*, 1999
Chromobacterium aquaticum (9)	Spring-water	NPR	NPR	Young *et al.*, 2008
Chryseobacterium bovis (3)	Cow's milk	NPR	NPR	Hantsis-Zacharov *et al.*, 2008
Comamonas koreensis (4)	Forest sediment, wetland	NPR	NPR	Chang *et al.*, 2002
Phyllobacterium myrsinacearum (5)	Leaf nodules of tropical plants	NPR	NPR	Mergaert *et al.*, 2002
Pseudomonas brenneri (6)	Natural mineral waters	NPR	NPR	Baïda *et al.*, 2001
Pseudomonas nitroreducens (10)	Rhizospheric soil	NPR	NPR	Korade *et al.*, 2009
Shinella yambaruensis (7)	Soil	NPR	NPR	Matsui *et al.*, 2009
Sphingomonas pseudosanguinis (8)	Water reservoir of air humidifier	NPR	NPR	Kämpfer *et al.*, 2007a
Chryseobacterium indologenes (3)	Water, soil, hospital environment	Various	NPR	Lin *et al.*, 2010
Delftia tsuruhatensis (16-18)	Agricultural soil, bioreactor, activated sludge, rhizoplane	Catheter	NPR	Preiswerk *et al.*, 2011
Microbacterium sp.[a] (3)	Rhizosphere, mosquito, medical wastes	Various	NPR	Gneiding *et al.*, 2008
Nocardia cyriacigeorgica[b] (12-15)	Soil, animals (bovin, cat, dog)	Various	NPR	Schlaberg *et al.*, 2008
Tsukamurella sp.[c] (4)	Activated sludge	Blood, RTS, brain, cornea	NPR	Sheng *et al.*, 2009
Wautersiella falsenii (11)	Poultry	Various	NPR	Kämpfer *et al.*, 2006
Cupriavidus metallidurans (19)	Industrial biotopes	NPR	2 isolates	Coenye *et al.*, 2005
Cupriavidus respiraculi (20, 21)	NPR	NPR	23 isolates	Coenye *et al.*, 2005
Pandoraea apista (22)	NPR	NPR	22 isolates	Atkinson *et al.*, 2006
Pandoraea pulmonicola (23)	NPR	NPR	2 isolates	Coenye *et al.*, 2000
Bordetella petrii (24)	Polluted soil, river sediment, marine sponges, grass root	Bone, RTS	5 isolates	Spilker *et al.*, 2008
Brevundimonas diminuta (25)	Water, marine soil, petroleum oil, food	Various	1 isolate	Menuet *et al.*, 2008
Nocardia farcinica[b] (22)	Activated sludge, animals	Various	3 isolates	Bittar *et al.*, 2010

[a] 16S rRNA gene sequencing did not allow discrimination between *Microbacterium oxydans* and *Microbacterium paraoxydans*.

[b] Species identification was achieved by the Observatoire National des Nocardioses laboratory, Lyon, France, due to lack of discrimination between several nocardial species using 16S rRNA gene sequencing.

[c] No discrimination between *Tsukamurella tyrosinosolvens* and *Tsukamurella pulmonis*.

NPR, not previously reported; RTS, respiratory tract sample

Patients' designation in bold type indicated patients with other samples positive for atypical species listed either in Table 1 or in Table 3.

Table 1. Atypical bacterial species identified by 16S rDNA sequencing in CFRTS from patients attending the center of the University Hospital of Montpellier and general data on isolation in non-human specimens, in non-CF and CF patients.

2.2 *Inquilinus*

I. limosus is a gram-negative bacilli that grew slowly with non-pigmented and extremely mucoid colonies (Figures 1C and 1E) (Coenye *et al.*, 2002). This alphaproteobacteria belongs to the order *Rhodospirillales* and to the family *Rhodospirillaceae* that groups environmental non-sulfur purple bacteria (Table 2). Members of this family were never isolated in man except for *I. limosus* that appeared human-associated. Since its characterization from CFRTS in 2002, *I. limosus* was regularly reported, mainly from CFRT (Bittar *et al.*, 2008a; Chiron *et al.*, 2005; Coenye *et al.*, 2002). Most patients with *Inquilinus* were chronically colonized by *P. aeruginosa* and *Inquilinus* chronic colonization appeared usual in CF patients (Chiron *et al.*, 2005; Hayes *et al.*, 2009; Schmoldt *et al.*, 2006). Typing *Inquilinus* strains by random amplified polymorphic DNA (RAPD) and pulsed-field gel electrophoresis (PFGE) revealed no cross-transmission within centers and a diversity of contamination sources (Chiron *et al.*, 2005; Schmoldt *et al.*, 2006).

In our center, a 21-year-old patient is chronically colonized by *Inquilinus* sp. since the age of 12 years (Chiron *et al.*, 2005). The patient has chronic colonization by a methicillin-susceptible *S. aureus* and was transiently colonized by *P. aeruginosa* (3 *P. aeruginosa* strains isolated since *Inquilinus* recovery and no *P. aeruginosa* isolated since 4 years). *Inquilinus* sp. bacterial load ranged from 10^4 to up to 10^8 CFU/ml depending on the sample, representing the dominant or one of the major species in the sputum samples. Despite environmental investigation, the source for infection remained unknown for this patient. Environmental sources for *Inquilinus* contamination are highly suspected but they were never traced. More generally, no environmental niche for *I. limosus* is detected when screening sequences deposited for environmental clones in the GenBank database (http://www.ncbi.nlm.nih.gov/genbank/).

2.3 Acetic acid bacteria

Members of the genus *Acetobacter*, *Gluconobacter* and *Asaia* were recently isolated from the respiratory tract of CF patients. These gram-negative bacilli belong to the family *Acetobacteraceae*, the second family forming the order *Rhodospirillales* in the alphaproteobacteria together with *Rhodospirillaceae*, the family of *Inquilinus* (Table 2). *Acetobacter*, *Gluconobacter* and *Asaia* are Acetic Acid Bacteria (AAB) characterized by their ability to oxidize alcohols or sugars, leading to the production of acetic acid. AAB are commonly found in soil or are associated with plants. They have been used in industrial food processing throughout human history, especially to convert wine to vinegar and to produce tropical fermented products (Yamada & Yukphan, 2008). The first report of human infection involving AAB dates from 2004, i.e. a case of peritonitis associated with *Asaia bogorensis* (Snyder *et al.*, 2004). Since then, AAB have increasingly been reported as organisms potentially infecting humans and were firstly recognized in a CF patient in 2008 (Alauzet *et al.*, 2010; Bittar *et al.*, 2008a).

We reported four additional AAB isolates in 3 CF patients as follows: (i) successive isolation of an *Asaia* sp. and of two unrelated *Gluconobacter* sp. in a 2-year-old CF patient, (ii) a *Gluconobacter* sp. isolate unrelated to the strains from previous patient and recovered in a 3-year-old CF patient followed at the same CF center, (iii) an *A. fabarum* isolate in a 19.5-year-old CF patient (Alauzet *et al.*, 2010; Jumas-Bilak *et al.*, 2011). In these cases, AAB were recovered at low bacterial load in the sputum samples ($\leq 8 \times 10^3$ CFU/ml). AAB strains usually grew in 24 to 72 h at 30°C on various agar media selective for gram-negative bacteria except MacConkey agar whereas culture on the same media at 37°C yielded very tiny colonies (Figure 1D) (Alauzet *et al.*, 2010; Bittar *et al.*, 2008a). More generally, reports of *A. fabarum*, an AAB species recently characterized from fermented Ghanaian cocoa beans, and of *Gluconobacter* sp. increased the list of AAB, recently recognized as emerging opportunistic human pathogens, recovered from human samples (Alauzet *et al.*, 2010; Cleenwerck *et al.*, 2008).

2.4 Agrobacterium

Members of the order *Rhizobiales* and of the family *Rhizobiaceae*, *Agrobacterium* spp. are gram-negative, non-fastidious, non-fermentative short rods that form mucoid or non-mucoid colonies on agar media (Dunne *et al.*, 1993). *Agrobacterium* are recovered from soil rhizosphere and are well-known plant-associated bacteria that may be phytopathogens. Modified strains of *Agrobacterium tumefaciens* are widely used in plant engineering. In the past two decades, *Agrobacterium radiobacter* has been recognized as an opportunistic human pathogen responsible for nosocomial infections, mainly bacteremia, peritonitis, and urinary tract infections despite virulence considered to be low (Chen *et al.*, 2008; Edmond *et al.*, 1993). In 2002, four *A. radiobacter* strains have been isolated from the respiratory tract of CF patients and it has been suggested that *A. radiobacter* may have the potential to spread from patient to patient (Coenye *et al.*, 2002).

In 2010, we reported 19 additional isolates of *Agrobacterium* sp. from 17 CF patients; strains were analyzed by multilocus sequence typing (MLST) showing 11 different Sequence Types (STs), 17 of the 19 strains belonging to the genovar A7, a genovar that contained only clinical strains and probably adapted to human beings. Diversity in a single ST was demonstrated by PFGE showing that cross-contamination between patients did not occur in our center (Aujoulat *et al.*, 2010). *A. radiobacter* was mainly recognized during transient colonization, no other isolate being recovered in the follow-up of most patients (19 patients out of the 22 currently colonized in our center, 86.4%). Patients' age at *A. radiobacter* isolation ranged from 6 months to 29 years (mean age, 9 years). Successive episodes of colonization occurred in 3 patients, from 2 months to 1.5 year apart. One of these cases was investigated by typing methods showing 2 unrelated isolates recovered 1.5 year apart. In three patients, two *A. radiobacter* isolates with different cultural characteristics were observed in a sample. One of these cases was further investigated showing the patient to be colonized by two genetically different and genomically unrelated strains. Bacterial load in samples was relatively low for most cases comprised between 10^2 and 10^3 CFU/ml except for three samples where the load was higher (from 10^4 to 2×10^6 CFU/ml) but *A. radiobacter* was not the dominant species. These samples were taken during scheduled consultation for two patients and during exacerbation attributed to *H. influenzae* for the third patient. Bacterial species mainly co-isolated are the usual pathogens *S. aureus* (9 patients) and *H. influenzae* (5 patients) while co-isolation of *P. aeruginosa* was noted in one patient only. Of note, *A. radiobacter* is usually recovered in highly diversified polymicrobial cultures associated with other rarely isolated organisms like *Acinetobacter* spp., *B. diminuta*, *Comamonas acidovorans*, *C. indologenes*, *C. respiraculi*, *D. tsuruhatensis*, *Enterobacteriaceae* (9 different species), *Ochrobactrum anthropi*, *Tsukamurella* sp. or *Roseomonas* sp. (16 out of 22 patients).

2.5 Ochrobactrum

Another member of the order *Rhizobiales* in alphaproteobacteria, the genus *Ochrobactrum* groups bacteria increasingly reported in CF (Menuet *et al.*, 2008; Yagüe-Muñoz *et al.*, 2010). First considered as an emerging pathogen by Menuet *et al.*, *O. anthropi* was responsible for a bacteremia in CF. *Ochrobactrum* spp. are gram-negative non-fermentative oxidase-positive short rods recovered from a wide variety of environmental sources (water, soil, rhizosphere) as well as from plants, animals and human. Five species, *O. anthropi*, *O. intermedium*, *O. pseudintermedium*, *O. haematophilum* and *O. pseudogrignonense* were recovered from human samples; the first two species being increasingly reported as opportunistic pathogens mainly during nosocomial infections, particularly bacteremia and endocarditis (Kämpfer *et al.*, 2007b; Teyssier *et al.* 2005, 2007). *Ochrobactrum* spp. do not present exigent cultural requirements and colony morphology depends on the species (Teyssier & Jumas-Bilak, 2011).

In our center, 14 patients are colonized by *Ochrobactrum* spp. strains (mean age, 3 years [10 months-18 years]) and 35 isolates were recovered (one to 10 isolates per patient). Serial isolates were isolated in seven patients. *O. anthropi* was the major species recovered in CF patients, all the isolates except three being identified as *O. anthropi*. Moreover, *O. intermedium* (n=1) and *O. pseudogrignonense* (n=2) were isolated from patients also colonized by *O. anthropi*. The relative importance of species observed in CF did not reflect the distribution of species in the general population where *O. intermedium* was more frequently represented (Teyssier *et al.*, 2003). In a collection of 66 *Ochrobactrum* spp. from the non-CF population attending the University Hospital of Montpellier, species identified by molecular means were distributed as follows: *O. anthropi* (n=37, 56.1%), *O. intermedium* (n=25, 37.9%), *O. pseudogrignonense* (n=1, 1.5%), and *O. pseudintermedium* (n=3, 4.5%) (unpublished data). Two strains of *O. pseudogrignonense* recovered from human clinical samples (blood and ear) supported the description of the species in 2007, then this recently described species was recovered from CFRTS, two patients attending our center being colonized by unrelated *O. pseudogrignonense* strains. Main associated bacteria were *S. maltophilia* (8 patients), *Enterobacteriaceae* (7 patients), and *S. aureus* and *H. influenzae* (6 patients each). Concomitant isolation of *P. aeruginosa* was observed for 6 samples from 4 patients while co-isolation of atypical species like *A. radiobacter*, *Acinetobacter* spp., *Alcaligenes* spp., *A. kashmirensis*, *C. acidovorans*, *C. indologenes*, *D. tsuruhatensis* and *S. paucimobilis* was frequently observed. Bacterial load was comprised between 10^2 and 4×10^4 CFU of *Ochrobactrum* spp./ml and in most samples *Ochrobactrum* spp. were not the dominant species. Molecular typing based on PFGE and MLST revealed a high level of diversity among isolates showing that no epidemic strains spread occurred in our center (Romano *et al.*, 2009). The same typing methods showed that serial isolates recovered from a patient could correspond to successive colonization by unrelated strains. Such successive episodes of colonization were observed in 5 patients. By contrast, chronic colonization was noted over a 10-month period (4 serial isolates) for one patient with intercurrent isolation of unrelated *O. anthropi* strains and for a 3-year period in a second patient (2 isolates). Complex route of colonization by *Ochrobactrum* spp. in CF is revealed here and warrants further investigation to search for the diversity of sources.

2.6 How unusual are atypical CF-associated bacteria?

2.6.1 Incidence of atypical species in CF

When looking at the isolation frequency of the atypical bacteria described by Hauser *et al.* in our CF center, we found that most of the taxa cited were recovered from sputum samples of the patients thereby underlining that these species were not exceptionally isolated from CFRTS (Hauser *et al.*, 2011).

Strains whose identification was confirmed by 16S rRNA gene sequencing were listed in Table 1. Regarding other taxa detailed herein, AAB have been recovered from the respiratory tract of about 1% of the patients attending our CF center and are still to be considered as an unusual isolation in CF. *Agrobacterium* and *O. anthropi* isolates were found in about 10% and 7% of the patients, respectively and should not be considered anymore as unusual species in CFRT. Other species of *Ochrobactrum* are still to be considered as very unusually isolated in CF. A unique patient was chronically colonized by *Inquilinus* sp. in our CF center (0.5% of the patients) while higher incidence was reported in other CF centers. Notably, a higher incidence is reported in a neighbor region in South of France because *Inquilinus* was reported in 2.8% out of 145 CF patients, incidence varying according to age from 1.2% in children to 4.9% in adult patients (Bittar *et al.*, 2008a). *Inquilinus* sp. was not found in the respiratory tract of non-CF patients (Bittar *et al.*, 2008a). Interestingly, we observed that patients colonized by one of the previous taxa are often simultaneously or successively colonized by other of these species. For example, among the 22 patients with at least one isolate of *Agrobacterium* sp., 9 had at least one episode of colonization by another environmental alphaproteobacteria. The two patients with AAB were also colonized by *A. radiobacter* alone or associated with *O. anthropi* colonization. Other species or genera cited by Hauser *et al.* that were isolated in our center but not detailed here are *Acinetobacter* spp., *Chryseobacterium* spp. and members of the family *Enterobacteriaceae*.

2.6.2 Atypical or underestimated species?

Modification in cultivation and identification methods applied for CFRTS processing may explain an increasing rate of recovery of some species during CF. For example, AAB are increasingly recognized as emerging human opportunistic pathogens and their frequency may probably be underestimated because of their growth characteristics, particularly their faint growth at 37°C, a default temperature setting in routine medical microbiology, and because of the difficulty with identifying these microorganisms. For instance, the recovery of AAB in CF was related to the use of *Burkholderia cepacia* complex selective agar that is incubated for a prolonged incubation time (5 days) at 30°C. Therefore, the recovery of *Asaia* and *Gluconobacter* is enhanced because they resisted to antibiotics included in the medium and they grew in such cultivation conditions while no growth is observed on MacConkey agar plates incubated for 3 days at 30°C or 37°C (Alauzet *et al.*, 2010) (Figure 1D).

Growth of atypical bacteria on different media and at different incubation temperatures is shown in Figure 1.

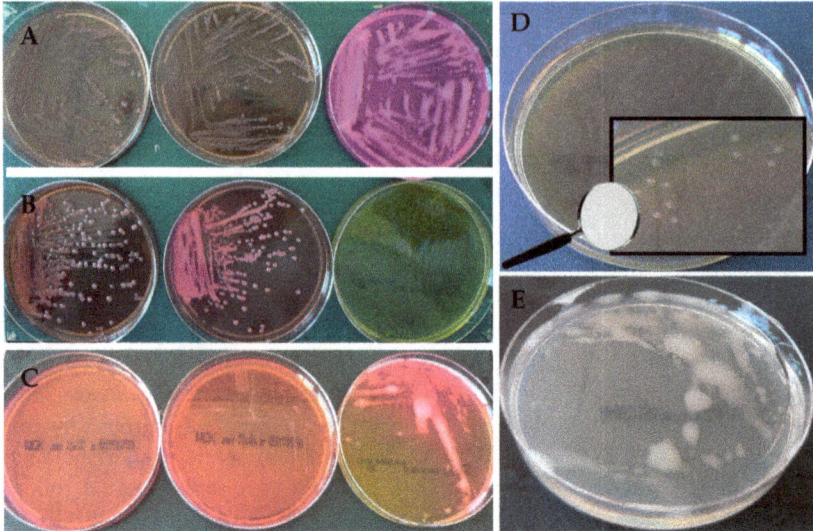

Fig. 1. Growth of *O. anthropi* (A), *A. radiobacter* (B) and *Inquilinus* sp. (C) on MacConkey agar plates (bioMérieux) incubated at 37°C (left) or 30°C (middle) and on the *Burkholderia cepacia*-selective medium Cepacia agar (AES) incubated at 30°C (right); growth of *Gluconobacter* sp. on *B. cepacia*-selective medium Cepacia agar (D), and growth of *Inquilinus* sp. on Mueller-Hinton agar (bioMérieux) (E) (incubation time was 3 days in all cases).

In addition to limitation related to cultivation conditions, recovery of atypical species could also be impaired by the routine practice of CFRT sampling. Indeed, the unique sample usually submitted to bacteriological analysis was shown to be insufficient for recognition of all bacteria that may colonize the patient, including CF pathogens (Rogers *et al.*, 2010).

Regarding identification, molecular-based methods revealed up to 25% of isolates without correct phenotypic identification (Bittar *et al.*, 2008b). *A. radiobacter* strains are accurately identified with API 20NE strip or VITEK2 GN card (bioMérieux) but *A. radiobacter* is named *Rhizobium radiobacter* in API and VITEK2 databases due to confusing taxonomy in these genera (Aujoulat *et al.*, 2010; Otto-Karg *et al.*, 2009; Teyssier *et al.*, 2009). Identification could be more difficult for other taxa. *O. anthropi* is the sole species of the genus included in API and VITEK2 databases. Both systems permit genus-level identification and sequencing of either 16S rRNA gene or another housekeeping gene should be performed for species identification. Although *Inquilinus* sp. showed several notable characteristics that will be discussed below, i.e. mucoid phenotype, characteristic multiresistant pattern to antibiotics and ability to persist in the CF airways, its identification remains difficult. This emerging pathogen was either not detected or misclassified by laboratories (Bittar *et al.*, 2008b; Hogard *et al.*, 2009). Since 2011, a second species has been described in the genus, *Inquilinus ginsengisoli*, isolated from soil (Jung *et al.*, 2011). This species could be differentiated from *I. limosus* by a careful 16S rRNA gene analysis. Similarly, both genera of AAB recovered in CF patients, i.e. *Asaia* and *Gluconobacter* required molecular methods for their identification. However, some closely related species belonging to these genera might remain unidentified despite sequencing housekeeping genes in addition to 16S rRNA gene (Alauzet *et al.*, 2010).

Recently, matrix-assisted laser desorption ionization–time of flight mass spectrometry (MALDI-TOF-MS) was used for identification of non-fermentative gram-negative bacilli isolated from CF patients (Degand *et al.*, 2008). A few atypical species covered by this chapter were included, i.e. 1 *B. hinzii*, 1 *I. limosus*, 1 *C. respiraculi*. The three isolates were correctly identified by the system. Another study evaluating the system for identification of environmental members of the family *Rhizobiaceae* including *Agrobacterium* (= *Rhizobium*) *radiobacter* showed comparable performances to housekeeping gene sequence analysis suggesting that this species might be correctly identified by the system if included in the "CF" database (Ferreira *et al.*, 2011). Additional studies on a larger panel of isolates are needed to precisely evaluate the performance of the system for identifying all the diversity of atypical bacteria that may be encountered in CF samples.

2.7 Taxonomic diversity of atypical bacteria in CF

Atypical taxa isolated from CFRTS in our center and identified by 16S rRNA gene sequencing are distributed among 3 phyla, the phylum *Proteobacteria* being the most represented. The Table 2 gives the taxonomic repartition of the atypical taxa in the 3 major phyla. In the *Proteobacteria*, gram-negative bacilli of the class *Alphaproteobacteria* account for the majority of atypical taxa identified (Table 2). This may suggest that patients are more frequently in contact with the environmental niches of these species and/or that these taxa have an increased potential to colonize the CFRT.

Phylum	Class	Order	Family	Taxon
Actinobacteria	*Actinobacteria*	*Actinomycetales*	*Actinomycetaceae*	*Actinomyces graevenitzii*
			Microbacteriaceae	*Microbacterium* sp.
			Nocardiaceae	*Nocardia* spp.
			Tsukamurellaceae	*Tsukamurella* sp.
Bacteroidetes	*Flavobacteria*	*Flavobacteriales*	*Flavobacteriaceae*	*Chryseobacterium* spp.
				Wautersiella falsenii
Proteobacteria	*Alphaproteobacteria*	*Caulobacterales*	*Caulobacteraceae*	*Brevundimonas diminuta*
		Rhizobiales	*Brucellaceae*	*Ochrobactrum* spp.
			Phyllobacteriaceae	*Aquamicrobium lusatiense*
				Phyllobacterium myrsinacearum
			Rhizobiaceae	*Agrobacterium* sp.
				Shinella yambaruensis
		Rhodospirillales	*Acetobacteraceae*	*Acetobacter fabarum*
				Asaia sp.
				Gluconobacter sp.
			Rhodospirillaceae	*Inquilinus limosus*
		Sphingomonadales	*Sphingomonadaceae*	*Sphingomonas pseudosanguinis*
	Betaproteobacteria	*Burkholderiales*	*Alcaligenaceae*	*Advenella kashmirensis*
				Bordetella spp.
			Burkholderiaceae	*Cupriavidus* spp.
				Pandoraea spp.
			Comamonadaceae	*Comamonas koreensis*
				Delftia tsuruhatensis
		Neisseriales	*Neisseriaceae*	*Chromobacterium aquaticum*
	Gammaproteobacteria	*Pseudomonadales*	*Pseudomonadaceae*	*Pseudomonas brenneri*
				Pseudomonas nitroreducens

Table 2. Taxonomic lineages for atypical bacteria identified from CFRTS in our center using 16S rRNA gene sequencing.

2.8 Unknown cultivated bacterial taxa in CF

Diversity of the cultivable part of the CFRT microbiota remains underestimated. In the past decade, 12 novel species were characterized based on isolates recovered in CFRTS, i.e. 7 *Burkholderia* species, 3 *Ralstonia* species (of which 2 are yet reclassified in the genus *Cupriavidus*), *Advenella incenata* and *I. limosus* (PubMed search on August the 1st, 2011 with key words "sp. nov." and "cystic fibrosis"). In our center, identification based on 16S rDNA revealed 5 potential novel taxa cultivated from CFRTS (Table 3). Of note, 2 patients had other samples positive for atypical species listed in Table 1. Altogether these data illustrate the diversity not fully explored of bacteria that could be cultivated from CFRTS.

Isolate reference	Patient no.	16S rDNA sequence similarity with the closest known species (%, name of the species)	Taxonomic interpretation*
29 dec. 2009, 2320	26	96%, *Corynebacterium durum*	Novel species in the genus *Corynebacterium*
15 jun. 2007, 5197	**19**	96.5%, *Cupriavidus metallidurans*	Novel species in the genus *Cupriavidus*
21 jul. 2009, 2477	27	97.6%, *Roseomonas cervicalis*	Probable novel species in the genus *Roseomonas*
20 nov. 2009, 5248	28	98.2%, *Cupriavidus respiraculi*	Probable novel species in the genus *Cupriavidus*
15 apr. 2005, 5138	**6**	98.5%, *Cupriavidus respiraculi*	Probable novel species in the genus *Cupriavidus*

* Isolates showing less than 97% of sequence similarity with the closest known species were considered as novel taxa (Stackebrandt & Goebel, 1994); isolates showing between 97% and 98.7% of sequence similarity with the closest known species were considered as probable novel taxa (Stackebrandt & Ebers, 2006). Bold type indicated patients with other samples positive for atypical species as listed in Table 1.

Table 3. Unknown taxa in the CFRTS from patients attending the CF center of the University Hospital of Montpellier.

3. Atypical pathologic communities in CF

3.1 Microbial diversity in CFRT assessed by cultivation-independent studies

Over the last decade, our knowledge of the bacterial diversity in CFRT microbiota has evolved due to cultivation-independent methods. Terminal Restriction Fragment Length Polymorphism Profiling, Temporal Temperature Gradient gel Electrophoresis or sequencing were employed to characterize 16S ribosomal DNA in CFRT community and revealed both a higher biodiversity than previously presumed and several atypical organisms (Bittar *et al.*, 2008b; Guss *et al.*, 2011; Kolak *et al.*, 2003; Rogers *et al.*, 2004).

Comparison between cultivation-based methods and cultivation independent methods revealed the overlooked part of bacteria present in CFRTS including species recovered from the oral microbiota during health and diseases, atypical species of unknown pathogenicity and well-known bacterial species pathogenic for CF patients (Bittar *et al.*, 2008b; Rogers *et al.*, 2009; van Belkum *et al.*, 2000). For example, Bittar *et al.*, studying 25 CF sputum samples showed that 53 species were found using the PCR-cloning-sequencing approach while only 13 were cultivated (Bittar *et al.*, 2008b). Sixteen species only found by the molecular method corresponded to anaerobes not covered by the cultivation conditions used in the study. Nevertheless, several aerobic and anaerobic species detected by the genomic method corresponded to species unusually or firstly detected in CF (Bittar *et al.*, 2008b).

Additional unexpected bacteria were described in other cultivation-independent studies. For example, Harris *et al.* reported in a 14-year-old CF patient the first occurrence in man of sequences corresponding to the alphaproteobacteria *Chelatococcus asaccharovorans* (Harris *et al.*, 2007). These sequences represented 5% of the total sequences found in the corresponding specimen. Some of the other unexpected bacteria overlooked by cultivation-based methods and revealed by cultivation-independent methods may be clinically relevant in CF. Indeed, CF candidate pathogens were identified by Harris *et al.* comparing microbiota from CF and non-CF patients as follows: *Prevotella denticola*, *Lysobacter* sp., and *Rickettsiales* sp. (Harris *et al.*, 2007). Interestingly, members of the genus *Lysobacter* are gram-negative bacilli showing similar environmental lifestyle as *Agrobacterium* and *Ochrobactrum*, i.e. isolated from soil, rhizosphere and plant-associated samples. *Lysobacter* spp. were also found as dominant species on the human tongue dorsum and recovered from the surface of prosthetic hip joints (Dempsey *et al.*, 2007; Riggio *et al.*, 2008). Unless additional arguments are given, *Lysobacter* sp. should be considered with caution as a CF potential pathogen. Finally, cultivation-independent studies revealed the occurrence of several unknown taxa in the CFRTS like novel members of the order *Rickettsiales* and of the family *Coxiellaceae* (the latter representing 11% of the sequences found in association with those of *Chelatococcus asaccharovorans*) (Harris *et al.*, 2007). Regarding bacterial taxa developed in this chapter, i.e. *Inquilinus*, acetic acid bacteria, *Agrobacterium* and *Ochrobactrum*, sequences of *Inquilinus* sp. were recovered in some cultivation-independent studies while the other taxa were not found (Bittar *et al.*, 2008b). In addition to patients' sampling methods, these taxa may be overlooked in molecular-based approaches due to their minority in the CFRT microbiota, a hypothesis congruent with the low bacterial load observed in culture for these bacteria.

3.2 Dysbiosis in the CF polymicrobial disease and example of anaerobes

Comparison of microbiota diversity in CF patients and in control groups, as well as cultivation-independent studies suggested that CF should be considered as a polymicrobial disease (Klepac-Ceraj *et al.*, 2010; Sibley *et al.*, 2006). A major recent finding revealed that lung function is significantly and positively correlated with the bacterial species richness of the global microbiota (van der Gast *et al.*, 2011). Considering the inter-individual variations in the microbiota composition, van der Gast *et al.* studying microbiota composition of sputum samples from 14 adult CF patients further showed that both core and satellite taxa are significantly correlated with lung function (van der Gast *et al.*, 2011). Moreover, any disequilibrium in the consortium of microorganisms found in the CFRT may have clinical consequences on the clinical status as previously observed in other dysbiosis-associated diseases like bacterial vaginosis (Oakley *et al.*, 2008). Although the total number of bacterial species observed in a population of CF patients was shown significantly more diverse than that observed in a control group including bronchiectasis patients (Bittar *et al.*, 2008b), at the individual level, libraries of lower complexity were observed in CF compared to a control group (Harris *et al.*, 2007). Such a low diversity observed in CF patients may reflect the enrichment of a pathogenic species and/or the consequence of dysbiosis and so possibly signify bacterial involvement in disease (Harris *et al.*, 2007). For example, among the 28 CF patients included in the study, more than the half (53.6%) had less than 5 organisms detected and one of these microorganisms dominated the poorly diversified microbiota (from 63 to 98% of the sequences). For 8 patients, all sequences corresponded to a unique bacterial taxon (*S. aureus*, *Lysobacter* sp., *S. maltophilia*, *P. aeruginosa* and *Mycobacterium abscessus*). Atypical bacteria proposed as CF candidate pathogens and cited above, i.e. *P. denticola*, *Lysobacter* sp., and *Rickettsiales* sp. were all encountered in dysbiotic environment. Indeed, these sequences were each recovered in a CF patient as a major or as the unique sequence among sequences of the patient's microbiota, representing 56%, 100% and 36% of the total sequences, respectively (Harris *et al.*, 2007). Based on the example of *P. denticola*, we will discuss further on the role of anaerobes, particularly those belonging to the genus *Prevotella*, in the dysbiosis that may occur in CF (for a review on anaerobic bacteria infection in cystic fibrosis airway disease, see Lambiase *et al.*, 2010).

In both cultivation-based and cultivation-independent studies, particular attention was recently paid to anaerobic microflora, which had received little attention before (Bittar *et al.*, 2008b; Harris *et al.*, 2007; Tunney *et al.*, 2008). Indeed, anaerobic cultures are not performed in the routine practice of sputum samples and thus anaerobic bacteria are totally ignored except when specifically studied (Jewes & Spencer, 1990). Tunney *et al.* assessing anaerobic bacteria in CF children by means of culture of bronchoalveolar lavage fluid samples demonstrated that anaerobic bacteria are: (i) frequently present in the airway specimens, (ii) in higher numbers than in healthy volunteers, and (iii) generally different species compared with those detected in the non-CF control group (Tunney *et al.*, 2008). Identification of the anaerobes isolated revealed 14 different genera with the genus *Prevotella*, being the most frequently isolated before *Veillonella*, *Propionibacterium*, and *Actinomyces*. *Prevotella* spp. were present in 22% to > 80% of the CF patients depending on the study while found in 10% of healthy patients (Field *et al.*, 2010; Tunney *et al.*, 2008). Based on cultivation-independent methods, Bittar *et al.* showed the anaerobes to represent 30.2% of the detected species in CF sputum specimens (16/53 species) with *Prevotella* sequences being dominant (48.7%) among sequences corresponding to anaerobes (Bittar *et al.*, 2008b). *Prevotella melaninogenica* is usually the most common species identified in these studies. Strict anaerobes are well-known oral species. However, they were not regarded to be simply contaminants because of their diversity and abundance within the CF airways compared to non-CF population (Jones, 2011). Among them, *Prevotella* spp., already known as contributing to the consortia of microorganisms involved in several human pathologies attributed to dysbiosis, may contribute to CF airway disease (Alauzet *et al.*, 2010; Field *et al.*, 2010).

What remains also unknown is how the quantitative and/or qualitative modification in the composition of the microbiota would affect interactions between organisms. These interactions were previously demonstrated in complex microbiota like modulation of *P. aeruginosa* gene expression by host microflora through interspecies communication (Duan *et al.*, 2003; Sibley *et al.*, 2008b). It was hypothesized that *Prevotella* spp. may also modulate *P. aeruginosa* virulence gene expression as well as growth and virulence of the potential CF pathogen of the *Streptococcus milleri* group (Field et al., 2010; Shinzato *et al.*, 1994; Sibley *et al.*, 2008a). Unfortunately, *Prevotella* spp. were not included by Sibley *et al.* in the 40 oropharyngeal species tested for both microbe–microbe and polymicrobe–host interactions in *Drosophila melanogaster* infection model (Sibley *et al.*, 2008b).

4. Pathogenesis and clinical consequences of colonization by atypical bacteria

Harris *et al.* previously hypothesized that atypical bacteria may explain inflammation in the absence of documented pathogens as well as failure to standard treatment in CF (Harris *et al.*, 2007). The clinical significance in CF of bacteria detailed in this chapter remains unclear, as it is still the case for more frequently isolated species like *A. xylosoxidans* (Hauser *et al.*, 2011).

Regarding anaerobes, Worlitzsch *et al.* showed that patients with and without obligate anaerobes in sputum specimens did not differ in lung function (Worlitzsch *et al.*, 2009). AAB, *Agrobacterium*, *Inquilinus* and *Ochrobactrum* members are considered as opportunistic human pathogens, being involved in systemic or severe infections in immunocompromised patients or patients with underlying diseases/conditions (Alauzet *et al.*, 2010; Chen *et al.*, 2008; Cieslak *et al.*, 1996; Kiratisin *et al.*, 2006).

Case reports documented potential virulence in CF for some of these atypical bacteria. For AAB, the first case report in CF documented *Acetobacter indonesiensis* isolation during pneumonia occurring after lung transplant. The bacterium was considered to be the primary cause of the infection because of clinical improvement after adapted antimicrobial therapy (Bittar *et al.*, 2008a). By contrast, *Gluconobacter* and *Asaia* sp. could not be incriminated in the evolution of the disease because of a favorable clinical evolution without any specific treatment (Alauzet *et al.*, 2010). Case reports also witnessed for a potential pathogenic power of *Ochrobactrum* sp. in CF patients because *O. anthropi* was previously involved: (i) in association with *B. diminuta* in a case of acute pneumonia in a 17-year-old CF patient showing clinical improvement after adapted antimicrobial therapy including imipenem and tobramycin (Menuet *et al.*, 2008), (ii) in a case of bacteremia in children (Yagüe-Muñoz *et al.*, 2010). *Inquilinus* isolation was associated either with acute pulmonary exacerbation, respiratory decline without signs of acute exacerbation or stable respiratory status (Chiron *et al.*, 2005; Schmoldt *et al.*, 2006). To date, the patient chronically colonized by *Inquilinus* sp. in our center has stable respiratory status. *Inquilinus* sp. was also responsible for prosthetic valve endocarditis in a tetralogy of Fallot patient (Kiratisin *et al.*, 2006). Additional arguments in favor of pathogenic potential of *Inquilinus* sp. are: (i) specific serum antibody response found in patients with *Inquilinus* sp. (Schmoldt *et al.*, 2006), (ii) mucoid characteristic of *Inquilinus* sp. that could be related to exopolysaccharides, recognised as important virulence factors in lung infections, showing novel structures with usual components and similarity with *P. aeruginosa* exopolysaccharides (Herasimenka *et al.*, 2007). Finally, no clinical data associated with *A. radiobacter* isolation in CF are currently available. From our personal data, *A. radiobacter* was mainly a transient colonizer of the CFRT while *Ochrobactrum* spp. displayed more complex relationships with CF host. These species were usually recovered at low bacterial load and in mixed cultures from the respiratory secretions sampled in patients during scheduled consultations. Their recovery was mainly associated with stable respiratory status but in some cases, respiratory decline with or without signs of acute exacerbation were noted. In these cases, multiple species were simultaneously isolated from the CFRTS, making it difficult to attribute signs and symptoms to a specific bacterium.

Treatment against these species was usually not started except in one case of *A. radiobacter* isolation that was recovered at low bacterial load but in pure culture in a context of respiratory decline in a 4-year-old patient. Trimethoprim/sulfamethoxazole treatment for 15 days led to eradication of the species from the airways and clinical improvement in this patient. In another patient with deteriorated respiratory status, antimicrobial treatment associating ciprofloxacin and trimethoprim/sulfamethoxazole was established. According to the antibiograms, this treatment was effective against all bacteria cultured from the sputum specimen, i.e. *A. radiobacter* but also *D. tsuruhatensis*, two enterobacteria and *S. aureus*, the major species in the sample and showed efficacy on the clinical status of the patient.

Of note, *Agrobacterium* and/or *Ochrobactrum* spp. were relatively frequently isolated after antimicrobial treatment against *P. aeruginosa* or *S. aureus* due to their resistance to amoxicillin/clavulanic acid, ceftazidime, tobramycin and/or colistin. Indeed, as previously described for other mild opportunistic pathogens of environmental origin like *S. maltophilia*; acetic acid bacteria, *Inquilinus* and *Ochrobactrum* spp. displayed a high level of resistance to antibacterial compounds (Alauzet *et al.*, 2010; Berg *et al.*, 2005; Bittar *et* al, 2008a; Thoma *et al.*, 2009) (Figure 2).

Multiresistance-encoding genetic determinant has only been characterized for *O. anthropi* as a chromosomal class C beta-lactamase named OCH-1 while remaining unknown for *Agrobacterium*, AAB, *Inquilinus* sp. and other *Ochrobactrum* species (Nadjar *et al.*, 2001). Moreover, majority of these species displayed intrinsic resistance to colistin. *Agrobacterium* sp. resisted to several drugs used in CF patients like ceftazidime and tobramycin but displayed resistance to less drugs than AAB, *Inquilinus* and *Ochrobactrum*.

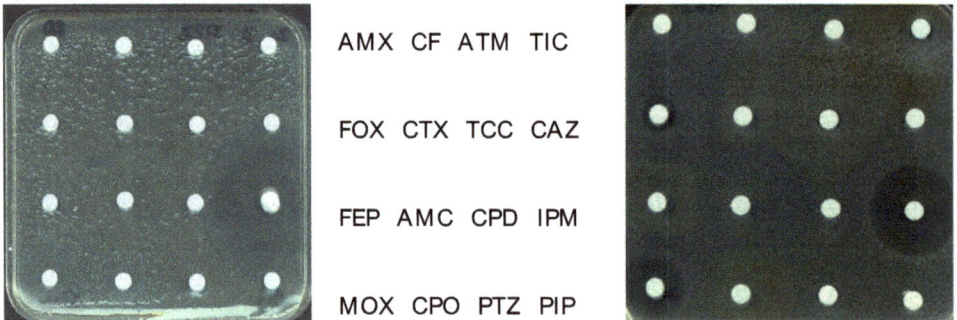

AMX CF ATM TIC

FOX CTX TCC CAZ

FEP AMC CPD IPM

MOX CPO PTZ PIP

Fig. 2. Multiresistance pattern to β-lactam agents observed for *Inquilinus* sp. (left) and *O. intermedium* (right) by disk diffusion assay (antibiotic disk position is indicated by corresponding drug abbreviation in the middle).

Abbreviations and concentrations for antibiotics indicated according to disk position are: AMX, amoxicillin (25 µg); CF, cephalotin (30 µg); ATM, aztreonam (30 µg); TIC, ticarcillin (75 µg); FOX, cefoxitin (30 µg); CTX, cefotaxime (30 µg); CAZ, ceftazidime (30µg); TCC, ticarcillin/clavulanic acid (75 µg /10 µg); FEP, cefepime (30 µg); AMC, amoxicillin/clavulanic acid (20 µg /10 µg); CPD, cefpodoxime (30 µg); IPM, imipenem (10 µg); MOX, latamoxef (30 µg); CPO, cefpirome (30 µg); PTZ, piperacillin/tazobactam (75 µg /10 µg); PIP, piperacillin (75 µg).

There are too few isolates reported in the literature and even fewer CF case reports involving these atypical bacteria to drawn conclusion on their clinical relevance in CF. Moreover, interactions between these atypical species and other organisms within the CFRT microbiota is unknown. Knowledge on the virulence of these atypical bacteria required rigorous description and follow-up of cases involving such bacteria. Moreover, case control studies will also be needed to determine their clinical implication in CF patients as well as risk factors for acquisition. From our experience, it could be hypothesized that these species may be selected by antimicrobial therapy against pathogens due to their resistance or multidrug resistance. This has been previously suggested for *S. maltophilia,* which has a predilection to infect CF patients with more advanced disease and consequently more frequently exposed to broad-spectrum antibiotics (Hauser *et al.*, 2011). Similarly, the increased use of nebulized colistin in CF patients may select specific colistin-resistant bacteria as previously suggested for *B. diminuta* (Menuet *et al.*, 2008).

Besides intrinsic resistance, several bacteria present in the CFRT microbiota may acquire additional resistance mechanisms. Development of multidrug resistance is a frequent finding in CF and is usually mediated by combination of several resistance mechanisms (Poole, 2011). Acquired multidrug resistance may also be encoded by extended spectrum β-lactamases (ESBLs) and carbapenemases, which are increasingly reported in pathogens commonly found in CF (*P. aeruginosa, S. maltophilia*). *Enterobacteriaceae* can harbor ESBL-encoding genes localized on mobile genetic elements that may be transferable between members of the community. Although such observations remain rare (Cantón *et al.*, 1997; 2 unpublished isolates in our centre), microbiologists have to be aware of multidrug resistant enterobacteria in CF due to pandemic dissemination of some enzymes like CTX-M ESBLs in the global population (Cantón *et al.*, 2006). In this context, atypical bacteria from environmental origin, even transiently colonizing CFRT may constitute a reservoir of resistance determinants that can be mobilized into the microbial community, thereby contributing to the global increase of the microbiota resistance (Wright, 2010). Moreover, antibiotic degrading diffusible enzymes that may be secreted by atypical bacteria are a matter of concern. Indeed, antimicrobial treatment against pathogens associated with these atypical bacteria may become ineffective due to antibiotic hydrolysis by these enzymes. Altogether, bacteria showing multidrug resistance whether this resistance is innate or acquired contribute to the increase of the global resistome of the CFRT microbiota.

5. Adaptation of atypical bacteria to the CF airways niche

5.1 Adaptation to CFRT conditions

Airways of CF patients represent an ecological niche recognized as a model system for studies on bacterial adaptation. Indeed, in this specific niche, the bacteria incoming from the outer environment are submitted to complex selective forces from microbiological, immunological, physiological and biochemical environment of the CF airways that may drive the evolution of the corresponding microorganism (Yang *et al.*, 2011a, 2011b). Several microbial species appear to be well adapted to survival within the CF airways (Hauser *et al.*, 2011). Some species may adapt by forming colony variants, i.e. small-colony variants for *S. aureus* and *P. aeruginosa* or mucoid colony variants for *P. aeruginosa*, favoring resistance to antibiotics, evasion to immune system and then long-term persistence in the CF airways. *P. aeruginosa*, the most studied pathogen, may adapt by a wide range of mechanisms that were recently reviewed (Hauser *et al.*, 2011).

For atypical bacteria considered herein, little is known about the mechanisms of adaptation to host environment i.e. to CFRT. Extrapolating from *P. aeruginosa*, mucoid phenotype (*Inquilinus*, *Ochrobactrum*), antibiotic resistance (*Inquilinus*, *Ochrobactrum*, *Agrobacterium*), modifications in lipopolysaccharide (gram-negative genera) or existence of subsets of host-adapted strains (*Ochrobactrum*, *Agrobacterium*) are traits that may favor adaptation to CFRT. Although not yet further investigated, we observed diversification in both colonial morphology and antibiotype (susceptibility/resistance to fluoroquinolones) after a 6-year period of *Inquilinus* sp. colonization. Moreover, population genetics revealed lineages of *Agrobacterium* and *O. anthropi* adapted to man but not specifically CF-adapted in contrast to *P. aeruginosa* for which two genotypes were shown as specifically-associated with CF (Aujoulat *et al.*, 2010; Romano *et al.*, 2009; van Mansfeld *et al.*, 2010). In addition, some other mechanisms of adaptation may be suspected for bacteria covered by this chapter. As far as AAB are concerned, it was previously hypothesized that they might specifically colonize the CFRT in relation to their ability to grow in acidic conditions. Indeed, this particular metabolic trait may confer a selective advantage to these bacteria in the acidified CF airways (Alauzet *et al.*, 2010; Poschet *et al.*, 2002).

5.2 Adaptative evolution in the CFRT

CFRT is a compartimentalized niche, which is spatially and temporally heterogeneous according to the anatomic site and to the period of disease evolution. A variable but relatively closed niche could drive diversification and adaptative evolution of the microbiota. In addition, mortality agents such as host immunity, antibiotics and lysogenic phages could lead to the diversification of a bacterial population that contribute to the persistence of the infection, as previously described for *P. aeruginosa* in the CF lung (Brockhurst *et al.*, 2005).

The ability to switch to hypermutable phenotypes by rapid acquisition of mutations at an unusually high rate lead to phenotypic diversification as observed for *H. influenzae*, *S. aureus* and *P. aeruginosa* (Hauser *et al.*, 2011). Besides hypermutation, genome plasticity is a mechanism for a bacterium to diversify its population and to adapt in various environments. Genomic rearrangements have been described in *P. aeruginosa* to switch from a saprophytic to a pathogenic lifestyle. Large chromosomal inversions are associated with insertion sequences duplication in *P. aeruginosa* strains isolated in CF. These events, by disrupting genes, have been shown to be involved in phenotypic adaptation of the strains to their particular environment (Coyne *et al.*, 2010).

Genomic macrorestriction followed by PFGE is an efficient tool to follow genomic rearrangements, particularly in bacterial species poorly investigated at the genetic level, as atypical species isolated from CFRT. Genomic evolution was previously demonstrated in serial isolates recovered from the respiratory tract of a non-CF patient chronically colonized over a 1.5-year period by *O. intermedium* (Teyssier *et al.*, 2003). The clone evolved *in vivo* by a deletion of a 150 kb-genomic fragment, which included one copy of ribosomal operon. It was suggested that: (i) the new genomic organization gave a selective advantage to the strain *in vivo*, (ii) the genomic reduction may be an adaptive phenomenon of this free-living bacterium to the narrow ecological niche represented by the human respiratory tract. Indeed, the relation between host-restricted lifestyle and a small genome size is patent in bacteria, particularly in alphaproteobacteria (Moreno, 1998). We recently hypothesize that a phenomenon of genomic rearrangement might also be observed in *Inquilinus* sp. strains. Investigation was conducted on 21 serial isolates recovered during the 9-year follow-up of a CF patient chronically colonized by *Inquilinus* sp. PFGE analysis revealed the genomic stability of the strains while showing the existence of two closely related variants. Genomic reduction is suspected in one of the two co-existing variants suggesting that an adaptation process to human host is ongoing in these isolates but this should be further investigated (Teyssier *et al.*, 2011). This hypothesis was supported by comparison of sequential *Inquilinus* isolates recovered in one German patient revealing identical RAPD profiles but slightly different protein patterns. Expression of two antigens disappeared between successively isolated strains and was considered as suggestive of an adaptation of the *Inquilinus* clone during the course of infection (Schmoldt *et al.*, 2006). As observed by PFGE, the two variants co-existed in the respiratory tract.

6. Hypothesis: CFRT is a hotspot for emergence of human pathogens

The emergence of human pathogens from environment involves a dramatic jump in the lifestyle of bacteria. CFRT and atypical bacteria provide examples for different types of lifestyle switches. Bacteria like *Ochrobactrum* spp. have a very versatile behavior with no obvious pathogenicity except in man but with close association with diverse organisms, association that can be as close as symbiosis (Teyssier *et al.*, 2004). In the respiratory tract, *O. intermedium* can evolve by genomic reduction until displaying a genome structure similar to *Brucella*, an intracellular strict pathogen phylogenetically related to *Ochrobactrum* spp. (Teyssier *et al.*, 2003). In some cases, pathogenic microorganisms are capable to cause disease in a variety of organisms that may belong to different biological kingdoms of life. Such cross-kingdom pathogenesis could be illustrated by *A. radiobacter/tumefaciens* that causes both plant and human diseases. The virulence factors involved in phytopathogenicity are not found in clinical strains (unpublished data). However, multi-locus phylogeny showed that the clinical strains belonged to an epidemic clone among the *Agrobacterium* spp. population. This epidemic clone so-called genovar A7 could correspond to a new species in the genus and presented some phenotypic characters such as growth at 40 °C, which is a basic trait for human pathogenicity (Aujoulat *et al.*, 2011). The bacterial lifestyle needs basic requirements such as temperature, water, nutrients and pH optima. In human-associated *Agrobacterium*, growth at high temperature is an emergent character. In other cases, basic requirements may be similar in both pathogenic and harmless members of neighbor clades, hence considered to be pre-existing adaptations. Different members of the *Acetobacteraceae* could infect human suggesting that they shared common traits, such as ability to grow at acidic pH, that permits their opportunistic growth, particularly in CFRT.

One primary condition for colonization and pathogenicity is the probability to meet the bacteria that implies living in close proximity. AAB could be considered as "domestic" for human since they were used for a long time in food processing. This situation differed from that observed for *Inquilinus*, which is the sole genus to include human-adapted bacteria in

Rhodospirillaceae. I. limosus emerged from the family *Rhodospirillaceae*, a group found in soil and plant but totally unrelated to human beings. Association with coral, sponge and cuttlefish is also described, particularly in the neighborhood of the genus *Inquilinus*. It is noteworthy that, when associated with animals, *Rhodospirillaceae* are found in mucous or gelatinous environment, such as the egg capsule in sepia. 16S rDNA sequences of *I. ginsengisoli* described from the soil of ginseng fields differed slightly from that of *I. limosus* type strain (Jung *et al.*, 2011). 16S rDNA-based phylogeny showed a short robust branch (bootstrap value at 85) that groups all the clinical isolates and only one environmental isolate from roots of a perennial grass of Thar Desert in India (Figure 3). In a rooted tree, this branch appeared as supporting the most recently emerging species in the *Inquilinus* genus (data not shown). Finally, no relationship with human or other mammals was found for bacteria in the phylogenetic neighborhood of *Inquilinus*. Therefore, we could hypothetize that the association of *I. limosus* with CFRT resulted from a recent emergence by a speciation process of a human-adapted species from a group that experimented life in mucous environment.

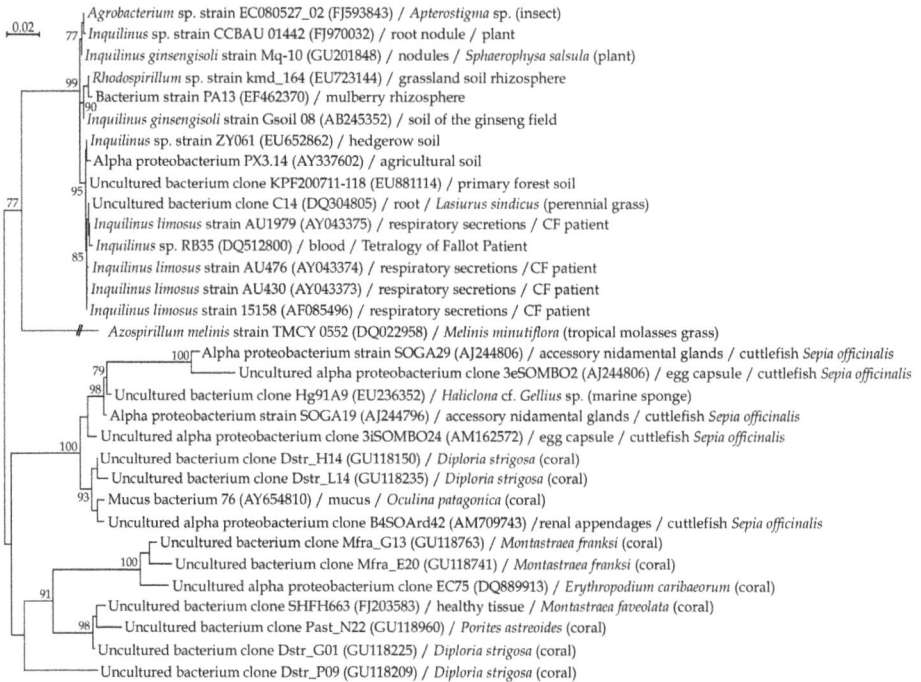

Fig. 3. Maximum-likelihood phylogenetic tree based on partial 16S rRNA gene sequences showing relationship among members of the genus *Inquilinus* and between *Inquilinus* spp. and selected close relatives from the family *Rhodospirillaceae*. Genbank accession numbers, isolation source and host follow sequence names. Numbers at nodes indicate percentage bootstrap support, based on analysis of 100 replicates. They are indicated for major nodes when >70. Bar, 0.02 substitutions per site.

We showed that the manner that CFRT niche drive the speciation and the adaptive evolution of bacteria is not univocal. However, the CFRT formed an abnormal human niche with basic conditions that allow the installation of environmental bacteria generally unrelated to human beings. Bacteria associated with CFRT, occupy two types of anatomical regions: i) the lower regions of the respiratory tract that are normally free of bacteria ii) the upper regions of the respiratory tract that are normally colonized by a resident microbiota. In CFRT, both dysbiosis and colonization by atypical environmental bacteria lead to a modified ecosystem where bacterial interactions may be unbalanced. The CFRT could be considered as an ecosystem with an emerging community where many bacteria belonging to different phyla interact and exchange genes at an increased rate. Lateral gene exchange is recognized as main innovation source for bacteria. They can acquire new genomic repertoires from which clonal specialists could emerge. Hotspots of interaction and exchange such as amoeba and rhizosphere have been previously described (Berg *et al.*, 2005; Saisongkorh *et al.*, 2010). The hypothesis that CFRT could play this role is reinforced by the number of atypical bacteria observed in this niche and by the probable emergence of specific sub-populations or species. Thus, emergence of opportunistic human pathogens from environmental origin may be first recognized from the CF airways model, a niche for bacterial adaptation and emergence (Yang *et al.*, 2011b).

7. Conclusion

Atypical bacteria are increasingly recognized in CF. These bacteria may be considered as emerging from both biological and methodological points of view in CF. Recognition of these atypical bacteria should be encouraged in the perspective of a more complete description of their prevalence, relative importance of encountered species, antimicrobial susceptibility patterns and clinical relevance.

Despite some candidate pathogens were proposed, the role of these atypical bacteria in the disease evolution is unknown. More than considering individual pathogenic species, the diversity of the microbiota is more and more considered as an important marker in the evolution of the disease. Klepac-Ceraj *et al.* recently suggested that community composition might be a better predictor of disease progression than the presence of *P. aeruginosa* alone (Klepac-Ceraj *et al.*, 2010) and van der Gast *et al.* showed that taxa richness decreased with a reduction in lung function (van der Gast *et al.*, 2011). From this point of view, each taxon contributing to increase the global diversity of the microbiota appeared important whatever its identification.

Finally, whether these species may interact with other members of the CFRT microbiota and with more common pathogens to influence the onset and/or the evolution of colonization/infection by typical pathogens like *P. aeruginosa* are great questions for future advances in CF-associated infectious diseases.

8. Acknowledgments

The authors sincerely thank Dr Corinne Teyssier and Fabien Aujoulat for their help with data summary. We are also very grateful to Linda Aleyrangues, Marie-Pierre Servent and Isabelle Zorgniotti for their excellent technical assistance in isolating and identifying atypical bacteria. Finally, we thank Dr Raphaël Chiron, pulmonary physician specialist for CF, for fruitful collaboration.

9. References

Alauzet, C.; Teyssier, C.; Jumas-Bilak, E.; Gouby, A.; Chiron, R.; Rabaud, C.; Counil, F.; Lozniewski, A. & Marchandin, H. (2010). *Gluconobacter* as well as *Asaia* species, newly emerging opportunistic human pathogens among acetic acid bacteria. *Journal of Clinical Microbiology*, Vol.48, No.11, (November 2010), pp. 3935-3942, ISSN 1098-660X

Atkinson, RM.; Lipuma, JJ.; Rosenbluth, DB. & Dunne, WM Jr. (2006). Chronic colonization with *Pandoraea apista* in cystic fibrosis patients determined by repetitive-element-sequence PCR. *Journal of Clinical Microbiology*, Vol.44, No.3, (March 2006), pp. 833-836, ISSN 1098-660X

Aujoulat, F.; Jumas-Bilak, E.; Masnou, A.; Sallé, F.; Faure, D.; Segonds, C.; Marchandin, H. & Teyssier, C. (2011). Multilocus sequence-based analysis delineates a clonal population of *Agrobacterium* (*Rhizobium*) *radiobacter* (*Agrobacterium tumefaciens*) of human origin. *Journal of Bacteriology*, Vol.193, No.10, (May 2011), pp. 2608-2618, ISSN 1098-5530

Baïda, N.; Yazourh, A.; Singer, E. & Izard, D. (2001). *Pseudomonas brenneri* sp. nov., a new species isolated from natural mineral waters. *Research in Microbiology*, Vol.152, No.5, (June 2001), pp. 493-502, ISSN 0923- 2508

Beringer, PM. & Appleman, MD. (2000). Unusual respiratory bacterial flora in cystic fibrosis: microbiologic and clinical features. *Current Opinion in Pulmonary Medicine*, Vol.6, No.6, (November 2000), pp. 545-550, ISSN 1531-6971

Berg, G.; Eberl, L. & Hartmann, A. (2005). The rhizosphere as a reservoir for opportunistic human pathogenic bacteria. *Environmental Microbiology*, Vol.7, No.11, (November 2005), pp. 1673-1685, ISSN 1462-2920

Bittar, F.; Reynaud-Gaubert, M.; Thomas, P.; Boniface, S.; Raoult, D. & Rolain JM. (2008). *Acetobacter indonesiensis* pneumonia after lung transplant. *Emerging Infectious Diseases*, Vol.14, No.6, (June 2008), pp. 997-998, ISSN 1080-6059

Bittar, F.; Richet, H.; Dubus, JC.; Reynaud-Gaubert, M.; Stremler, N.; Sarles, J.; Raoult, D. & Rolain, JM. (2008). Molecular detection of multiple emerging pathogens in sputa from cystic fibrosis patients. *Public Library of Science One*, Vol.3, No.8, (August 2008), e2908, ISSN 1932-6203

Bittar, F.; Stremler, N.; Audié, JP.; Dubus, JC.; Sarles, J.; Raoult, D. & Rolain, JM. (2010). *Nocardia farcinica* lung infection in a patient with cystic fibrosis: a case report. *Journal of Medical Case Reports*, Vol.4, (March 2010), p. 84, ISSN 1752-1947

Brockhurst, MA.; Buckling, A. & Rainey, PB. (2005) The effect of a bacteriophage on diversification of the opportunistic bacterial pathogen, *Pseudomonas aeruginosa*. *Proceedings in Biological Sciences*, Vol.272, No.1570 (July 2005), pp. 1385-1391, ISSN 1471-2954.

Cantón, R.; Morosini, MI.; Ballestero, S.; Alvarez, ME.; Escobar, H.; Máiz, L & Baquero, F. (1997). Lung colonization with *Enterobacteriaceae* producing extended-spectrum beta-lactamases in cystic fibrosis patients. *Pediatric Pulmonology*, Vol.24, No.3, (September 1997), pp. 213-217, ISSN 1099-0496

Cantón, R. & Coque, TM. (2006). The CTX-M beta-lactamase pandemic. *Current Opinion in Microbiology*, Vol.9, No.5, (October 2006), pp. 466-75, ISSN 1879-0364

Chang, YH.; Han, JI.; Chun, J.; Lee, KC.; Rhee, MS.; Kim, YB. & Bae, KS. (2002). *Comamonas koreensis* sp. nov., a non-motile species from wetland in Woopo, Korea. *International*

Journal of Systematic and Evolutionary Microbiology, Vol.52, No.2, (March 2002), pp. 377-381, ISSN 1466-5034

Chen, CY.; Hansen, KS. & Hansen, LK. (2008). *Rhizobium radiobacter* as an opportunistic pathogen in central venous catheter associated bloodstream infection: case report and review. *Journal of Hospital Infection*, Vol.68, No.3, (March 2008), pp. 203-207, ISSN 1532-2939

Chiron, R.; Marchandin, H.; Counil, F.; Jumas-Bilak, E.; Freydière, A-M.; Bellon, G.; Husson, M-O.; Turck, D.; Brémont, F.; Chabanon, G. & Segonds, C. (2005). Clinical and microbiological features of *Inquilinus* sp. isolates from five patients with cystic fibrosis. *Journal of Clinical Microbiology*, Vol.43, No.8, (August 2005), pp. 3938-3943, ISSN 1098-660X

Cieslak, TJ.; Drabick, CJ. & Robb, ML. (1996). Pyogenic infections due to *Ochrobactrum anthropi*. Clinical Infectious Diseases, Vol.22, No.5, (May 1996), pp. 845-847, ISSN 1537-6591.

Cleenwerck, I.; Gonzalez, A.; Camu, N.; Engelbeen, K.; De Vos, P.& De Vuyst, L. (2008). *Acetobacter fabarum* sp. nov., an acetic acid bacterium from a Ghanaian cocoa bean heap fermentation. *International Journal of Systematic and Evolutionary Microbiology*, Vol.58, No.9, (September 2008), pp. 2180-2185, ISSN 1466-5034

Coenye, T.; Falsen, E.; Hoste, B.; Ohlén, M.; Goris, J.; Govan, JR.; Gillis, M. & Vandamme, P. (2000). Description of *Pandoraea* gen. nov. with *Pandoraea apista* sp. nov., *Pandoraea pulmonicola* sp. nov., *Pandoraea pnomenusa* sp. nov., *Pandoraea sputorum* sp. nov. and *Pandoraea norimbergensis* comb. nov. *International Journal of Systematic and Evolutionary Microbiology*, Vol.50, No.2, (March 2000), pp. 887-899, ISSN 1466-5034

Coenye, T.; Goris, J.; Spilker, T.; Vandamme, P. & LiPuma, JJ. (2002). Characterization of unusual bacteria isolated from respiratory secretions of cystic fibrosis patients and description of *Inquilinus limosus* gen. nov., sp. nov *Journal of Clinical Microbiology*, Vol.40, No.6, (June 2002), pp. 2062-2069, ISSN 1098-660X

Coenye, T.; Spilker, T.; Reik, R.; Vandamme, P. & Lipuma, JJ. (2005). Use of PCR analyses to define the distribution of *Ralstonia* species recovered from patients with cystic fibrosis. *Journal of Clinical Microbiology*, Vol.43, No.7, (July 2005), pp. 3463-3466, ISSN 1098-660X

Coyne, S.; Courvalin, P. & Galimand, M. (2010). Acquisition of multidrug resistance transposon Tn*6061* and IS*6100*-mediated large chromosomal inversions in *Pseudomonas aeruginosa* clinical isolates. *Microbiology*,Vol.156, No.5, (May 2010), pp. 1448-1458, ISSN 1465-2080

Degand, N.; Carbonnelle, E.; Dauphin, B.; Beretti, JL.; Le Bourgeois, M.; Sermet-Gaudelus, I.; Segonds, C.; Berche, P.; Nassif, X. & Ferroni, A. (2008). Matrix-assisted laser desorption ionization-time of flight mass spectrometry for identification of nonfermenting gram-negative bacilli isolated from cystic fibrosis patients. *Journal of Clinical Microbiology*, Vol.46, No.10, (October 2008), pp. 3361-3367, ISSN 1098-660X

Dempsey, KE.; Riggio, MP.; Lennon, A.; Hannah, VE.; Ramage, G.; Allan, D. & Bagg, J. (2007). Identification of bacteria on the surface of clinically infected and non-infected prosthetic hip joints removed during revision arthroplasties by 16S rRNA gene sequencing and by microbiological culture. *Arthritis Research and Therapy*, Vol.9, No.3, (May 2007), R46, ISSN 1478-6354

Duan, K.; Dammel, C.; Stein, J.; Rabin, H. & Surette, MG. (2003). Modulation of *Pseudomonas aeruginosa* gene expression by host microflora through interspecies communication. *Molecular Microbiology*, Vol.50, No.5, (December 2003), pp. 1477-1491, ISSN 1365-2958

Dunne, WM. Jr; Tillman, J. & Murray, JC. (1993). Recovery of a strain of *Agrobacterium radiobacter* with a mucoid phenotype from an immunocompromised child with bacteremia. *Journal of Clinical Microbiology*, Vol.31, No.9, (September 1993), pp. 2541-2543, ISSN 1098-660X

Edmond, MB.; Riddler, SA.; Baxter, CM.; Wicklund, BM. & Pascuile, AW. (1993). *Agrobacterium radiobacter* a recently recognized opportunistic pathogen. *Clinical Infectious Diseases*, Vol.16, No.3, (March 1993), pp. 388-391, ISSN 1537-6591

Ferreira, L.; Sánchez-Juanes, F.; García-Fraile, P.; Rivas, R.; Mateos, PF.; Martínez-Molina, E.; González-Buitrago, JM. & Velázquez, E. (2011). Maldi-tof mass spectrometry is a fast and reliable platform for identification and ecological studies of species from family *rhizobiaceae*. *Public Library of Science One*, Vol.6, No.5, (May 2011), e20223, ISSN 1932-6203

Field, TR.; Sibley, CD.; Parkins, MD.; Rabin, HR. & Surette, MG. (2010). The genus *Prevotella* in cystic fibrosis airways. *Anaerobe*, Vol.16, No.4, (August 2010), pp. 337-344, ISSN 1075-9964

Foweraker, J. (2009). Recent advances in the microbiology of respiratory tract infection in cystic fibrosis. *British Medical Bulletin*, Vol.89, (January 2009), pp. 93-110, ISSN 1468-5833

Frank, DN.; St Amand, AL.; Feldman, RA.; Boedeker, EC.; Harpaz, N. & Pace, NR. (2007). Molecular-phylogenetic characterization of microbial community imbalances in human inflammatory bowel diseases. *Proceedings of the National Academy of Sciences of the United States of America*, Vol.104, No.34, (August 2007), pp. 13780-13785, ISSN 1091-6490

Fritsche, K.; Auling, G.; Andreesen, JR. & Lechner, U. (1999). *Defluvibacter lusatiae* gen. nov., sp. nov., a new chlorohenol-degrading member of the alpha-2 subgroup of proteobacteria. *Systematic and Applied Microbiology*, Vol.22, No.2, (May 1999), pp. 197-204, ISSN 0723-2020

Ghosh, W.; Bagchi, A.; Mandal, S.; Dam, B. & Roy, P. (2005). *Tetrathiobacter kashmirensis* gen. nov., sp. nov., a novel mesophilic, neutrophilic, tetrathionate-oxidizing, facultatively chemolithotrophic betaproteobacterium isolated from soil from a temperate orchard in Jammu and Kashmir, India. *International Journal of Systematic and Evolutionary Microbiology*, Vol.55, No.5, (September 2005), pp. 1779-1787, ISSN 1466-5034

Gneiding, K.; Frodl, R. & Funke, G. Identities of *Microbacterium* spp. encountered in human clinical specimens. (2008). *Journal of Clinical Microbiology*, Vol.46, No.11, (November 2008), pp. 3646-3652, ISSN 1098-660X

Grice, EA.; Kong, HH.; Conlan, S.; Deming, CB.; Davis, J.; Young, AC.; NISC Comparative Sequencing Program; Bouffard, GG.; Blakesley, RW.; Murray, PR.; Green, ED.; Turner, ML. & Segre, JA. (2009). Topographical and temporal diversity of the human skin microbiome. *Science*, Vol.324, No.5931, (May 2009), pp. 1190-1192, ISSN 1095-9203

Grice, EA.; Snitkin, ES.; Yockey, LJ.; Bermudez, DM.; NISC Comparative Sequencing Program; Liechty, KW. & Segre, JA. (2010). Longitudinal shift in diabetic wound microbiota correlates with prolonged skin defense response. *Proceedings of the National Academy of Sciences of the United States of America*, Vol.107, No.33, (August 2010), pp. 14799-14804, ISSN 1091-6490

Guss, AM.; Roeselers, G.; Newton, IL.; Young, CR.; Klepac-Ceraj, V.; Lory, S. & Cavanaugh, CM. (2011). Phylogenetic and metabolic diversity of bacteria associated with cystic fibrosis. *ISME Journal*, Vol.5, No.1 (January 2011), pp. 20-29, ISSN 1751-7370

Hall V. (2008). *Actinomyces*--gathering evidence of human colonization and infection. *Anaerobe*, Vol.14, No.1, (February 2008), pp. 1-7, ISSN 1075-9964

Hantsis-Zacharov, E.; Senderovich, Y. & Halpern, M. (2008). *Chryseobacterium bovis* sp. nov., isolated from raw cow's milk. *International Journal of Systematic and Evolutionary Microbiology*, Vol.58, No.4, (April 2008), pp. 1024-1028, ISSN 1466-5034

Harris, JK.; De Groote, MA.; Sagel, SD.; Zemanick, ET.; Kapsner, R.; Penvari, C.; Kaess, H.; Deterding, RR.; Accurso, FJ. & Pace, NR. (2007). Molecular identification of bacteria in bronchoalveolar lavage fluid from children with cystic fibrosis. *Proceedings of the National Academy of Sciences of the United States of America*, Vol.104, No.51, (December 2007), pp. 20529-20533, ISSN 1091-6490

Hauser, AR.; Jain, M.; Bar-Meir, M. & McColley, SA. (2011). Clinical significance of microbial infection and adaptation in cystic fibrosis. *Clinical Microbiology Reviews*, Vol.24, No.1, (January 2011), pp. 29-70, ISSN 1098-6618

Hayes, D Jr.; Murphy, BS.; Kuhn, RJ.; Anstead, MI. & Feola, DJ. (2009). Mucoid *Inquilinus limosus* in a young adult with cystic fibrosis. *Pediatric Pulmonology*, Vol.44, No.6, (June 2009), pp. 619-621, ISSN 1099-0496

Herasimenka, Y.; Cescutti, P.; Impallomeni, G. & Rizzo R. (2007). Exopolysaccharides produced by *Inquilinus limosus*, a new pathogen of cystic fibrosis patients: novel structures with usual components. Carbohydrate Research, Vol.342, No.16, (November 2007), pp. 2404-2415, ISSN 0008-6215

Hogardt, M.; Ulrich, J.; Riehn-Kopp, H. & Tümmler, B. (2009). EuroCareCF quality assessment of diagnostic microbiology of cystic fibrosis isolates. *Journal of Clinical Microbiology*, Vol.47, No.11, (November 2009), pp. 3435-3438, ISSN 1098-660X

Hyman, RW.; Fukushima, M.; Diamond, L.; Kumm.; Giudice, LC. & Davis, RW. (2005). Microbes on the human vaginal epithelium. *Proceedings of the National Academy of Sciences of the United States of America*, Vol.102, No.22, (May 2005), pp. 7952-7957, ISSN 1091-6490

Jewes, LA. & Spencer RC. (1990). The incidence of anaerobes in the sputum of patients with cystic fibrosis. *Journal of Medical Microbiology*, Vol.31, No.4, (April 1990), pp. 271-274, ISSN 1473-5644

Jones, AM. (2011). Anaerobic bacteria in cystic fibrosis: pathogens or harmless commensals? *Thorax*, Vol.66, No.7, (July 2011), pp. 558-599, ISSN 1468-3296

Jumas-Bilak, E.; Chiron, R.; Michon, AL.; Filleron, A.; Aleyrangues, L.; Teyssier, C. & Marchandin, H. (2011). CF airways, a particular ecological niche for bacterial species as-yet non-reported in man. 34th European Cystic Fibrosis Conference, Hamburg, Germany, June 2011

Jung, HM.; Lee, JS.; Bae, HM.; Yi, TH.; Kim, SY.; Lee, ST. & Im, WT. (2011). *Inquilinus ginsengisoli* sp. nov., isolated from soil of a ginseng field. *International Journal of*

Systematic and Evolutionary Microbiology, Vol.61, No.1, (January 2011), pp. 201-204, ISSN 1466-5034

Kämpfer P.; Avesani, V.; Janssens, M.; Charlier, J.; De Baere, T. & Vaneechoutte, M. (2006). Description of *Wautersiella falsenii* gen. nov., sp. nov., to accommodate clinical isolates phenotypically resembling members of the genera *Chryseobacterium* and *Empedobacter*. *International Journal of Systematic and Evolutionary Microbiology*, Vol.56, No.10, (October 2006), pp. 2323-2329, ISSN 1466-5034

Kämpfer, P.; Meurer, U.; Esser, M.; Hirsch, T. & Busse, HJ. (2007). *Sphingomonas pseudosanguinis* sp. nov., isolated from the water reservoir of an air humidifier. *International Journal of Systematic and Evolutionary Microbiology*, Vol.57, No.6, (June 2007), pp. 1342-1345, ISSN 1466-5034

Kämpfer, P.; Scholz, HC.; Huber, B.; Falsen, E. & Busse, H. (2007). *Ochrobactrum haematophilum* sp. nov. and *Ochrobactrum pseudogrignonense* sp. nov., isolated from human clinical specimens. *International Journal of Systematic and Evolutionary Microbiology*, Vol.57, No.11, (November 2007), pp. 2513-2518, ISSN 1466-5034

Kiratisin, P.; Koomanachai, P.; Kowwigkai, P.; Pattanachaiwit, S.; Aswapokee, N. & Leelaporn, A. (2006). Early-onset prosthetic valve endocarditis caused by *Inquilinus* sp. *Diagnostic Microbiology and Infectious Disease*, Vol.56, No.3, (November 2006), pp. 317-320, ISSN 0732-8893

Klepac-Ceraj, V.; Lemon, KP.; Martin, TR.; Allgaier, M.; Kembel, SW.; Knapp, AA.; Lory, S.; Brodie, EL.; Lynch, SV.; Bohannan, BJ.; Green, JL.; Maurer, BA. & Kolter, R. (2010). Relationship between cystic fibrosis respiratory tract bacterial communities and age, genotype, antibiotics and *Pseudomonas aeruginosa*. *Environmental Microbiology*, Vol.12, No.5, (May 2010), pp. 1293-1303, ISSN 1462-2920

Kolak, M.; Karpati, F.; Monstein, HJ. & Jonasson, J. (2003). Molecular typing of the bacterial flora in sputum of cystic fibrosis patients. *International Journal of Medical Microbiology*, Vol.293, No.4, (August 2003), pp. 309-317, ISSN 1438-4221

Korade, DL. & Fulekar, MH. (2009). Rhizosphere remediation of chlorpyrifos in mycorrhizospheric soil using ryegrass. *Journal of Hazardous Materials*, Vol.172, No.2-3, (December 2009), pp.1344-50, ISSN 1873-3336

Lambiase, A.; Catania, MR. & Rossano, F. (2010). Anaerobic bacteria infection in cystic fibrosis airway disease. *New Microbiologica*, Vol.33, No.3, (July 2010), pp. 185-194, ISSN 1121-7138

Lin, YT.; Jeng, YY.; Lin, ML.; Yu, KW.; Wang, FD. & Liu, CY. (2010). Clinical and microbiological characteristics of *Chryseobacterium indologenes* bacteremia. *Journal of Microbiology, Immunology and Infection*, Vol.43, No.6, (December 2010), pp. 498-505, ISSN 1995-9133

Matsui, T.; Shinzato, N.; Tamaki, H.; Muramatsu, M. & Hanada, S. (2009). *Shinella yambaruensis* sp. nov., a 3-methyl-sulfolane-assimilating bacterium isolated from soil. *International Journal of Systematic and Evolutionary Microbiology*, Vol.59, No.3, (March 2009), pp. 536-539, ISSN 1466-5034

Menuet, M.; Bittar, F.; Stremler, N.; Dubus, JC.; Sarles, J.; Raoult, D. & Rolain, J-M. (2008). First isolation of two colistin-resistant emerging pathogens, *Brevundimonas diminuta* and *Ochrobactrum anthropi*, in a woman with cystic fibrosis: a case report. *Journal of Medical Case Reports*, Vol.2, (December 2008), p. 373, ISSN 1752-1947

Mergaert, J.; Cnockaert, MC. & Swings, J. (2002). *Phyllobacterium myrsinacearum* (subjective synonym *Phyllobacterium rubiacearum*) emend. *International Journal of Systematic and Evolutionary Microbiology*, Vol.52, No.5, (September 2002), pp. 1821-1823, ISSN 1466-5034

Moreno, E. (1998). Genome evolution within the alpha Proteobacteria: why do some bacteria not possess plasmids and others exhibit more than one different chromosome? *FEMS Microbiology Reviews*, Vol.22, No.4, (October 1998), pp. 255–275, ISSN 1574-6976

Nadjar, D.; Labia, R.; Cerceau, C.; Bizet, C.; Philippon, A. & Arlet, G. (2001). Molecular characterization of chromosomal class C beta-lactamase and its regulatory gene in *Ochrobactrum anthropi*. *Antimicrobial Agents and Chemotherapy*, Vol.45, No.8, (August 2001), pp. 2324-2330, ISSN 1098-6596

Oakley, BB.; Fiedler, TL.; Marrazzo, JM. & Fredricks, DN. (2008). Diversity of human vaginal bacterial communities and associations with clinically defined bacterial vaginosis. *Applied and Environmental Microbiology*, Vol.74, No.15, (August 2008), pp. 4898-4909, ISSN 1098-5336

Otto-Karg, I.; Jandl, S.; Müller, T.; Stirzel, B.; Frosch, M.; Hebestreit, H. & Abele-Horn, M. (2009). Validation of Vitek 2 nonfermenting gram-negative cards and Vitek 2 version 4.02 software for identification and antimicrobial susceptibility testing of nonfermenting gram-negative rods from patients with cystic fibrosis. *Journal of Clinical Microbiology*, Vol.47, No.10, (October 2009), pp. 3283-3288, ISSN 1098-660X

Poole, K. (2011). *Pseudomonas aeruginosa*: resistance to the max. *Frontiers in Microbiology*, Vol.2, (April 2011), 65, ISSN 1664-302X

Poschet, J.; Perkett, E. & Deretic, V. (2002). Hyperacidification in cystic fibrosis: links with lung disease and new prospects for treatment. *Trends in Molecular Medicine*, Vol.8, No.11, (November 2002), pp. 512-519, ISSN 1471-4914

Preiswerk, B.; Ullrich, S.; Speich, R.; Bloemberg, GV. & Hombach, M. (2011). Human infection with *Delftia tsuruhatensis* isolated from a central venous catheter. *Journal of Medical Microbiology*, Vol.60, No.2, (February 2011), pp. 246-248, ISSN 1473-5644

Riggio, MP.; Lennon, A.; Rolph, HJ.; Hodge, PJ.; Donaldson, A.; Maxwell, AJ. & Bagg, J. (2008). Molecular identification of bacteria on the tongue dorsum of subjects with and without halitosis. *Oral Diseases*, Vol.14, No.3, (April 2008), pp. 251-258, ISSN 1354-523X

Rogers, GB.; Carroll, MP.; Serisier, DJ.; Hockey, PM.; Jones, G. & Bruce, KD. (2004). Characterization of bacterial community diversity in cystic fibrosis lung infections by use of 16s ribosomal DNA terminal restriction fragment length polymorphism profiling. *Journal of Clinical Microbiology*, Vol.42, No.11, (November 2004), pp. 5176-5183, ISSN 1098-660X

Rogers, GB.; Daniels, TW.; Tuck, A.; Carroll, MP.; Connett, GJ.; David, GJ. & Bruce, KD. (2009). Studying bacteria in respiratory specimens by using conventional and molecular microbiological approaches. *BMC pulmonary medicine*, Vol.9, (April 2009), 14, ISSN 1471-2466

Rogers, GB.; Skelton, S.; Serisier, DJ.; van der Gast, CJ. & Bruce KD. (2010). Determining cystic fibrosis-affected lung microbiology: comparison of spontaneous and serially induced sputum samples by use of terminal restriction fragment length polymorphism profiling. *Journal of Clinical Microbiology*, Vol.48, No.1, (January 2010), pp. 78-86, ISSN 1098-660X

Romano, S.; Aujoulat, F.; Jumas-Bilak, E.; Masnou, A.; Jeannot, JL.; Falsen, E.; Marchandin, H. & Teyssier C. (2009). Multilocus sequence typing supports the hypothesis that *Ochrobactrum anthropi* displays a human-associated subpopulation. BMC Microbiology, Vol.9, No.267 (December 2009), ISSN 1471-2180

Saisongkorh, W.; Robert, C.; La Scola, B.; Raoult, D. & Rolain, JM. (2010). Evidence of transfer by conjugation of type IV secretion system genes between *Bartonella* species and *Rhizobium radiobacter* in amoeba. *Public Library of Science One*, Vol.5, No.9, (September 2010), e12666, ISSN 1932-6203

Schlaberg, R.; Huard, RC. & Della-Latta, P. (2008). *Nocardia cyriacigeorgica*, an emerging pathogen in the United States. *Journal of Clinical Microbiology*, Vol.46, No.1, (January 2008), pp. 265-273, ISSN 1098-660X

Schmoldt, S.; Latzin, P.; Heesemann, J.; Griese, M.; Imhof, A. & Hogardt M. (2006). Clonal analysis of *Inquilinus limosus* isolates from six cystic fibrosis patients and specific serum antibody response. *Journal of Medical Microbiology*, Vol.55, No.19, (October 2006), pp. 1425-1433, ISSN 1473-5644

Sheng, WH.; Huang, YT.; Chang, SC.& Hsueh, PR. (2009). Brain abscess caused by *Tsukamurella tyrosinosolvens* in an immunocompetent patient. *Journal of Clinical Microbiology*, Vol.47, No.5, (May 2009), pp. 1602-1604, ISSN 1098-660X

Shinzato, T. & Saito, A. (1994). A mechanism of pathogenicity of "*Streptococcus milleri* group" in pulmonary infection: synergy with an anaerobe. *Journal of Medical Microbiology*, Vol.40, No.2, (February 1994), pp. 118-123, ISSN 1473-5644

Sibley, CD.; Rabin, H. & Surette, MG. (2006). Cystic fibrosis: a polymicrobial infectious disease. *Future Microbiology*, Vol.1, No.1, (June 2006), pp. 53-61, ISSN 1746-0913

Sibley, CD.; Parkins, MD.; Rabin, HR.; Duan, K.; Norgaard, JC. & Surette, MG. (2008). A polymicrobial perspective of pulmonary infections exposes an enigmatic pathogen in cystic fibrosis patients. *Proceedings of the National Academy of Sciences of the United States of America*, Vol.105, No.39, (September 2008), pp. 15070-15075, ISSN 1091-6490

Sibley, CD.; Duan, K.; Fischer, C.; Parkins, MD.; Storey, DG.; Rabin, HR. & Suretten MG. (2008). Discerning the complexity of community interactions using a *Drosophila* model of polymicrobial infections. *Public Library of Science One* Pathogens, Vol.4, No.10, (October 2008), e1000184, ISSN 1553-7374

Snyder, RW.; Ruhe, J.; Kobrin, S.; Wasserstein, A.; Doline, C.; Nachamkin, I. & Lipschutz JH. (2004). *Asaia bogorensis* peritonitis identified by 16S ribosomal RNA sequence analysis in a patient receiving peritoneal dialysis. *American Journal of Kidney Diseases*, Vol.44, No.2, (August 2004), e15-17, ISSN 1523-6838

Spilker, T.; Liwienski, AA. & LiPuma, JJ. (2008). Identification of *Bordetella* spp. in respiratory specimens from individuals with cystic fibrosis. *Clinical Microbiology and Infection*, Vol.14, No.5, (May 2008), pp. 504-506, ISSN 1469-0691

Stackebrandt, E. & Goebel, BM. (1994). Taxonomic note: a place for DNA–DNA reassociation and 16S rRNA sequence analysis in the present species definition in bacteriology. *International Journal of Systematic Bacteriology*, Vol.44, No.4, (October 1994), pp. 846-849, ISSN 0020-7713

Stackebrandt, E. & Ebers, J. (2006). Taxonomic parameters revisited: tarnished gold standards. *Microbiology Today*, Vol.33, (November 2006), pp. 152–155, ISSN 1464-0570

Teyssier, C.; Marchandin, H.; Siméon de Buochberg, M.; Ramuz, M. & Jumas-Bilak E. (2003). Atypical 16S rRNA gene copies in *Ochrobactrum intermedium* strains reveal a large genomic rearrangement by recombination between *rrn* copies. *Journal of Bacteriology*, Vol.185, No.9, (May 2003), pp. 2901-2909, ISSN 1098-5530

Teyssier, C.; Marchandin, H. & Jumas-Bilak, E. (2004). The genome of alpha-proteobacteria : complexity, reduction, diversity and fluidity. *Canadian Journal of Microbiology*, Vol.50, No.6, (June 2004), pp. 383-396, ISSN 1480-3275

Teyssier, C.; Marchandin, H.; Jean-Pierre, H.; Diego, I.; Darbas, H.; Jeannot, JL.; Gouby, A. & Jumas-Bilak, E. (2005). Molecular and phenotypic features for identification of the opportunistic pathogens *Ochrobactrum* spp. *Journal of Medical Microbiology*, Vol.54, No.10, (October 2005), pp. 945-953, ISSN 1473-5644

Teyssier, C.; Marchandin, H.; Jean-Pierre, H.; Masnou, A.; Dusart, G. & Jumas-Bilak E. (2007). *Ochrobactrum pseudintermedium* sp. nov., a novel member of the family *Brucellaceae*, isolated from human clinical samples. *International Journal of Systematic and Evolutionary Microbiology*, Vol.57, No.5, (May 2007), pp. 1007-1013, ISSN 1466-5034

Teyssier, C.; Jumas-Bilak, E.; Counil, F.; Masnou, A.; Aleyranges, L.; Chiron, R. & Marchandin H. (2009). *Ochrobactrum* and *Agrobacterium* spp.: emerging opportunistic pathogens in cystic fibrosis patients? 32nd European Cystic Fibrosis Conference, Brest, France, June 2009

Teyssier, C. & Jumas-Bilak, E. (2011). *Ochrobactrum*, In: *Molecular detection of human bacterial pathogens*, Liu D., pp. 659-670, CRC press, ISBN 978-1-4398-1238-9, USA

Teyssier, C.; Kypraios, S.; Aujoulat, F.; Chiron, R.; Jumas-Bilak, E. & Marchandin H. (2011). Remarkable persistence of genomically stable isolates of *Inquilinus* sp. in the respiratory tract of a cystic fibrosis patient. 4th congress of the Federation of European Microbiological Societies, Genève, Switzerland, June 2011

Thoma, B.; Straube, E.; Scholz, HC.; Al Dahouk, S.; Zöller, L.; Pfeffer, M.; Neubauer, H. & Tomaso, H. (2009). Identification and antimicrobial susceptibilities of *Ochrobactrum* spp. *International Journal of Medical Microbiology*, Vol.299, No.3, (March 2009), pp. 209-220, ISSN 1438-4221

Tunney, MM.; Field, TR. & Moriarty, TF. (2008). Detection of anaerobic bacteria in high numbers in sputum from patients with cystic fibrosis. *American Journal of Respiratory and Critical Care Medicine*, Vol.177, No.9, (May 2008), pp. 995-1001, ISSN 1535-4970

van Belkum, A.; Renders, NH.; Smith, S.; Overbeek, SE. & Verbrugh, HA. (2000). Comparison of conventional and molecular methods for the detection of bacterial pathogens in sputum samples from cystic fibrosis patients. *FEMS immunology and medical microbiology*, Vol.27, No.1, (January 2000), pp. 51-57, ISSN 1574-695X

van der Gast, CJ.; Walker, AW.; Stressmann, FA.; Rogers, GB.; Scott, P.; Daniels, TW.; Carroll, MP.; Parkhill, J. & Bruce, KD. (2011). Partitioning core and satellite taxa from within cystic fibrosis lung bacterial communities. *The ISME journal*, Vol.5, No.5, (May 2011), pp. 780-789, ISSN 1751-7370 van Mansfeld, R.; Jongerden, I.; Bootsma, M.; Buiting, A.; Bonten, M. & Willems, R. (2010). The population genetics of *Pseudomonas aeruginosa* isolates from different patient populations exhibits high-level host specificity. *Public Library of Science One*, Vol.5, No.10, (October 2010), e13482, ISSN 1932-6203

Worlitzsch, D.; Rintelen, C.; Böhm, K.; Wollschläger, B.; Merkel, N.; Borneff-Lipp, M. & Döring, G. (2009). Antibiotic-resistant obligate anaerobes during exacerbations of cystic fibrosis patients. *Clinical Microbiology and Infection*, Vol.15, No.5, (May 2009), pp. 454-460, ISSN 1469-0691

Wright, GD. (2010). Antibiotic resistance in the environment: a link to the clinic? *Current Opinion in Microbiology*, Vol.13, No.5, (October 2010), pp. 589-594. ISSN 1879-0364

Yagüe-Muñoz, A.; Gregori-Roig, P.; Valls-López, S. & Pantoja-Martínez, J. (2010). *Ochrobactrum anthropi* bacteremia in a child with cystic fibrosis. *Enfermedades Infecciosas y Microbiología Clínica*, Vol.28, No.2, (February 2010), pp. 137-138, ISSN 0213-005X

Yamada, Y. & Yukphan P. (2008). Genera and species in acetic acid bacteria. *International Journal of Food Microbiology*, Vol.125, No.1, (June 2008), pp. 15–24, ISSN 0168-1605

Yang, L.; Jelsbak, L.; Marvig, RL.; Damkiær, S.; Workman, CT.; Rau, MH.; Hansen, SK.; Folkesson, A.; Johansen, HK.; Ciofu; O.; Høiby, N.; Sommer, MO. & Molin, S. (2011). Evolutionary dynamics of bacteria in a human host environment. *Proceedings of the National Academy of Sciences of the United States of America*, Vol.108, No.18, (May 2011), pp. 7481-7486, ISSN 1091-6490

Yang, L.; Jelsbak, L. & Molin, S. (2011). Microbial ecology and adaptation in cystic fibrosis airways. *Environmental Microbiology*, Vol.13, No.7, (July 2011), pp. 1682-1689, ISSN 1462-2920

Young, CC.; Arun, AB.; Lai, WA.; Chen, WM.; Chou, JH.; Shen, FT.; Rekha, PD. & Kämpfer P. (2008). *Chromobacterium aquaticum* sp. nov., isolated from spring water samples. *International Journal of Systematic and Evolutionary Microbiology*, Vol.58, No.4, (April 2008), pp.877-880, ISSN 1466-5034

11

Immune Dysfunction in Cystic Fibrosis

Yaqin Xu and Stefan Worgall

Weill Cornell Medical College, Department of Pediatrics, New York, NY, USA

1. Introduction

Absence of the cystic fibrosis transmembrane regulator (CFTR) function leads to chronic lung disease characterized by inflammation and persistent infections. The mechanisms for the increased susceptibility of the respiratory tract for infections in CF are most likely complex and only partially understood. Most attention has been focused on the effect of the defective expression of CFTR in epithelial cells and submucosal gland cells and the increased susceptibility of the respiratory tract to infections was was mostly thought to be related to the abnormal chloride channel function (Welsh MJ, 2011, Ratjen F 2003). However, numerous studies over the past years have shown that the absence of CFTR affects the immune system and that dysfunctional immune responses contribute to pathological processes in the CF lung. In addition, it has become increasingly evident that the chloride channel dysfunction alone cannot completely explain the pathology of CF lung disease and that other pathways known to be regulated by CFTR play a role in the immune dysregulation in the CF lung (Mehta A 2008). This chapter reviews both soluble factors in the CF milieu that modify immune cell function and specific alterations in the cellular components of the innate and adaptive immune system that contribute to the impaired immune defense in CF lung disease.

2. The role of immune responses in CF

Innate host defenses are defective in CF. It is still not entirely clear how defective CFTR results in an impaired host response in the CF lung. Three general components comprise the innate and adaptive immune defenses in the respiratory tract: (1) the mucociliary escalator; (2) a humoral component of surfactant proteins, defensins, and other antimicrobial compounds; and (3) a cellular component that includes epithelial cells, neutrophils, macrophages, monocytes, dendritic cells, and lymphocytes.

2.1 Abnormal humoral responses in CF

The respiratory tract epithelium and the cells of the submucosal glands in the airways constitute a major part of the innate immune defense system of the lung that responds primarily to incoming pathogens with the release of various mediators. They are influenced and/or amplified in their responses by factors such as cytokines derived from neighboring inflammatory and immune cells (Bartlett J 2008). The defective chloride channel function in CF leads to alterations in the physical properties of the airway mucus and the composition of the airway surface liquid that are linked to impairment of innate defense mechanisms. These affect the shield of antimicrobial factors such as lysozyme, lactoferrin, defensins, and other antimicrobial peptides, as well as disturb the mechanical clearance of inhaled particles and pathogens by the mucociliary escalator. **Table 1** summarizes the known alterations in soluble innate immune factors in the CF lung. One school of thought has pursued the concept that alterations in the chloride secretion and sodium hyperabsorption in the airways lead to the subsequent entrapment of pathogens that then lead to recruitment and activation of neutrophils and macrophages. This has also been supported by the lung phenotype of a mouse model with genetic over-expression of the sodium channel ENac that mimics CF with thick mucus and inflammation in the absence of infection (Mall MA 2010). Salt-sensitive antimicrobials such as defensins were initially thought to be defective in the human CF lung. However, as the exact concentrations of chloride and sodium in the airway liquid are still not entirely clear, and so the degree of impairment of these innate defense mechanisms in CF is not exactly known.

Mediator	Abnormality	Reference
Defensins	Impaired activity	Goldman MJ et al. 1997, Bals R et al. 2001
Surfactant proteins	Decreased or inactive	Hartl D, Griese M 2006, Meyer KC et al. 2000, Noah TL et al. 2003
Antioxidants	Reduced glutathione availability in airways	Gao L et al. 1999, Roum JH et al. 1993, Day BJ 2005, Childers M et al. 2007, Hudson VM 2001
Opsonins	Proteolytic degradation	Eichler I et al. 1989
Cytokines		
IFN-γ [1]	Decreased secretion	Moss RB et al.1996 and 2000
IL-1[2]	Increased secretion	Bonfield TL et al. 1995
IL-4[3]	Increased secretion	Moss RB et al.1996 and 2000, Mueller C et al.2010
IL-6[4]	Increased secretion	Black HR et al. 1998, Becker MN et al. 2004, Andersson C et al. 2007, Vandivier RW et al. 2009,
IL-8[5]	Increased secretion	Bonfield TL et al. 1995, Black HR et al. 1998, Becker MN et al. 2004, Vandivier RW et al. 2009,
IL-10[6]	Altered secretion	Bonfield TL et al. 1995, Moss RB et al. 1996 and 2000, Armstrong DS et al. 2005
IL-13[7]	Increased secretion	Mueller C et al.2010
IL-17[8]	Increased secretion	McAllister F et al.2005, Tan HL et al.2011
TNF- α[9]	Increased secretion	Bonfield TL et al. 1995, Andersson C et al. 2007,
Chemokines		
MIP-1β[10]	Increased secretion	Brennan S et al. 2009
MCP-1[11]	Increased secretion	Brennan S et al. 2009

Notes: [1] IFN-γ (interferon-gamma); [2] IL-1β (interleukin-1 beta), [3] IL-4 (interleukin-4), [4] IL-6 (interleukin-6), [5] IL-8 (interleukin-8), [6] IL-10 (interleukin-10), [7] IL-13 (interleukin-13), [8] IL-17(interleukin-17), [9] TNF-α (tumor necrosis factor-alpha), [10] MIP-1β (macrophage inflammatory protein-1 beta), [11] MCP-1 (macrophage chemotactic protein-1)

Table 1. Altered humoral mediators in the respiratory tract in CF

2.1.1 Soluble mediators

Numerous humoral factors that affect pulmonary innate immune response have been studied in the CF lung. These include the collectins and surfactant proteins (Hartl D 2006, Noah TL 2003, Meyer KC 2000), defensins (Goldman MJ 1997, Bals 2001), glutathione (Gao TJ 1999, Kogan I 2003, Roum JH 1993, Hudson VM 2001) and antiproteases such as secretory leukoprotease inhibitor (SLPI) and tissue inhibitor of metalloproteinase 1 (TIMP-1) (Gaggar 2007, Cantin AM 1991, Vandivier 2002). Initially, it was thought that defensins in the CF lung were impaired due to the altered salt concentration in the CF airway (Goldmann 1997). Subsequent studies showed the impairment of defensins is not only related to an altered salt concentration, but also to increased inflammation (Bals 2001, Chen CI 2004). The Levels of β-defensin were even found to be similar in bronchial brushings in CF and non CF patients (Dauletbaev N 2002). Surfactant proteins, besides their surface-tension regulating properties, also have immuno-modulatory and anti-inflammatory functions were shown to be degraded (Hartl D 2006, Noah TL 2003) and structurally altered in CF (Meyer KC 2000). Glutathione, a critical component of the antioxidant defense system in the lung, was found to be reduced in the CF lung (Roum JH 1993). Importantly, this seemed to be directly related to the function of CFTR as a channel for the transmembrane transport of glutathione (Gao 1999, Kogan 2003). As glutathione deficiency also leads to activation of nucleic factor kappa B (NFκB)-mediated inflammation, aerosolized glutathione has been studied as a potential anti-inflammatory therapeutic in CF (Roum 1999).

Antiprotease, which plays an important role in the lung to counter the proteolytic products released by activated neutrophils, did not seem to be altered in the CF lung at baseline (Cartin AM 1991). However, these normal baseline levels were probably insufficient to neutralize the massive invasion of neutrophils and have thus been considered to be relatively deficient in the CF lung.

2.1.2 Defective CFTR leads to release of inflammatory cytokines

One of the dominant features of CF lung disease is the exaggerated inflammatory response. Numerous studies have linked the CFTR defect to activation of inflammatory cytokines, in particular interleukin-8 (IL-8). IL-8 is closely related to the CF inflammation as it is one of the major chemoattractants for neutrophils. Neutrophils dominate the inflammatory milieu in the CF lung. The importance of the vast number of neutrophils has been underscored by the successful use of recombinant DNAse to break down DNA released from neutrophils as one of the few effective therapeutics to ameliorate CF lung disease (Suri R 2002). Although it is still debated if inflammation precedes infection in the lungs of infants and young children with CF, it is undisputed that CFTR is linked to the NFκB pathway, a crucial transcription activator for inflammatory and immune responses. These intrinsic activations of NFκB and cytokines, such as IL-8 and tumor necrosis factor alpha (TNF-α), have been observed both in naïve lung macrophages from CFTR knockout mice (CF mice) and in un-stimulated human macrophages with decreased CFTR expression (Bruscia EM 2008, Xu Y 2010). It seems that the intrinsic activation of NFκB-mediated inflammatory cytokine release is independent of the chloride channel function of the CFTR protein. Neutrophil elastase and other products of neutrophils, that are abundant in the CF lung, also induce IL-8 expression in epithelial cells (McElvaney NG 1992). Besides an increase in inflammatory cytokines, the CFTR defect has also been associated with a decrease in the anti-inflammatory cytokine interleukin-10 (IL-10). Increased susceptibility to CF pathogens such as *Pseudomonas aeruginosa* (*P. aeruginosa*) has been demonstrated in IL-10 deficient mice (Soltys J 2002).

2.2 Abnormal cellular immune response in CF

Cells of the innate and adaptive immune system have been studied in CF. The main findings are outlined in **Table 2**. As the role of epithelial cells in CF will be discussed in other chapters, the following details the functions and abnormalities seen in the neutrophils, macrophages, monocytes, dendritic cells, and lymphocytes that are likely playing a part in the pathogenesis of CF lung disease.

2.2.1 Neutrophils

Neutrophils are the dominating cell type in the inflammatory milieu of the CF airways. The content of their granules and products, in particular DNA and neutrophil elastase, contribute significantly to the CF lung damage. The increase in the serum and lung cytokine levels, especially of IL-8, preactivates neutrophils and lowers their threshold for granule release (Swain SD 2002). A number of abnormalities have been observed in CF neutrophils, including defective phagocytosis and oxidative burst (Alexis NE 2006), increased degranuation (myeloperoxidase) (Koller DY 1995), augmented proteolytic activity with elevated elastase and matrix metalloprotein release (Brockbank S 2005, Ratjen F 2002, Sagel SD 2005), increased apoptosis and chemotaxis (Brennan S 2001, Watt AP 2005), decreased acidification of phagolysosomes and reduced antimicrobial activity (Painter RG 2006), defective protein kinase C (Graff I 1991), and dysregulated cytokine secretion (Corvol H 2003).Blood neutrophils from CF patients were impaired in chlorination of ingested bacteria due to defective hypochlorous acid (HOCl) production within phagolysosomes, whereas extracellular HOCl production was normal (Painter RG 2006). Profound functional and signaling changes have been shown in viable inflammatory neutrophils collected from airways of CF patients compared to their blood counterparts (Tirouvanziam R 2007). On CF airway neutrophils, the surface expression of phagocytosis receptors CD16 and CD14 was lost, whereas other lineage markers such as CD80 and MHCII appeared, indicating potential functional reprogramming (Tirouvanziam R 2007).

The study by Hartl D *et al.* has provided another pathophysiologic mechanism showing unopposed proteolytic cleavage of chemokine receptor CXCR1 on CF neutrophils and subsequent failure of their bacterial-killing capacity (Hartl D 2007). One of the most important features of the neutrophils in CF is their delayed apoptosis, which could be even measured in CF heterozygous individuals (Moriceau S 2010).

Toll-like receptors (TLRs) play crucial roles in the innate host defense against *P. aeruginosa* Neutrophils express all human TLRs except for TLR3. TLR2 and TLR5 present the main TLRs for the recognition of *P. aeruginosa*. TLR2 and TLR4 are involved in the cytokine response to *P. aeruginosa* infection. Intact flagellin/TLR5 signaling is a prerequisite for an efficient clearance of acute *P. aeruginosa* infection. The expression levels of TLRs in CF neutrophils have been investigated (Koll B 2008, Petit-Bertron AF 2008). Circulating and airway neutrophils from CF patients displayed a distinct pattern of surface markers as compared to the cells from healthy controls (Petit-Bertron AF 2008). CF blood neutrophils

Cell type	Function	Reference
Epithelial cells	Bacterial killing	Moskwa P et al. 2007
	Transport of GSH[1]	Velsor LW et al. 2001
	Redox balance	Xu Y et al. 2006
	Cytokine production	Tabary O et al. 2000
Neutrophils	Phagocytosis	Morris MR et al. 2005, Alexis NE et al. 2006
	Degranulation	Gaggar A et al. 2007, Koller DY et al. 1995, Brockbank S et al. 2005, Ratjen F et al. 2002, Sagel SD et al. 2005
	Apoptosis	Vandivier RW et al. 2002, Watt AP et al. 2005
	Chemotaxis	Brennan S et al. 2001
	Chlorination of phagolysosomes	Painter RG et al. 2006
	Anti-microbial activity	Painter RG et al. 2006, Moraes TJ et al. 2006
	Cytokine production	Corvol H et al. 2003, Tirouvanziam R et al. 2007
	CXCR1[2] cleavage	Hartl D et al. 2007
	TLR[3]-2, 4, 5 expression	Petit Bertron AF et al. 2008
Macrophages	Clearance of apoptotic cells	Vandiview RW et al. 2002a, 2002b
	Cytokine production	Bonfield TL et al. 1995, Bruscia EM et al. 2009, Brennan S et al. 2009, Xu Y et al. 2010
	Phagocytosis	Knight RA et al. 1997, Di A et al. 2006
	Acidification of lysosomes	Di A et al. 2006, Haggie PM, Verkman AS 2007 and 2009
	Antigen presentation	Knight RA et al. 1997
	PPAR[4]/LXR[5] regulation	Andersson C et al. 2007
Dendritic cells	CD1d-restricted natural killer T cells activation	Rzemienaik SE et al. 2010
	Differentiation and maturation	Xu Y et al. 2009
	Activation, antigen presentation, and cytokine secretion	Roghanian A et al. 2006, Xu Y et al. 2009
Monocytes	Phagocytosis	del Fresno C et al. 2009
	Antigen presentation	Sorio C et al. 2011
	MHCII expression	del Fresno C et al. 2008
	TREM-1[6] expression	del Fresno C et al. 2008
	Cytokine production	del Fresno C et al. 2008
	Toll-2, 4 expression	Sturge N C et al. 2010
Lymphocytes	Chloride channel function	McDonald TV et al.1992, Dong YJ et al.1995, Moss RB et al.1996
	Cytokine production	Knutsen AP et al.1989 and 1990, Lahat N et al.1989, Moss RB et al.1996 and 2000, Hubeau C et al.2004, Hartl D et al.2005 Muller C et al.2010, Tan HL et al.2011

Notes: [1] GSH (glutathione); [2] CXCR (C-X-C chemokine receptor), [3] TLR (toll like receptor), [4] PPAR (peroxisomal proliferator activated receptors), [5] LXR (liver X receptors), [6] TREM-1 (triggering receptor expressed on myeloid cells-1)

Table 2. Cellular immune dysfunction in CF

expressed elevated levels of CD64, an activation marker, and lower levels of TLR2 compared to blood neutrophils from healthy controls (Petit-Bertron AF 2008). In contrast, CF airway neutrophils expressed an elevated level of TLR4 and spontaneously released IL-8 that was neither enhanced by microbial activators nor inhibited by recombinant human IL-10, indicating intrinsic resistance to anti-inflammatory signals delivered by IL-10 (Petit-Bertron AF 2008). A similar study by Koller B *et al.* investigated the expression levels of TLR2, TLR4, TLR5, and TLR9 on airway neutrophils compared to circulating neutrophils in CF patients infected with *P. aeruginosa*. TLR5 was the only TLR that was significantly higher expressed in CF airway neutrophils compared to the controls (Koller B 2008).

2.2.2 Macrophages

Alveolar macrophages (AM) are important as a first line host defense in the lung. Besides the phagocytosis of inhaled pathogens and apoptotic cells and the release of inflammatory mediators they play an important role in orchestrating innate immune defenses (Takabayshi 2006). One of the important regulatory functions of AM may be to dampen immune responses (Lambrecht 2006), so that dysfunction of AM in CF could be related to increased inflammation. The antigen-presenting capacity of AM is low, compared to other macrophages and a majority of their function is related to phagocytosis. Dysfunctional CFTR in macrophages has been linked to impaired clearance of apoptotic cells, pro-inflammatory cytokines production, deficient antigen presentation, abnormal TLR4 trafficking, decreased bactericidal activity, and defective phagocytosis (Bonfield TL 1995, Bruscia EM 2009 and 2011, del Porto P 2011, Di A 2006, Knight RA 1997, Vandivier RW 2002a and 2002b, Xu Y 2010). Lipopolysaccharide (LPS) stimulated peritoneal macrophages from CF mice showed increased TNF-α and IL-6 secretion as well as NFκB p65 activity. It also demonstrated attenuated induction of peroxisomal proliferator activated receptors (PPAR) and liver X receptors (LXR), those are two mediators known as the inhibitory regulators of pro-inflammatory cytokines (Andersson C 2007). Bruscia *et al.* showed that macrophages directly contributed to the exaggerated inflammatory response following LPS administration in CF mice with increased secretion of cytokines including IL-6 and keratinocyte chemoattractant (Bruscia EM 2009). The same group also demonstrated that abnormal trafficking and degradation of TLR4 might underlie the elevated inflammatory response in CF (Bruscia EM 2011). Macrophages isolated from lavage samples from CF patients were not able to stimulate allogeneic lymphocytes and to present antigen, while peripheral blood monocytes from the same patients were functional in both assays (Knight RA 1997). Macrophages derived from peripheral blood from CF patients did not differ in phagocytic activity when infected with *P. aeruginosa*, whereas the percentage of surviving bacteria was significantly higher inside CF cells compared to the controls (del Porto P 2011). As AM in human CF lungs are highly activated by the inflammatory milieu, our group assessed the direct influence of CFTR on the function of AM by knockdown CFTR expression in normal human AM with siRNA silencing. A pro-inflammatory phenotype and increased apoptosis were seen in human AM with defective CFTR, possibly due to increased expression of the lipid raft protein Caveolin-1 (Xu Y 2010). The CFTR defect has been linked to augmented apoptosis with an abnormal cellular ceramide composition which is thought to be dependant on alteration in the lipid rafts in CF cells (Becker KA 2010). Altered pH of lysosome in CF macrophages has been suggested to induce defective acidification and bactericidal activity (Di A 2006). These findings have been disputed by others as the pH in the CF lysosomes was not altered using pH sensitive fluorescent probes (Haggie PM 2007 and 2009).

Macrophages may be part of an abnormal priming process in CF during fetal development. This has been suggested by the analysis of fetal lungs for early features of immune dysregulation, which showed that the number of macrophages in the lung was higher in CF fetal lungs compared to non-CF lungs during the later stages of lung development (Hubeau 2001). Findings in the lungs of young infants with CF also point to the presence of increased macrophages as the macrophage recruiting CC chemokines elevated (Brennan S 2008; Starner 2003).

2.2.3 Monocytes

Peripheral blood monocytes, the precursors of AM, represent a pool of cells available to migrate to the lungs in response to bacterial infection. Abnormal functions of monocytes in peripheral blood from CF patients have been shown despite of absence of systemic infection in CF (del Fresno C 2008 and 2009, Sturges NC 2010, Zaman MM 2004). Augmented IL-8 secretions at baseline and in response to LPS were seen in monocytes of adult subjects heterozygous for ΔF508 mutation, with no increased expression of LPS receptors including CD14 and TLR4 but possible association with alterations in mitogen activated phosphate kinase (MAPK) signaling (Zaman MM 2004). Blood peripheral monocytes isolated from CF patients were found to be locked in an endotoxin tolerance state in comparison to those exacted from healthy volunteers, not due to a deficient TLR activation but likely resulted from down-regulation of Triggering Receptor Expressed on Myeloid cells-1 (TREM-1) (del Fresno C 2008). Further investigation demonstrated potent phagocytic activity with impaired antigen presentation in LPS-tolerant monocytes from CF patients, possible by reason of decreased expression of MHCII and co-stimulatory molecules CD80, CD83, and CD86 (del Fresno C 2008). Contradictory to Zaman's finding, Sturge *et al.* have shown enhanced expression of TLR4 but similar TLR2 levels in monocytes from young CF patients with median age of 3.3 compared to healthy controls (Sturges NC 2010). The conflicting results may be due to difference in the age of subjects, and longitudinal studies are required to determine TLR4 expression as CF lung disease progresses.

2.2.4 Dendritic cells

Dendritic cells (DC), the most potent antigen presenting cells, are critical at the interface of innate and adaptive immune response. It is not known if DC function is affected in CF in humans. Only one study assessed blood-derived DC from CF patients in their capacity to activate CD1d-restricted natural killer T cells (NKT cells). The finding was that CF and non CF DC could comparably stimulate NKT cells with no apparent impact from defective CFTR chloride channel function (Rzemieniak SE 2010). Normal murine bone marrow derived DC (BMDC) were cultured in sputum from CF patients. These DC showed down-regulated expression of co-stimulatory molecules CD40, CD80, and CD86 (but not MHCII), inhibited LPS-induced activation, and defective antigen-presenting ability, partially owing to the inflammatory mediator neutrophil elastase (Roghanian A 2006). In our study, BMDC from CF mice expressed CFTR but were delayed in the early phase of differentiation. The expression levels of a number of genes related to lipid metabolism including caveolin-1, 3β-hydroxysterol-Δ7 reductase (Dhcr7), and stearoyl-CoA desaturase 2 (Scd2) were altered (Xu Y 2009). The roles of pulmonary DC, crucial in orchestrating innate and adaptive immune responses, have been investigated in lungs from CF mice in our laboratory (Xu Y 2009).

Phenotypic and functional abnormalities in CF lung DC were found including decreased numbers, altered maturation and activation profiles, and an impaired T cell-stimulation capacity. In response to respiratory syncytial virus infection, recruitment to the lung and T cell stimulatory potential of lung DC of CF mice were impaired in comparison to controls (Xu Y 2009). The dysfunctional CFTR might play a direct role in impaired lung DC. Indirect influence from the environment, where DC reside, on the phenotype and function of lung DC could not be excluded, although inflammation in lungs of CF mice at baseline is considerably mild compared to lungs of CF patients. Further investigation is undertaken to elucidate the mechanism of mal-functional DC in CF lungs.

2.2.5 Lymphocytes

Like the other immune cells, lymphocytes express CFTR and CF lymphocytes have a defective cAMP-regulated chloride channel function (Dong YJ 1995, McDonald TV 1992). B-lymphocytes from CF patients produced similar amounts of IgG compared to non-CF cells, but showed resistance to dexamethasone. This was proposed as a potential factor for the susceptibility to bacterial bronchopulmonary infections (Emilie D 1990). Selective cytokine dysregulation has been shown in CF CD4+ T cells after maximal activation with anti-CD3 or phorbol myristate acetate. It included decreased IFN-γ secretion and reduced IL-10 production, whereas the levels of IL-2, IL-4, and IL-5 remained similar to controls (Moss RB 1996 and 2000). IL-2 has been known to stimulate the growth, differentiation and survival of antigen-selected cytotoxic T cells. IL-4 is a cytokine that induces differentiation of naïve helper T cells (Th0 cells) to Th2 cells. The functions of IL-5 are to stimulate B cell growth and increase immunoglobulin secretion.

Lymphocytes from CF patients or CF mice showed a profile skewed towards T_H2 (Hartl D 2005, Mueller C 2010). In CF patients with *P. aeruginosa* infection, the prevalence of a pulmonary T_H2 immune response has been shown with higher levels of CCR4+CD4+ (T_H2) cells, increased levels of IL-4, IL-13, and lower levels of IFN-γ compared with non-infected patients with CF and healthy controls (Hartl D 2005). Comparably, CF mice mounted an exaggerated IgE response upon *Aspergillus fumigatus* infection in the lung with increased levels of IL-4 and IL-13, mimicking both the T_H2 biased immune responses seen in CF patients (Mueller C 2010). Similar findings are also reported in studies with peripheral blood derived monocytes or whole blood cultures from CF patients infected with *P. aeruginosa* (Brazova J 2005, Moser C 2000). A dysregulated $T_H1/2$ response might contribute to the impaired clearance of pathogens in CF.

Recently, more attention has been focused on the role of T_H17 cells and interleukin-17 (IL-17) in the CF lung disease (McAllister F 2005, Tan HL 2011). IL-17 receptor signaling is critical for pulmonary neutrophil recruitment and host defense against Gram-negative bacteria through the coordinated release of granulocyte-colony stimulating factor (G-CSF) and CXC chemokine elaboration (Steinman L 2007, Bettelli 2007). Significantly elevated levels of IL-17A, IL-17F and IL-17R were found in the sputum of patients with CF who were colonized with *P. aeruginosa* at the time of pulmonary exacerbation. These levels were declined with therapy directed against *P. aeruginosa* (McAllister F 2005). T_H17 lymphocytes and other T_H17+ cells, including neutrophils, $\gamma\delta$ T cells, and natural killer T cells, have been shown to be present in the airway sub-mucosa in CF patients even in a young, newly diagnosed group. Highest levels of IL-17 were found in bronchoalveolar lavage from established CF compared to the controls, with a significant correlation between IL-17 and neutrophil counts as well as IL-4 (Tan HL 2011). IL-17 pathway could serve as a new therapeutic candidate for CF, while the exact pathogenic mechanisms of IL-17 in CF still remain to be elucidated.

3. Conclusion

Augmented inflammation, increased susceptibility of the respiratory tract for infections and lack of efficient clearance of the pathogens are features of a defective immune function. Abnormal CFTR chloride channel function (and potentially associated sodium hyperabsorption) in epithelial and mucous gland cells in the lung can only partially explain the pathophysiology of CF lung disease. Members of the innate and adaptive immune system are clearly affected by the milieu created by the altered salt and water composition. There is also evidence that CFTR dysfunction directly affects immune responses, probably beyond the stimulation of inflammatory cytokines. CFTR is expressed and is functional in a variety of immune cells. CFTR-related abnormalities have been shown in neutrophils, macrophages, monocytes, dendritic cells, and lymphocytes independent of exposure to the CF milieu of the respiratory tract as demonstrated in **Fig 1.** Thus, direct CFTR-mediated dysfunction of these cells may play a role in the enigmatic CF lung disease.

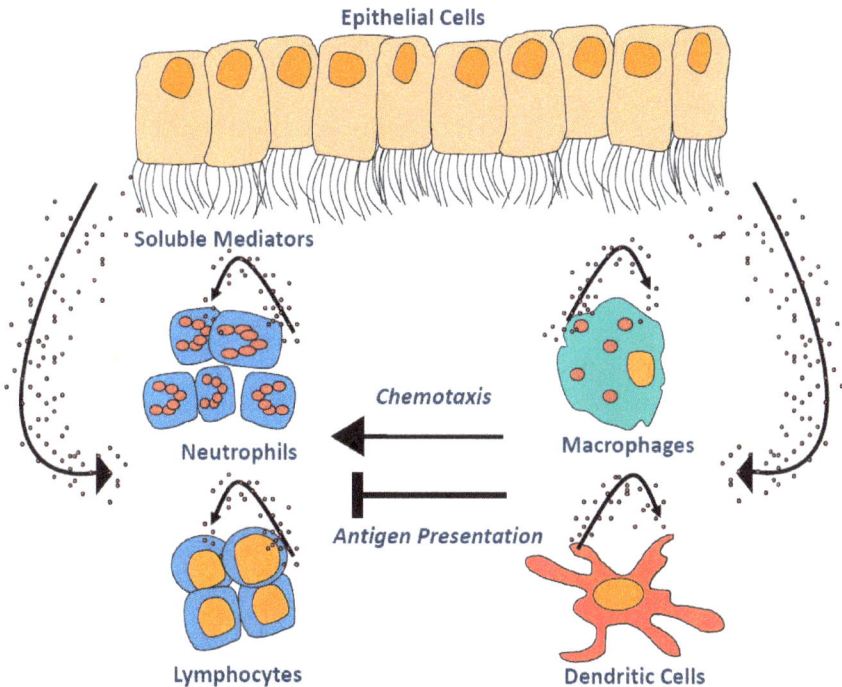

Fig. 1. Model of abnormal humoral and cellular immune responses in the CF lung. Altered humoral responses are comprised of soluble mediators including cytokines, chemokines, antioxidants, and antiproteases. Neutrophils, macrophages, dendritic cells, and lymphocytes are either affected by the altered soluble mediators from the CFTR-deficient epithelial and immune cells or by their own defective CFTR function.

4. Acknowledgment

We thank Ms. Christine Filner for excellent assistance in the preparation of this manuscript. Our studies were supported by R21 HL077557 and the Cystic Fibrosis Foundation XU09F0, Bethesda, MD.

5. References

Alexis, N.E., M.S.Muhlebach, D.B.Peden, and T.L.Noah. (2006). Attenuation of Host Defense Function of Lung Phagocytes in Young Cystic Fibrosis Patients. *Journal of Cystic Fibrosis* 5:17-25. ISSN 1569-1993

Andersson, C., M.M.Zaman, A.B.Jones, and S.D.Freedman. (2008). Alterations in Immune Response and PPAR/LXR Regulation in Cystic Fibrosis Macrophages. *Journal of Cystic Fibrosis* 7:68-78. ISSN 1569-1993

Armstrong, D.S., S.M.Hook, K.M.Jamsen, G.M.Nixon, R.Carzino, J.B.Carlin, C.F.Robertson, and K.Grimwood. (2005). Lower Airway Inflammation in Infants with Cystic Fibrosis Detected by Newborn Screening. *Pediatr. Pulmonol.* 40:500-510. ISSN 8755-6863

Armstrong, D., K.Grimwood, J.Carlin, R.Carzino, J.Gutièrrez, J.Hull, A.Olinsky, E.Phelan, C.Robertson, and P.Phelan. (1997). Lower Airway Inflammation in Infants and Young Children with Cystic Fibrosis. *Am. J. Respir. Crit. Care Med.* 156:1197-1204. ISSN 1073-449X

Assef, Y.A., A.E.Damiano, E.Zotta, C.Ibarra, and B.A.Kotsias. (2003). CFTR in K562 Human Leukemic Cells. *Am J Physiol Cell Physiol* 285:C480-C488. ISSN 0363-6143

Bals, R., D.J.Weiner, R.L.Meegalla, F.Accurso, and J.M.Wilson. (2001). Salt-independent Abnormality of Antimicrobial Activity in Cystic Fibrosis Airway Surface Fluid. *Am. J. Respir. Cell Mol. Biol.* 25:21-25. ISSN:1044-1549

Bals, R., D.J.Weiner, and J.M.Wilson. (1999). The Innate Immune System in Cystic Fibrosis Lung Disease. *J Clin Invest* 103:303-307. ISSN 0021-9738

Bartlett J, Fischer A, and J.McCray PB. (2008). Innate Immune Functions of the Airway Epithelium. *In* Trends in Innate Immunity.Contrib Microbiol. Egesten A, Schmidt A, and Herwald H, editors. S Karger, ISBN 3805585489, Basel. 147-163.

Bhattacharyya, S., U.Gutti, J.Mercado, C.Moore, H.B.Pollard, and R.Biswas. (2010). MAPK Signaling Pathways Regulate IL-8 mRNA Stability and IL-8 Protein Expression in Cystic Fibrosis Lung Epithelial Cells Lines. *Am J Physiol Lung Cell Mol Physiol* doi:10.1152/ajplung.00051.2010. ISSN 1040-0605

Black, H.R., J.R.Yankaskas, L.G.Johnson, and T.L.Noah. (1998). Interleukin-8 Production by Cystic Fibrosis Nasal Epithelial Cells after Tumor Necrosis Factor-alpha and Respiratory Syncytial Virus Stimulation. *Am. J. Respir. Cell Mol. Biol.* 19:210-215. ISSN:1044-1549

Bonfield, T.L., J.R.Panuska, M.W.Konstan, K.A.Hilliard, J.B.Hilliard, H.Ghnaim, and M.Berger. (1995). Inflammatory Cytokines in Cystic Fibrosis Lungs. *Am. J. Respir. Crit. Care Med.* 152:2111-2118. ISSN: 1073-449X

Brazova, J., A.Sediva, D.Pospisilova, V.Vavrova, P.Pohunek, J.Macek, J.Bartunkova, and H.Lauschmann. (2005). Differential Cytokine Profile in Children with Cystic Fibrosis. *Clin Immunol* 115:210-215. ISSN:1521-6616

Brennan, S., D.Cooper, and P.D.Sly. (2001). Directed Neutrophil Migration to IL-8 is Increased in Cystic Fibrosis: a Study of the Effect of Erythromycin. *Thorax* 56:62-64. ISSN 0040-6376

Brennan, S., P.D.Sly, C.L.Gangell, N.Sturges, K.Winfield, M.Wikstrom, S.Gard, J.W.Upham, and on behalf of AREST CF. (2009). Alveolar Macrophages and CC Chemokines are Increased in Children with Cystic Fibrosis. *European Respiratory Journal* 34:655-661. ISSN 0903-1936

Brennan, S. (2008). Innate Immune Activation and Cystic Fibrosis. *Paediatric Respiratory Reviews* 9:271-280. ISSN 1526-0542

Brockbank, S., D.Downey, J.S.Elborn, and M.Ennis. (2005). Effect of Cystic Fibrosis Exacerbations on Neutrophil Function. *International Immunopharmacology* 5:601-608. ISSN 1567-5769

Bruscia, E.M., P.X.Zhang, A.Satoh, C.Caputo, R.Medzhitov, A.Shenoy, M.E.Egan, and D.S.Krause. (2011). Abnormal Trafficking and Degradation of TLR4 Underlie the Elevated Inflammatory Response in Cystic Fibrosis. *J Immunol* 186:6990-6998. ISSN 0022-1767

Bruscia, E.M., P.X.Zhang, E.Ferreira, C.Caputo, J.W.Emerson, D.Tuck, D.S.Krause, and M.E.Egan. (2008). Macrophages Directly Contribute to the Exaggerated Inflammatory Response in CFTR-/- Mice. *Am. J. Respir. Cell Mol. Biol.* 40:295-304. ISSN 1044-1549

Bubien, J. (2001). CFTR may Play a Role in Regulated Secretion by Lymphocytes: a New Hypothesis for the Pathophysiology of Cystic Fibrosis. *Pflugers Arch* 443:S36-S39. ISSN 0031-6768

Buchanan, P.J., R.K.Ernst, J.S.Elborn, and B.Schock. (2009). Role of CFTR, Pseudomonas aeruginosa and Toll-like Receptors in Cystic Fibrosis Lung Inflammation. *Biochem Soc Trans* 37:863-867. ISSN 0300-5127

Cantin, A.M., S.Lafrenaye, and R.O.Begin. (1991). Antineutrophil Elastase Activity in Cystic Fibrosis Serum. *Pediatr. Pulmonol.* 11:249-253. ISSN 8755-6863

Chen CI, Schaller-Bals S, Paul KP, Wahn U, and Bals R. (2004). Beta-defensins and LL-37 in Bronchoalveolar Lavage Fluid of Patients with Cystic Fibrosis. *Journal of Cystic Fibrosis* 3:45-50. ISSN 1569-1993

Childers, M., G.Eckel, A.Himmel, and J.Caldwell. (2007). A New Model of Cystic Fibrosis Pathology: Lack of Transport of Glutathione and its Thiocyanate Conjugates. *Medical Hypotheses* 68:101-112. ISSN 0306-9877

Conese, M. (2011). Cystic Fibrosis and the Innate Immune System: Therapeutic Implications. *Endocr. Metab Immune. Disord. Drug Targets.* 11:8-22. ISSN 1871-5303

Corvol, H., C.Fitting, K.Chadelat, J.Jacquot, O.Tabary, M.Boule, J.M.Cavaillon, and A.Clement. (2003). Distinct Cytokine Production by Lung and Blood Neutrophils from Children with Cystic Fibrosis. *American Journal of Physiology - Lung Cellular and Molecular Physiology* 284:L997-L1003. ISSN 1522-1504

Day, B.J. (2005). Glutathione: a Radical Treatment for Cystic Fibrosis Lung Disease? *Chest* 127:12-14. ISSN 0012-3692

Deriy, L.V., E.A.Gomez, G.Zhang, D.W.Beacham, J.A.Hopson, A.J.Gallan, P.D.Shevchenko, V.P.Bindokas, and D.J.Nelson. (2009). Disease Causing Mutations in the Cystic Fibrosis Transmembrane Conductance Regulator Determine the Functional Responses of Alveolar Macrophages. *Journal of Biological Chemistry*. ISSN 0021-9258 del Fresno, C., F.Garcia-Rio, V.Gomez-Pina, A.Soares-Schanoski, I.Fernandez-Ruiz, T.Jurado, T.Kajiji, C.Shu, E.Marin, A.Gutierrez del Arroyo, C.Prados, F.Arnalich, P.Fuentes-Prior, S.K.Biswas, and E.Lopez-Collazo. (2009). Potent Phagocytic Activity with Impaired Antigen Presentation Identifying Lipopolysaccharide-tolerant Human Monocytes: Demonstration in Isolated Monocytes from Cystic Fibrosis Patients. *J Immunol* 182:6494-6507. ISSN 0022-1767

del Fresno, C., V.Gomez-Pina, V.Lores, A.Soares-Schanoski, I.Fernandez-Ruiz, B.Rojo, R.varez-Sala, E.Caballero-Garrido, F.Garcia, T.Veliz, F.Arnalich, P.Fuentes-Prior, F.Garcia-Rio, and E.Lopez-Collazo. 2008. Monocytes from Cystic Fibrosis Patients are Locked in an LPS Tolerance State: Down-Regulation of TREM-1 as Putative Underlying Mechanism. *PLoS ONE* 3:e2667. ISSN 1932-6203

Di, A., M.E.Brown, L.V.Deriy, C.Li, F.L.Szeto, Y.Chen, P.Huang, J.Tong, A.P.Naren, V.Bindokas, H.C.Palfrey, and D.J.Nelson. (2006). CFTR Regulates Phagosome Acidification in Macrophages and Alters Bactericidal Activity. *Nat Cell Biol* 8:933-944. ISSN 1465-7392

dib-Conquy, M., T.Pedron, A.F.Petit-Bertron, O.Tabary, H.Corvol, J.Jacquot, A.Clement, and J.M.Cavaillon. (2008). Neutrophils in Cystic Fibrosis Display a Distinct Gene Expression Pattern. *Mol Med* 14:36-44. ISSN 1432-1440

Dong, Y.J., A.C.Chao, K.Kouyama, Y.P.Hsu, R.C.Bocian, R.B.Moss, and P.Gardner. (1995.) Activation of CFTR Chloride Current by Nitric Oxide in Human T Lymphocytes. *EMBO J* 14:2700-2707. ISSN 0261-4189

Gaggar, A., A.Hector, P.E.Bratcher, M.A.Mall, M.Griese, and D.Hartl. (2011). The Role of Matrix Metalloproteinases in Cystic Fibrosis Lung Disease. *European Respiratory Journal* 38:721-727. 0903-1936

Gaggar, A., Y.Li, N.Weathington, M.Winkler, M.Kong, P.Jackson, J.E.Blalock, and J.P.Clancy. (2007). Matrix Metalloprotease-9 Dysregulation in Lower Airway Secretions of Cystic Fibrosis Patients. *American Journal of Physiology Lung Cellular and Molecular Physiology* 293:L96-L104. ISSN 1040-0605

Gao, L., K.J.Kim, J.R.Yankaskas, and H.J.Forman. (1999). Abnormal Glutathione Transport in Cystic Fibrosis Airway Epithelia. *American Journal of Physiology - Lung Cellular and Molecular Physiology* 277:L113-L118. ISSN 1040-0605

Goldman, M.J., G.M.Anderson, E.D.Stolzenberg, U.P.Kari, M.Zasloff, and J.M.Wilson. (1997). Human [beta]-Defensin-1 Is a Salt-Sensitive Antibiotic in Lung That Is Inactivated in Cystic Fibrosis. *Cell* 88:553-560. ISSN 0092-8674

Haggie, P.M. and A.S.Verkman. (2009). Unimpaired Lysosomal Acidification in Respiratory Epithelial Cells in Cystic Fibrosis. *J Biol Chem* 284:7681-7686. ISSN 0021-9258

Hampton, T.H. and B.A.Stanton. (2010). A Novel Approach to Analyze Gene Expression Data Demonstrates that the {Delta}F508 Mutation in CFTR Downregulates the Antigen Presentation Pathway. *Am J Physiol Lung Cell Mol Physiol* 298:L473-L482. ISSN 1040-0605

Hartl, D. and M.Griese. (2006). Surfactant Protein D in Human Lung Diseases. *European Journal of Clinical Investigation* 36:423-435. ISSN 1526-0542

Hartl, D., M.Griese, M.Kappler, G.Zissel, D.Reinhardt, C.Rebhan, D.J.Schendel, and S.Krauss-Etschmann. (2006). Pulmonary TH2 Response in Pseudomonas aeruginosa-infected Patients with Cystic Fibrosis. *J Allergy Clin Immunol* 117:204-211. ISSN 0091-6749

Hauber, H.P., M.K.Tulic, A.Tsicopoulos, B.Wallaert, R.Olivenstein, P.Daigneault, and Q.Hamid. (2005). Toll-like Receptors 4 and 2 Expression in the Bronchial Mucosa of Patients with Cystic Fibrosis. *Can. Respir J* 12:13-18. ISSN 1198-2241

Hausler, M., K.Schweizer, S.Biesterfeld, T.Opladen, and G.Heimann. (2002). Peripheral Decrease and Pulmonary Homing of CD4+CD45RO+ Helper Memory T cells in Cystic Fibrosis. *Respiratory Medicine* 96:87-94. ISSN 0954-6111

Hubeau, C., E.Puchelle, and D.Gaillard. (2001). Distinct Pattern of Immune Cell Population in the Lung of Human Fetuses with Cystic Fibrosis. *Journal of Allergy and Clinical Immunology* 108:524-529. ISSN 0091-6749

Hudson, V.M. (2001). Rethinking Cystic Fibrosis Pathology: the Critical Role of Abnormal Reduced Glutathione (GSH) Transport Caused by CFTR Mutation. *Free Radical Biology and Medicine* 30:1440-1461. ISSN 0891-5849

Jacquot, J., O.Tabary, P.Le Rouzic, and A.Clement. (2008). Airway Epithelial Cell Inflammatory Signalling in Cystic Fibrosis. *The International Journal of Biochemistry & Cell Biology* 40:1703-1715. ISSN 1357-2725

Kerby, G.S., V.Cottin, F.J.Accurso, F.Hoffmann, E.D.Chan, V.A.Fadok, and D.W.H.Riches. (2002). Impairment of Macrophage Survival by NaCl: Implications for Early Pulmonary Inflammation in Cystic Fibrosis. *American Journal of Physiology - Lung Cellular and Molecular Physiology* 283:L188-L197. ISSN 1040-0605

Khan, T.Z., J.S.Wagener, T.Bost, J.Martinez, F.J.Accurso, and D.W.Riches. (1995). Early Pulmonary Inflammation in Infants with Cystic Fibrosis. *Am. J. Respir. Crit. Care Med.* 151:1075-1082. ISSN 1073-449X

Knight, R.A., S.Kollnberger, B.Madden, M.Yacoub, and M.E.Hodson. (1997). Defective Antigen Presentation by Lavage Cells from Terminal Patients with Cystic Fibrosis. *Clin Exp Immunol* 107:542-547. ISSN 0009-9104

Knutsen, A.P. and R.G.Slavin. (1989). In vitro T cell Responses in Patients with Cystic Fibrosis and Allergic Bronchopulmonary Aspergillosis. *J Lab Clin Med.* 113:428-435. ISSN 0022-2143

Knutsen, A.P., K.R.Mueller, P.S.Hutcheson, and R.G.Slavin. (1990). T- and B-cell Dysregulation of IgE Synthesis in Cystic Fibrosis Patients with Allergic Bronchopulmonary Aspergillosis. *Clinical Immunology and Immunopathology* 55:129-138. ISSN 0090-1229

Kogan, I., M.Ramjeesingh, C.Li, J.F.Kidd, Y.Wang, E.M.Leslie, S.P.C.Cole, and C.E.Bear. (2003). CFTR Directly Mediates Nucleotide-regulated Glutathione Flux. *EMBO J* 22:1981-1989. I SSN 0261-4189

Koller, B., M.Kappler, P.Latzin, A.Gaggar, M.Schreiner, S.Takyar, M.Kormann, M.Kabesch, D.Roos, M.Griese, and D.Hartl. (2008). TLR Expression on Neutrophils at the Pulmonary Site of Infection: TLR1/TLR2-Mediated Up-Regulation of TLR5 Expression in Cystic Fibrosis Lung Disease. *J Immunol* 181:2753-2763. ISSN 0022-1767

Koller, D.Y., R.Urbanek, and M.Gotz. (1995). Increased Degranulation of Eosinophil and Neutrophil Granulocytes in Cystic Fibrosis. *Am J Respir Crit Care Med* 152:629-633. ISSN 1073-449X

Lahat, N., J.Rivlin, and T.C.Iancu. (1989). Functional Immunoregulatory T-cell Abnormalities in Cystic Fibrosis Patients. *J Clin Immunol* 9:287-295. ISSN 0271-9142

Mall, M.A., B.Button, B.Johannesson, Z.Zhou, A.Livraghi, R.A.Caldwell, S.C.Schubert, C.Schultz, W.K.O'Neal, S.Pradervand, E.Hummler, B.C.Rossier, B.R.Grubb, and R.C.Boucher. (2010). Airway Surface Liquid Volume Regulation Determines Different Airway Phenotypes in Liddle Compared with betaENaC-overexpressing Mice. *Journal of Biological Chemistry* 285:26945-26955. ISSN 0021-9258

McAllister, F., A.Henry, J.L.Kreindler, P.J.Dubin, L.Ulrich, C.Steele, J.D.Finder, J.M.Pilewski, B.M.Carreno, S.J.Goldman, J.Pirhonen, and J.K.Kolls. (2005). Role of IL-17A, IL-17F, and the IL-17 Receptor in Regulating Growth-Related Oncogene-+¦ and Granulocyte Colony-Stimulating Factor in Bronchial Epithelium: Implications for Airway Inflammation in Cystic Fibrosis. *J Immunol* 175:404-412. ISSN 022-1767

McDonald, T.V., P.T.Nghiem, P.Gardner, and C.L.Martens. (1992). Human Lymphocytes Transcribe the Cystic Fibrosis Transmembrane Conductance Regulator Gene and Exhibit CF-defective cAMP-regulated Chloride Current. *Journal of Biological Chemistry* 267:3242-3248. ISSN 0021-9258

McElvaney, N.G., H.Nakamura, P.Birrer, C.A.H+¬bert, W.L.Wong, M.Alphonso, J.B.Baker, M.A.Catalano, and R.G.Crystal. (1992). Modulation of Airway Inflammation in Cystic Fibrosis. In vivo Suppression of Interleukin-8 Levels on the Respiratory Epithelial Surface by Aerosolization of Recombinant Secretory Leukoprotease Inhibitor. *J Clin Invest* 90:1296-1301.ISSN 0021-9738

Meyer, K.C., A.Sharma, R.Brown, M.Weatherly, F.R.Moya, J.Lewandoski, and J.J.Zimmerman. (2000). Function and Composition of Pulmonary Surfactant and Surfactant-derived Fatty Profiles are Altered in Young Adults with Cystic Fibrosis. *Chest* 118:164-174. ISSN 0012-3692

Meyer, M., F.Huaux, X.Gavilanes, S.van den Brule, P.Lebecque, S.Lo Re, D.Lison, B.Scholte, P.Wallemacq, and T.Leal. (2009). Azithromycin Reduces Exaggerated Cytokine Production by M1 Alveolar Macrophages in Cystic Fibrosis. *Am. J. Respir. Cell Mol. Biol.* 41:590-602. ISSN 1044-1549

Moraes, T.J., J.Plumb, R.Martin, E.Vachon, V.Cherepanov, A.Koh, C.Loeve, J.Jongstra-Bilen, J.H.Zurawska, J.V.Kus, L.L.Burrows, S.Grinstein, and G.P.Downey. (2006). Abnormalities in the Pulmonary Innate Immune System in Cystic Fibrosis. *Am. J. Respir. Cell Mol. Biol.* 34:364-374. ISSN 1044-1549

Morris, M.R., I.J.M.Doull, S.Dewitt, and M.B.Hallett. (2005). Reduced iC3b-mediated Phagocytotic Capacity of Pulmonary Neutrophils in Cystic Fibrosis. *Clinical & Experimental Immunology* 142:68-75. ISSN 1365-2249

Moskwa, P., D.Lorentzen, K.J.D.A.Excoffon, J.Zabner, P.B.McCray, Jr., W.M.Nauseef, C.Dupuy, and B.Banfi. (2007). A Novel Host Defense System of Airways is Defective in Cystic Fibrosis. *Am. J. Respir. Crit. Care Med.* 175:174-183. ISSN 1073-449X

Moss, R.B., R.C.Bocian, Y.P.Hsu, Y.J.Dong, M.KEMNA, T.WEI, and P.Gardner. (1996). Reduced IL-10 Secretion by CD4+ T Lymphocytes Expressing Mutant Cystic Fibrosis Transmembrane Conductance Regulator (CFTR). *Clinical & Experimental Immunology* 106:374-388. ISSN 1365-2249

Moss, R.B., Y.P.Hsu, and L.Olds. (2000). Cytokine Dysregulation in Activated Cystic Fibrosis (CF) Peripheral Lymphocytes. *Clinical & Experimental Immunology* 120:518-525. ISSN 1365-2249

Mueller, C., S.A.Braag, A.Keeler, C.Hodges, M.Drumm, and T.R.Flotte. (2010). Lack of Cftr in CD3+ Lymphocytes Leads to Aberrant Cytokine Secretion and Hyper-inflammatory Adaptive Immune Responses. *Am. J. Respir. Cell Mol. Biol.*doi:10.1165/rcmb.2010-0224OC. ISSN 1044-1549

Noah, T.L., P.C.Murphy, J.J.Alink, M.W.Leigh, W.M.Hull, M.T.Stahlman, and J.A.Whitsett. (2003). Bronchoalveolar Lavage Fluid Surfactant Protein-A and Surfactant Protein-D Are Inversely Related to Inflammation in Early Cystic Fibrosis. *Am. J. Respir. Crit. Care Med.* 168:685-691. ISSN 1073-449X

Nurlan Dauletbaev, Roswitha Gropp, Michaela Frye, Stefan Loitsch, Thomas-Otto-Friedrich Wagner, and Joachim Bargon. (2002). Expression of Human Beta Defensin (HBD-1 and HBD-2) mRNA in Nasal Epithelia of Adult Cystic Fibrosis Patients, Healthy Individuals, and Individuals with Acute Cold. *Respiration* 69:46-51. ISSN 1423-0356

Painter, R.G., R.W.Bonvillain, V.G.Valentine, G.A.Lombard, S.G.LaPlace, W.M.Nauseef, and G.Wang. (2008). The Role of Chloride Anion and CFTR in Killing of Pseudomonas aeruginosa by Normal and CF Neutrophils. *J Leukoc Biol* 83:1345-1353. ISSN 0741-5400

Petit-Bertron, A.F., O.Tabary, H.Corvol, J.Jacquot, A.Clqment, J.M.Cavaillon, and M.dib-Conquy. (2008). Circulating and Airway Neutrophils in Cystic Fibrosis Display Different TLR Expression and Responsiveness to Interleukin-10. *Cytokine* 41:54-60. ISSN 1043-4666

Ratjen, F. and G.Doring. (2003). Cystic Fibrosis. *The Lancet* 361:681-689. ISSN 0140-6736

Roghanian, A., E.M.Drost, W.MacNee, S.E.M.Howie, and J.M.Sallenave. (2006). Inflammatory Lung Secretions Inhibit Dendritic Cell Maturation and Function via Neutrophil Elastase. *Am. J. Respir. Crit. Care Med.* 174:1189-1198. ISSN 1073-449X

Roum, J.H., R.Buhl, N.G.McElvaney, Z.Borok, and R.G.Crystal. (1993). Systemic Deficiency of Glutathione in Cystic Fibrosis. *Journal of Applied Physiology* 75:2419-2424. ISSN 8750-7587

Rzemieniak, S.E., A.F.Hirschfeld, R.E.Victor, M.A.Chilvers, D.Zheng, P.Van Den Elzen, and S.E.Turvey. (2010). Acidification-dependent Activation of CD1d-restricted Natural Killer T cells is Intact in Cystic Fibrosis. *Immunology* 130:288-295. ISSN 1365-2567

Sagel, S.D., R.K.Kapsner, and I.Osberg. (2005). Induced Sputum Matrix Metalloproteinase-9 Correlates with Lung Function and Airway Inflammation in Children with Cystic Fibrosis. *Pediatr. Pulmonol.* 39:224-232. ISSN 1099-0496

Soltys, J., T.Bonfield, J.Chmiel, and M.Berger. (2002). Functional IL-10 Deficiency in the Lung of cystic fibrosis (cftr-/-) and IL-10 Knockout Mice causes Increased Expression and Function of B7 Costimulatory Molecules on Alveolar Macrophages. *J Immunol* 168:1903-1910. ISSN 0022-1767

Sturges, N.C., M.E.Wikstrim, K.R.Winfield, S.E.Gard, S.Brennan, P.D.Sly, and J.W.Upham. (2010). Monocytes from Children with Clinically Stable Cystic Fibrosis Show Enhanced Expression of Toll-like Receptor 4. *Pediatr. Pulmonol.* 45:883-889. ISSN 8755-6863

Suri, R., L.J.Marshall, C.Wallis, C.Metcalfe, A.Bush, and J.K.Shute. (2002). Effects of Recombinant Human DNase and Hypertonic Saline on Airway Inflammation in Children with Cystic Fibrosis. *Am. J. Respir. Crit. Care Med.* 166:352-355. ISSN 1073-449X

Tabary, O., S.Escotte, J.Couetil, D.Hubert, D.Dusser, E.Puchelle, and J.Jacquot. (2001). Relationship Between IkappaBa Deficiency, NFkappaB Activity and Interleukin-8 Production in CF Human Airway Epithelial Cells. *Pflugers Archiv European Journal of Physiology* 443:S40-S44. ISSN 0031-6768

Tan, H.L., N.Regamey, S.Brown, A.Bush, C.M.Lloyd, and J.C.Davies. (2011). The Th17 Pathway in Cystic Fibrosis Lung Disease. *Am. J. Respir. Crit. Care Med.* 184:252-258. ISSN 1073-449X

Tirouvanziam, R. (2006). Neutrophilic Inflammation as a Major Determinant in the Progression of Cystic Fibrosis. *Drug News Perspect.* 19:609-614. ISSN 0214-0934

Vandivier, R.W., V.A.Fadok, P.R.Hoffmann, D.L.Bratton, C.Penvari, K.K.Brown, J.D.Brain, F.J.Accurso, and P.M.Henson. (2002a). Elastase-mediated Phosphatidylserine Receptor Cleavage Impairs Apoptotic Cell Clearance in Cystic Fibrosis and Bronchiectasis. *Journal of Clinical Investigation* 109:661. ISSN 0021-9738

Vandivier, R.W., V.A.Fadok, C.A.Ogden, P.R.Hoffmann, J.D.Brain, F.J.Accurso, J.H.Fisher, K.E.Greene, and P.M.Henson. (2002b). Impaired Clearance of Apoptotic Cells From Cystic Fibrosis Airways. *Chest* 121:89S. ISSN 0012-3692

Velsor, L.W., A.van Heeckeren, and B.J.Day. (2001). Antioxidant Imbalance in the Lungs of Cystic Fibrosis Transmembrane Conductance Regulator Protein Mutant Mice. *American Journal of Physiology - Lung Cellular and Molecular Physiology* 281:L31-L38. ISSN 1522-1504

Watt, A.P., J.Courtney, J.Moore, M.Ennis, and J.S.Elborn. (2005). Neutrophil Cell Death, Activation and Bacterial Infection in Cystic Fibrosis. *Thorax* 60:659-664. ISSN 0040-6376

Welsh MJ, Ramsey BW, Accurso F, and Cutting GR. (2011). Cystic Fibrosis. *In* the Online Metabolic & Molecular Bases of Inherited Disease. Charles R.Scriver, editor. McGraw-Hill, ISBN 0079130356, New York.

Xu, Y., C.Liu, J.C.Clark, and J.A.Whitsett. (2006). Functional Genomic Responses to Cystic Fibrosis Transmembrane Conductance Regulator (CFTR) and CFTRdeltaF508 in the Lung. *Journal of Biological Chemistry* 281:11279-11291. ISSN 0021-9258

Xu Y, Krause A, Wu W, Joh J, Limberis MP, and Worgall S. Characterization of Pulmonary Dendritic Cell in the Lung Disease of Cystic Fibrosis Mice following Respiratory Syncytial Virus Infection. American Thoracic Society 2009 International Conference. The American Journal of Respiratory and Critical Care Medicine ISSN 1535-4970, San Diego, California, USA, May 15-20, 2009.

Xu, Y., A.Krause, H.Hamai, B.G.Harvey, T.S.Worgall, and S.Worgall. (2010). Proinflammatory Phenotype and Increased Caveolin-1 in Alveolar Macrophages with Silenced CFTR mRNA. *PLoS. One.* 5:e11004. ISSN 1932-6203

Xu, Y., C.Tertilt, A.Krause, L.Quadri, R.Crystal, and S.Worgall. (2009). Influence of the CysticFibrosis Transmembrane Conductance Regulator on Expression of Lipid Metabolism-related Genes in Dendritic Cells. *Respir Res* 10:26.ISSN 1465-9921

Zaman, M.M., A.Gelrud, O.Junaidi, M.M.Regan, M.Warny, J.C.Shea, C.Kelly, B.P.O'Sullivan, and S.D.Freedman. (2004). Interleukin 8 Secretion from Monocytes of Subjects Heterozygous for the deltaF508 Cystic Fibrosis Transmembrane Conductance Regulator Gene Mutation is Altered. *Clin Diagn Lab Immunol* 11:819-824. ISSN 1071-412X

12

Viral Respiratory Tract Infections in Cystic Fibrosis

Dennis Wat

Adult Cystic Fibrosis Unit, Papworth Hospital, Cambridge,
United Kingdom

1. Introduction

Cystic Fibrosis (CF) is the most commonly inherited potentially lethal disease amongst Caucasian children and young adults. In Europe, approximately 35,000 children and adults are affected by CF. The prevalence in the US and in Canada is approximately 30,000 and 3,000, respectively. CF is an autosomal recessive disorder and is caused by mutations in the Cystic Fibrosis Transmembrane Conductance Regulator gene (CFTR) (Riordan, Rommens et al. 1989). The main function of CFTR in many tissues is to regulate and participate in the transport of chloride ions across epithelial cell membranes. To date, more than 1,800 mutations have been described in this gene, but the most common mutation worldwide is caused by deletion of phenylalanine at position 508 (Delta F508) of the CFTR on chromosome 7. The dramatic improvement in survival from CF has taken great strides over the past 40 years with the introduction of specialist centre care, optimising nutritional status and preventing pulmonary inflammation. The median survival of children born in the 1990s is estimated to exceed 40 years of age with more than 85% of them achieving adulthood. CF is a multisystem disorder and is characterised by chronic suppurative lung disease and by exocrine pancreatic insufficiency which affects gastrointestinal function and causes restricted growth and maturation. CF also causes obstructive azoospermia and thus male infertility. However, in most individuals with CF the major burden is on the lungs. The absence of CFTR in airway epithelium leads to malfunction of chloride conductance and subsequent airway surface liquid (ASL) volume reduction, mucins are concentrated, the periciliary liquid depleted, and mucous clearance by ciliary and cough dependent mechanisms diminished, which leads to airflow obstruction and eventually bacterial colonisation. Bacteria implicated in the morbidity and mortality of CF include *Pseudomonas aeruginosa, Burkholderia cepacia complex, Achromobacter xylosoxidans, Staphylococcus aureus, Haemophilus influenzae, Stenotrophomonas maltophilia* and *non-tuberculous mycobacteria*. However despite the appropriate use of antibiotic therapy, chronic obstructive airway disease continues to develop in patients with CF and is the major cause of morbidity and mortality.

However, the use of appropriate antibiotic therapy has had a limited effect in slowing the progression of pulmonary disease. As a result, recent studies have hypothesised that respiratory viral infection may be a contributing factor to pulmonary exacerbations. Respiratory viruses implicated in the respiratory exacerbations of CF include *influenza A and*

B, respiratory syncytial virus (RSV), parainfluenza virus (PIV) types 1 to 4, rhinovirus, metapneumovirus, coronavirus and *adenovirus.*

The role of respiratory viruses in the aetiology of respiratory exacerbations in CF is not fully understood and may have been underestimated as many previous studies have used insensitive techniques to isolate respiratory viruses, therefore undermining their prevalence. New viral detection techniques have further enhanced the awareness of respiratory viral aetiology in CF exacerbations. A recent in vitro study illustrating the interaction of respiratory virus and *P. aeruginosa* may contribute to the pathogenesis of CF exacerbations. No doubt more work will be required in this area to further understand their relationship so as to allow the development of potential novel treatment. If respiratory viruses do lead to secondary bacterial infection in CF, this may rationalize the treatment of CF in future. Although there are commercially available vaccines and anti-virals for the prevention and treatment of respiratory viral infections, they are mainly limited to influenza viral infection. A number of studies are currently underway looking at the development of new vaccines and anti-virals, hopefully it will not be long before treatment becomes available for different types of respiratory viruses.

This chapter will provide an overview on the epidemiology of respiratory viruses in CF, the available detection techniques for viruses and their differences in sensitivities, the clinical implications of viral infection in CF, the interaction between viruses and bacteria, and the management of viral infections.

CF is the most commonly inherited, potentially lethal disease amongst Caucasian children and young adults (Mearns 1993). Pathological changes occur in all exocrine glands (Vawter and Shwachman 1979), however, in most individuals with CF the major impact is on the lungs (Oppenheimer and Esterly 1975). Chronic lung infections may start very early in the lives of patients with CF. It has been hypothesised that impaired mucociliary clearance and low airway surface liquid (ASL) volume is pivotal for the pathogenesis of lung infections. These in turn lead to impaired bacterial clearance from respiratory epithelial cells (Saiman and Siegel 2004). Pulmonary infections remain to be the greatest cause of morbidity and mortality leading to premature death in CF (Rajan and Saiman 2002).

The incidence of CF in the United Kingdom is around 1 in 2500 live births and 1 in 25 of the population carry a mutation in their CF genes (Dodge, Morison et al. 1993). CF is a multisystem disorder and is characterised by chronic suppurative lung disease and by exocrine pancreatic insufficiency which affects gastrointestinal function and causes restricted growth and maturation. CF also causes obstructive azoospermia and thus male infertility.

CF is an autosomal recessive disorder and is caused by mutations in the CFTR (Riordan, Rommens et al. 1989). The main function of CFTR in many tissues is to regulate and participate in the transport of chloride ions across epithelial cell membranes (Barasch and al-Awqati 1993). So far more than 1,800 mutations have been described in this gene (http://genet.sickkids.on.ca/cgi-bin/WebObjects/MUTATION), but the most common mutation worldwide is caused by deletion of phenylalanine at position 508 (Delta F508) of the CFTR on chromosome 7.

Survival from CF is increasing rapidly as exemplified by the median life expectancy of CF children born in 1990 to be around 40 years which is double that of 20 years ago (Elborn, Shale et al.). The prolonged life expectancy might be attributed to multi-disciplinary care, improved nutritional status, use of antibiotics and better understanding of disease pathology.

CF pulmonary exacerbations represent decreased host defences within the lungs leading to alterations in airway microbiology, airway obstruction related to increased sputum production and ventilatory failure (Goss and Burns 2007). Pulmonary exacerbations are associated with acquisition of new organisms and increased concentration of airway flora (Aaron, Ramotar et al. 2004). The presences of some organisms including S. aureus, P. aeruginosa and B. cepacia in the airways have been shown to lead to clinical deterioration (Thomassen, Demko et al. 1985; Nixon, Armstrong et al. 2001; Sawicki, Rasouliyan et al. 2008). The new acquisitions of *P. aeruginosa* in CF have been demonstrated to occur in the winter months coinciding with the peak of respiratory viral infections (Johansen and Hoiby 1992). *Influenza* is a substantial health threat, it is associated with approximately >36,000 deaths and 220,000 hospitalisations in the United States yearly (Thompson, Shay et al. 2004). The emergence of novel *influenza virus (H1N1)* further heightened the awareness of influenza-like illness. CF Pulmonary exacerbation rates have been shown to be significantly increased during the winter and are highly associated with the influenza season (Ortiz, Neuzil et al. 2010).

2. Viral respiratory infections in CF

Early studies looking at respiratory viruses in CF relied on repeated serological testing, either alone (Petersen, Hoiby et al. 1981) or in combination with viral cultures for viral detection (Wang, Prober et al. 1984; Ramsey, Gore et al. 1989; Pribble, Black et al. 1990; Armstrong, Grimwood et al. 1998; Hiatt, Grace et al. 1999). These methods are relatively insensitive and more recent studies have utilised PCR based methodologies (Smyth, Smyth et al. 1995; Collinson, Nicholson et al. 1996; Punch, Syrmis et al. 2004; Olesen, Nielsen et al. 2006; Wat, Gelder et al. 2008). All these studies produced different results in terms of prevalence of respiratory viruses in CF. The differences can be due to different methodologies. There are also likely to be differences in the populations studied as the prognosis for CF has improved with each successive birth cohort.

The viruses implicated in causing respiratory symptoms in CF include *RSV, adenovirus, PIV (Types 1 to 4) , influenza A&B, rhinovirus* (Ramsey, Gore et al. 1989; Smyth, Smyth et al. 1995; Collinson, Nicholson et al. 1996; Wat, Gelder et al. 2008) and more recently *metapneumovirus* (Garcia, Hiatt et al. 2007). RSV represents 9-58% of all reported viral infection in CF, with the highest incidence in young children (Armstrong, Grimwood et al. 1998). It is possible that RSV precipitates in the initial infection by *P. aeruginosa* of the CF airway(Petersen, Hoiby et al. 1981), the proposed mechanism of which will be discussed later. A new subtype of human *rhinovirus* was recently identified, *rhinovirus C*, and was shown by de Almeida et al (de Almeida, Zerbinati et al. 2010) that it is significantly associated with respiratory exacerbations in children with CF (Odd ratio- 1.213). *Influenza A and B* take 12-27%, but in one small study, it comprised of 77% of positive samples (Hordvik, Konig et al. 1989). *PIV* are found in lower frequencies with only one study showing a detection rate of 43% from positive samples (Petersen, Hoiby et al. 1981). *Metapneumovirus* has recently been detected in nasopharyngeal aspirates taken from hospitalised children and infants with respiratory tract infections who had signs and symptoms similar to those of RSV infection (van den Hoogen, de Jong et al. 2001). This virus is also associated with lower respiratory tract infections in patients with CF (Garcia, Hiatt et al. 2007).

It is now nearly 30 years since Wang et al (Wang, Prober et al. 1984) described the relationship between respiratory viral infections and deterioration in clinical status in CF. In this 2 year prospective study (Wang, Prober et al. 1984), viruses were identified through repeated serology and nasal lavage for viral isolation in 49 patients with CF (mean age 13.7 years). Although the CF patients had more respiratory illnesses than sibling controls (3.7 versus 1.7/year), there were no differences in virus identification rates (1.7/year). The rate of proven virus infection was significantly correlated with the decline in lung functions, radiology score, and frequency and duration of hospitalisation.

More recent studies suggest no difference in the frequency of either upper respiratory tract illness (URTI) episodes (Hiatt, Grace et al. 1999) or proven respiratory viral infections (Ramsey, Gore et al. 1989) between children with CF and healthy controls, but children with CF have significantly more episodes of lower airway symptoms than controls (Ramsey, Gore et al. 1989; Hiatt, Grace et al. 1999). Ramsey et al (Ramsey, Gore et al. 1989) prospectively compared the incidence and effect of viral infections on pulmonary function and clinical scores in 15 school-age patients with CF aged between 5 to 21 years and their healthy siblings. Over a two-year period, samples were taken at regular two monthly intervals and during acute respiratory illnesses (ARI) for pharyngeal culture and serology for respiratory viruses. There was a total of 68 ARI episodes occurred in the patients with CF and in 19 episodes there was an associated virus identified. A total of 49 infective agents were identified either during ARIs or at routine testing in the patients with CF; 14 were identified on viral isolation (*rhinovirus* on 11 occasions), whilst 35 were isolated on seroconversion (*PIV* on 12, *RSV* on 9 and *M. pneumoniae* on 6 occasions). There was no significant difference in the rate of viral infections between the patients with CF and their sibling controls, as measured either by culture or serology. The rate of viral infections was higher in younger children (both CF and controls), and the rate of decline in pulmonary function was greater in the younger children with CF with more viral infections. At the time of an ARI, the virus isolation and seroconversion (fourfold increase in titres) rates were 8.8% and 19.1%, respectively in children with CF compared to 15.0% and 15.0% respectively for the non-affected siblings. In contrast the rates of virus isolation and seroconversion at routine 2 monthly visits were 5.6% and 16.2 % respectively for children with CF and 7.7% and 20.2% respectively for the healthy siblings.

Similarly Hiatt (Hiatt, Grace et al. 1999) assessed respiratory viral infections over three winters in 22 infants less than two years of age with CF (30 patient seasons), and 27 age matched controls (28 patient seasons). The average number of acute respiratory illness per winter was the same in the control and CF groups (5.0 versus 5.0). However, only 4 of the 28 control infants had lower respiratory tract symptoms in association with the respiratory tract illness, compared with 13 out of the 30 infants with CF (Odd ratio- 4.6; 95% confidence interval 1.3 and 16.5; p-value <0.05). 7 of the infants with CF cultured *RSV*, of whom 3 required hospitalisation. In contrast, none of the controls required hospitalisation. Pulmonary function measured by rapid chest compression technique was significantly reduced in the infants with CF after the winter months and was associated with two interactions; *RSV* infection with lower respiratory tract infection and male sex with lower respiratory tract infection.

From previous reports, two viral agents appear to have the greatest effect on respiratory status in CF, namely *RSV and influenza*, possibly because the uses of viral culture and serology have underestimated the effects of rhinovirus. In younger children, *RSV* is a major pathogen resulting in an increased rate of hospitalisation. Abman et al (Abman, Ogle et al. 1991) prospectively followed up 48 children with CF diagnosed through newborn screening and documented the effect of *RSV* infection. Eighteen of the infants were admitted into hospital a total of 30 times over a mean follow-up of 28 months (range 5-59). In seven of these infants *RSV* was isolated, and their clinical course was severe with 3 requiring mechanical ventilation and 5 necessitating chronic oxygen therapy. Over the next 2 years these infants had significantly more frequent respiratory symptoms and lower Brasfield chest radiograph (Brasfield, Hicks et al. 1979) scores than *non-RSV* infected counterparts. Brasfield scores air trapping on the lateral chest film, and linear markings, nodular cystic lesions, large lesions, and general severity on the posteroanterior chest film. Twenty five points represent a normal chest radiograph with lower scores indicating increasing disease severity.

In older children and adults with CF, *influenza* seems to have the greatest effect. Pribble et al (Pribble, Black et al. 1990) assessed acute pulmonary exacerbation isolates from 54 patients with CF. Over the year of the study, 80 exacerbations were identified, of which 21 episodes were associated with an identified viral agent (*influenza A*- 5 episodes; *influenza B*- 4 episodes; *RSV*- 3 episodes) with most agents identified on serology. Compared to other respiratory viruses, infection with *influenza* was associated with a more significant drop in pulmonary function (FEV_1 declined by 26% compared with 6%). There were also a higher proportion of patients with a greater than 20% drop in FEV_1 within the *influenza* infected cohort. A retrospective study in older patients with chronic *P. aeruginosa* infection reported an acute deterioration in clinical status in association with *influenza A* virus infection (Conway, Simmonds et al. 1992).

Over a 1-year period, Smyth et al (Smyth, Smyth et al. 1995) prospectively investigated 108 patients with CF (mean age of 7.9 years) using a combination of viral immunofluorescence, culture and seroconversion (fourfold increase in titres) to identify respiratory viruses. With the exception of *rhinovirus*, a seminested reverse transcriptase PCR technique was used. During the study, 76 subjects had 157 respiratory exacerbations (1.5 episodes/patient/year) and a viral agent was identified in 44 episodes, 25 of which were *rhinovirus* and an equal distribution of other viruses identified almost always on seroconversion. Identification of a respiratory virus during the course of the year was associated with a significantly greater decline in Shwachman score (Shwachman and Kulczycki 1958) and days of intravenous antibiotics use. The Shwachman scoring system is an objective measurement of the clinical status of cystic fibrosis patients. This score is based on clinical and radiological evaluation and represented a milestone in the history of CF. Patients with scores of 90 to 100 are classified as 'excellent', 80 to 89 as 'good', 70 to 79 as 'fair', and 50 to 69 reflects a 'poor' clinical status. In addition, those children in whom a non-rhinovirus was identified had a significantly greater decrease in FEV_1 over the year of the study.

Collinson et al (Collinson, Nicholson et al. 1996) followed 48 children with CF over a 15 month period using viral cultures for viral detection, with the exception of *picornaviruses* where PCR was used. 38 children completed the study and there were 147 symptomatic upper respiratory tract infections (2.7 episodes/child/year), with samples available for 119 episodes. *Picornaviruses* were identified in 51 (43%) of these episodes, of which 21 (18%) were *rhinoviruses*. In those children old enough to perform spirometry, there were significant reduction in both FVC and FEV_1 in association with URTIs, with little difference in severity of reduction whether a picornavirus was identified or not. Maximal mean drop in FEV_1 was 16.5%, at 1-4 days after onset of symptoms, but a deficit of 10.3% persisted at 21-24 days. Those with more URTIs appeared to have greater change in total Shwachman score (Shwachman and Kulczycki 1958) and Chrispin-Norman score (Chrispin and Norman 1974) over the study. Chrispin-Norman score (Chrispin and Norman 1974)is a standardized scoring system to assess the severity of CF lung disease on chest radiograph and to allow longitudinal follow-up. Six children isolated a *P.aeruginosa* for the first time during the study, 5 at the time of a URTI and only 1 was asymptomatic at the time of first isolation. However, the data from this study has to be handled with care as the term 'upper respiratory tract illness-URTI' did not necessarily imply a positive viral isolation.

Punch et al (Punch, Syrmis et al. 2004) used a multiplex reverse transcriptase PCR (RT-PCR) assay combined with an enzyme-linked amplicon hybridization assay (ELAHA) for the identification of seven common respiratory viruses in the sputum of 38 CF patients. 53 sputum samples were collected over 2 seasons and 12 (23%) samples from 12 patients were positive for a respiratory virus (4 for *influenza B*, 3 for *parainfluenza type 1*, 3 for *influenza A* and 2 for *RSV*). There were no statistical associations between virus status and demographics, clinical variables or isolation rates for *P. aeruginosa, S. aureus or A. fumigatus*.

Olesen and colleagues (Olesen, Nielsen et al. 2006) obtained sputum/laryngeal aspirates from children with CF over a 12 month period in outpatient clinics. They achieved a viral detection rate of 16%, with *rhinovirus* being the most prevalent virus. FEV_1 was significantly reduced during viral infection (-12.5%, p=0.048), with the exception of *rhinovirus* infection. The authors were not able to demonstrate a positive correlation between respiratory viruses and bacterial infections in their studied population as the type or frequency of bacterial infection during or after viral infections were not altered. They also concluded that clinical viral symptoms had a very poor predictive value (0.39) for a positive viral test.

Wat et al (Wat, Gelder et al. 2008) utilised 'real-time' Nucleic Acid Sequenced Based Amplification to examine the role of respiratory viruses in CF. They achieved the highest detection rate of 46% amongst all existing literature concerning respiratory viruses in the CF population during reported episodes of respiratory illness. The results compare favourably with previous studies and this may be that earlier studies relied heavily on repeated serological testing, either alone(Petersen, Hoiby et al. 1981) or in combination with viral isolation (Wang, Prober et al. 1984; Ramsey, Gore et al. 1989; Pribble, Black et al. 1990; Armstrong, Grimwood et al. 1998; Hiatt, Grace et al. 1999). They also achieved a viral detection rate of 18.3% from routine nasal samples and this is comparable to the seroconversion rate of 12.3% as reported by Wang et al(Wang, Prober et al. 1984). This value is similar to the seroconversion rate of 16.2% from asymptomatic samples achieved by Ramsey and colleagues(Ramsey, Gore et al. 1989). Amongst stable asthmatic children, Johnston et al (Johnston, Pattemore et al. 1995) found a viral detection rate of 12% by PCR. Therefore, a laboratory method with a higher sensitivity for viral detection used in this study has not increased the detection rate in asymptomatic samples, implying that the high detection rate of respiratory viruses during exacerbations reinforces their pathogenicity. The authors also demonstrated that *influenza A and B* viruses are major viruses in causing respiratory exacerbations in CF and both viruses are more commonly detected during pulmonary exacerbations. 22 of 88 (23%) viruses found in this study are *influenza viruses (A & B)*. The result is consistent with majority of the previous studies which showed that *influenza* virus represented between 12 to 27% of all viruses detected. In relation to *influenza* vaccination, the uptake rate was up to 70% during the 2003/4 season (Wat, Gelder et al. 2008) and the significance is that the *influenza* detection rate in this study could easily have been higher had the vaccination uptake rate in the study not been this high.

In 2009, a novel swine pandemic *influenza A virus (H1N1)* was identified. To date very little data exists regarding its impact on patients with CF. Nash et al (Nash, Whitmill et al. 2011) showed the symptoms of CF patients infected with H1N1 tend to be mild. There was no significant reduction in FEV_1 % predicted, FVC % predicted and body mass index regardless of whether the patients were positive or negative for *H1N1*. Colombo et al (Colombo, Battezzati et al. 2011) performed a multi-centre survey showed that diagnostic testing did not identify clinical characteristics specifically associated with *H1N1* infections. Similarly, they did not show a significant decline in lung function associated with this infection.

Experimental data on the effects of viral infections in CF are limited. Toll-like receptors (TLRs) have recently been identified as key mediators of the innate response and they recognise pathogens through detection of conserved microbial structures that are absent from the host. Kurt-Jones et al (Kurt-Jones, Popova et al. 2000) found that *RSV* persisted longer in the lungs of infected TLR4-deficient mice compared to normal mice. Haynes et al (Haynes, Moore et al. 2001) also demonstrated that TLR4-deficient mice when challenged with *RSV* exhibited impaired natural killer cell trafficking and impaired virus clearance compared to normal ones. Limited human studies have demonstrated the important role of TLRs in host response against many major groups of mammalian pathogens(Qureshi and Medzhitov 2003). The relationship between TLR and respiratory virus including *RSV* in humans will require further studies before it can be established.

Some studies have suggested a higher viral replication when there is an impairment of the innate host defence in CF. *Influenza* titres were significantly increased in a mouse model which were chronically infected with *P. aeruginosa* compared to control model (Seki, Higashiyama et al. 2004). Increased virus replication was also found after *PIV* infection of CF human airway epithelial cells, compared to controls (Zheng, De et al. 2003). One of the possible causes of increased virus replication and of virus persistence might be a reduced production of respiratory nitric oxide (NO), which is a vital part of innate antiviral defence mechanism (Zheng, Xu et al. 2004). Increased production of NO protects against viral infections. In CF patients, expression of the NO producing enzyme NO synthase type 2 (NOS2) is considerably reduced.

3. Detection of respiratory viruses

The principal laboratory methods of respiratory virus diagnosis rely on their detection in respiratory secretions and another important factor in respiratory viral diagnosis is to submit an appropriate sample for testing. Inappropriate specimen collection and transport account for the largest source of error in the accuracy of viral detection results (Nutting, Main et al. 1996). Nasal swabs, nasopharyngeal aspirates, nasal wash and sputum specimens are generally considered as the specimens of choice for the detection of respiratory viruses (Hall and Douglas 1975; Schmid, Kudesia et al. 1998; Covalciuc, Webb et al. 1999; Punch, Syrmis et al. 2004). Performing a nasopharyngeal aspirate or suction can be unpleasant and requires the use of a suction device by a trained individual, which makes it unattractive in widespread clinical applications. In contrast, the collection of a nasal swab is simple, painless and quick and it does not require special equipment and skilled personnel. A prospective study by Heikkinen et al showed that the sensitivity of nasal swabs was comparable to nasopharyngeal aspirates for the detection of all major respiratory viruses by tissue culture with the exception of RSV (Heikkinen, Marttila et al. 2002). In non-sputum producing patients with CF, it has been shown that throat swab is not inferior to nasopharyngeal suction in detecting pathogens (Taylor, Corey et al. 2006).

Molecular techniques have superseded many 'conventional' methods utilised for respiratory viral detection such as viral culture and serology analysis due to their rapid turn-around of results. Traditional virus culture and serology analysis may require 1 to 2 weeks before results are available and direct antigen detection can have variable sensitivity and specificity (Swierkosz, Erdman et al. 1995). Molecular assays also have particular advantages where the starting material available is acellular (swab) or where surveillance samples have a low copy number of the viral target. The rapid turn-over of results allowing diagnostic virology to have an impact on patient management, avoiding the inappropriate prescription of antibiotics and allowing the proper use of anti-virals. It may also play an important role in infection control in the hospital setting.

More recently, Virochip has been shown to be a pan-virus microarray platform that is capable of detection of known as well as novel viruses in a single assay simultaneously (Chiu, Rouskin et al. 2006). The Virochip is very much a research tool at present, and several issues must be addressed before it can be used on a routine basis for virus detection in the clinical setting. These issues include cost, accuracy, reproducibility, and sensitivity/specificity for virus detection in comparison with traditional laboratory techniques. In addition, the implication of novel viruses in the human respiratory tract is not yet defined.

4. Interaction between respiratory viruses and bacteria

In a 25 year retrospective review from the Danish CF clinic, the first isolation of *P. aeruginosa* was most likely between October and March (Johansen and Hoiby 1992) coinciding with the peak of the *RSV* season. These findings must be interpreted with caution by the design of the study, as there are a number of other possible agents that would broadly fit the *RSV* season, most notably *influenza, rhinovirus* and *metapneumovirus*.

An increase in immunoglobulin A (IgA) antibodies to the O-antigen of *P. aeruginosa* is noted in 62% of viral infections (Przyklenk, Bauernfeind et al. 1988). This suggests a possible 'microbial synergism' between bacterial infections and infections with respiratory viruses in CF.

The first bacterial isolation of a given organism in CF has also been shown to often follow a viral infection. In the 17 month prospective study reported by Collinson et al (Collinson, Nicholson et al. 1996), five of the six first isolations of *P. aeruginosa* were made during the symptomatic phase of an upper respiratory tract infection or three weeks thereafter. In contrast only one of the six initial infections with *P. aeruginosa* was identified during the asymptomatic period. Similarly, *H. influenzae* was recovered for the first time from 3 children within 3 weeks of an upper respiratory tract infection and the one new *S. aureus* infection was identified immediately following a viral infection.

Armstrong and colleagues have reported that 50% of CF respiratory exacerbations requiring hospitalisation are associated with isolation of a respiratory virus (Armstrong, Grimwood et al. 1998). In their prospective study of repeated bronchoalveolar lavage (BAL) in infants over a 5 year period, a respiratory virus was identified in 52% of infants hospitalised for a respiratory exacerbation, most commonly *RSV*. 11 of the 31 hospitalised infants (35%) acquired *P. aeruginosa* in the subsequent 12-60 month follow up, compared to 3 of 49 (6%) non-hospitalised infants (Relative risk 5.8).

Respiratory viruses can disrupt the airway epithelium and precipitate bacterial adherence. *Influenza A* infection has been shown to cause epithelial shedding to basement membrane with submucosal oedema and neutrophil infiltrate (Walsh, Dietlein et al. 1961), while both influenza and adenovirus have a cytopathic effect on cultured nasal epithelium leading to destruction of the cell monolayer (Winther, Gwaltney et al. 1990). This epithelial damage results in an increase in the permeability of the mucosal layer (Igarashi, Skoner et al. 1993; Ohrui, Yamaya et al. 1998) and possibly facilitating bacterial adherence. Bacteria can also utilise viral glycoproteins and other virus induced receptors on host cell membrane as bacterial receptors in order to adhere to virus infected cells (Sanford, Shelokov et al. 1978; Raza, Essery et al. 1999).

Kim et al (Kim, Battaile et al. 2008) found that invariant natural killer T cells induce a type of macrophage activation driving the secretion of interleukin-13 leading to the production of globlet cell metaplasia and airway hyperactivity following infection with Sendai virus. The term 'invariant' stems from the fact that all invariant natural killer T cells in humans and mice use a unique T cell receptor that is essential for interaction with CD1d. CD1d molecules present lipid antigens to T lymphocytes rather than peptide antigens as in the case of major histocompatibility-complex (MHC) class I and II molecules. Historically, MHC class II dependent CD4 and T lymphocytes, through their response to stimulation by environmental allergens, are keys to the pathogenesis of human asthma. The findings by the authors lead to the notion of the use of anti-interleukin-13 therapy as a potential therapy in patients.

Viral infections might predispose to secondary bacterial infections by impairing mucociliary function and triggering host inflammatory receptors (Wilson and Cole 1988; Murphy and Sethi 1992). This phenomenon has been demonstrated both in vivo and in vitro (Jiang, Nagata et al. 1999; White, Gompertz et al. 2003). Avadhanula et al (Avadhanula, Rodriguez et al. 2006) showed that different respiratory viruses use different mechanisms to enhance the adherence of bacteria to respiratory epithelial cells. In particular *RSV* and *PIV type 3* upregulate intercellular adhesion molecule-1 (ICAM-1), carcinoembryonic adhesion molecule 1 (CEACAM1) and platelet activating factor receptor (PAFr) but not mucin on the surfaces of A549, BEAS-2B and NHBE but not SAE cell lines. Much of the increased bacterial adhesion following *RSV* infection could be blocked by antibodies directed against these receptors. A549 and BEAS-2B are transformed cell lines derived from type II alveolar and normal bronchial cells, respectively. NHBE and SAE cells and primary epithelial cells obtained from bronchi and distal bronchial tree and are likely to include a heterogeneous population of cells.

Mechanisms independent of the expression of conventional receptors for bacteria, such as binding to viral proteins, could be responsible for enhanced adhesion (Hament, Kimpen et al. 1999). Immunofluorescence microscopy demonstrates that bacteria binding to *RSV* infected A549 cells adhere not only to these cells expressing viral antigens but also to uninfected epithelial cells. These data suggest that the ability to augment bacterial adhesion may result from a factor served by infected cells that exert a paracrine effect on adjacent epithelium. Cytokines or other inflammatory molecules are potential good candidates for such a mediator.

Rhinovirus has been shown to potentiate bacterial infections by inhibiting the secretion of TNF alpha and interleukin-8 by macrophages in vitro following co-infection with gram negative bacterial products, lipopolysaccharide (LPS), and gram positive bacterial products, lipoteichoic acid (LTA) (Oliver, Lim et al. 2008). This rhinovirus dependent impairment of the macrophage immune response was not mediated by autocrine production of the anti-inflammatory cytokines interleukin-10 and PGE2, or by downregulation of the cell surface receptor for LTA and LPS. In addition, the authors also show that rhinovirus inhibit the phagocytosis of bacterial products by macrophages. These findings support the notion that *rhinovirus* exposure resulted in a reduced ability to innate and adaptive immune responses against bacterial products, hence promoting the occurrence of bacterial and viral co-infections.

The lower respiratory tract is protected by local mucociliary mechanisms that involve the integration of the ciliated epithelium, periciliary fluid and mucus. Mucus acts as a physical and chemical barrier onto which particles and organisms adhere. Cilia lining the respiratory tract propel the overlying mucus to the oropharynx where it is either swallowed or expectorated. *Influenza* viral infection has been shown to precipitate the loss of cilial beat, and shedding of the columnar epithelial cells generally within 48 hours of infection (Thompson, Barclay et al. 2006). Pittet et al (Pittet, Hall-Stoodley et al.) showed that a prior *influenza* infection of tracheal cells in vivo does not increase the initial number of *pneumococci* found during the first hour of infection, but it does significantly reduce mucociliary velocity, and thereby reduces *pneumococcal* clearance during the first 2 hours after *pneumococcal* infection at both 3 and 6 days after an *influenza* infection. The defects in *pneumococcal* clearance were greatest at 6 days after *influenza* infection. Changes to the tracheal epithelium induced by *influenza* virus may increase susceptibility to a secondary *S. pneumoniae* infection by increasing *pneumococcal* adherence to the tracheal epithelium and/or decreasing the clearance of *S. pneumoniae* via the mucociliary escalator of the trachea, and thus increasing the risk of secondary bacterial infection.

De Vrankrijker et al (de Vrankrijker, Wolfs et al. 2009) showed that mice that were co-infected with *RSV* and *P. aeruginosa* had a 2,000 times higher colony-forming units (CFU) counts of Pseudomonas aeruginosa in the lung homogenates compared to mice that were infected with *P. aeruginosa* alone. Co-infected mice also had more severe lung function changes. These results suggest that *RSV* can facilitate the initiation of acute *P. aeruginosa* infection.

Another study also showed that *H. influenzae* and *S. pneumoniae* bind to both free *RSV* virions and epithelial cells transfected with cell membrane-bound G protein, but not to secreted G protein. Pre-incubation with specific anti-G antibody significantly reduce bacterial adhesion to G protein-transfected cells (Avadhanula, Wang et al. 2007).

Stark et al (Stark, Stark et al. 2006) showed that mice that were exposed to *RSV* had significantly decreased *S. pneumonia, S. aureus* or *P. aeruginosa* clearance 1 to 7 days after *RSV* exposure. Mice that were exposed to both *RSV* and bacteria had a higher production of neutrophil-induced peroxide but less production of myeloperoxidase compared to mice that were exposed to *S. pneumoniae* alone. This suggests that functional changes in the recruited neutrophils may contribute to the decreased bacterial clearance.

More recently, Chattoraj et al (Chattoraj, Ganesan et al., 2011) demonstrated that acute infection of primary CF airway epithelial cells with rhinovirus liberates planktonic bacteria from biofilm. Superinfection with *rhinovirus* stimulates robust chemokine responses from CF airway epithelial cells that were pretreated with mucoid *P. aeruginosa*. The authors also showed that these chemokine responses lead to a liberation of bacteria from mucoid *P. aeruginosa* biofilm and transmigration of planktonic bacteria from the apical to the basolateral surface of mucociliary-differentiated CF airway epithelial cells. Planktonic bacteria, which are more proinflammatory than their biofilm counterparts, stimulate increased chemokine responses in CF airway epithelial cells which, in turn, may contribute to the pathogenesis of CF exacerbations and subsequent prolonged intravenous antibiotic use and hospitalisation.

Taken together, these findings suggest that respiratory viruses may lead to epithelial disruption, increased or decreased cytokine production, neutrophil influx, inhibition of macrophage phagocytosis, destruction of mucociliary escalator, increased cytokine production, and increased neutrophil induced peroxide release, indirectly facilitating bacterial infection of the airway.

5. Prevention and treatment for respiratory viruses

The existence of diverse viral serotypes in causing infection has made vaccine preparation very difficult. Frequent mutations of viral proteins of RNA viruses (for example genetic drift and shift of *influenza*) have further hampered the prevention of the illness.

Influenza associated death is between 13,000 to 20,000 per year in the winter months in the UK (Fleming 1996), though some of the deaths may be attributed to *RSV*. *Influenza* vaccines are the only commercially available vaccines against common respiratory viruses. They have been used since mid 1940s and they now have an established role in prevention of *influenza A and B* infections. Inactivated *influenza* vaccine is effective even in young children including those younger than 2 years (Heinonen, Silvennoinen et al. 2010). The waning of vaccine-induced immunity over time requires annual re-immunisation even if the vaccine antigens are unchanged.

Recent vaccines contain antigens of two *influenza A* subtypes, strains of the currently circulating *H3N2 and H1N1 (Swine flu)* subtypes, and one *influenza B* virus. The current recommendation for *influenza* vaccination in the UK is to offer it to those over the age of 65, those with chronic heart, respiratory (including CF) or renal diseases and those who are diabetic or immunosuppressed.

Wat et al (Wat, Gelder et al. 2008) recently showed that *influenza* vaccination provides protection against *influenza* acquisition in patients with CF, with 1 of 41 patients vaccinated had a positive nasal swab for influenza compared to 4 of the 22 non-vaccinated patients (p=0.046). Although *influenza* vaccination does not appear to have any impact on respiratory exacerbation rates, it does have a role in preventing live infections. In this study, respiratory exacerbation rates in the preceding 10 months before the study between the vaccinated and non-vaccinated groups were similar, indicating that these were unlikely to be the reasons influencing the decision on immunisation. The decision may be down to a combination of patient/ parent education, social background, awareness of vaccination and accessibility of vaccination.

Due to the lack of randomised controlled studies looking at the efficacy of *influenza* vaccine in CF, the Cochrane review recommends clinicians to make their own judgements on the benefits and risks of this therapy in this cohort of patients (Dharmaraj and Smyth 2009). In addition to vaccine, neuraminidase inhibitors have been shown to have a role in preventing *influenza A and B* infections (Harper, Bradley et al. 2009).

Rhinovirus has more than 100 serotypes; it is unlikely that a unifying vaccine will be developed. VP4, one of the nonenveloped capsids, is highly conserved among all of the rhinoviruses; anti-VP4 antibodies have recently been generated and been shown to have the potential for future vaccine development(Katpally, Fu et al. 2009).

The development of an *RSV* vaccine has been hampered by the experience with formalin-inactivated whole *RSV* vaccine in the 1960s, as it caused 80% of *RSV* vaccinees to become hospitalised compared with 5% of controls, as well as two fatalities (Kim, Canchola et al. 1969). Current major research work has focused on a prophylaxis using a humanised mouse monoclonal antibody, Palizivumab. In patients with CF, monthly Palizivumab injection significantly reduce the hospitalisation rate for acute respiratory illness during the *RSV* season compared to those who were not immunised (p<0.05). The former group also had fewer hospital days for acute respiratory illness (Giebels, Marcotte et al. 2008).

There is currently no licensed *PIV* vaccine to date. The formalin-inactivated vaccine generated in the 1960s was not able to prevent *PIV* infection and was soon abandoned. Recently, recombinant bovine *PIV type 3* and human *PIV type 3* attenuated vaccines are being evaluated in animal models as vectors for the delivery of other viral antigens such as *RSV*-G and *RSV*-F proteins. This bivalent vaccine combination provides high level of resistance to challenges with *PIV type 3* and *RSV* in animal models (Schmidt, McAuliffe et al. 2001).

The conventional methods of vaccination are via the intramuscular and subcutaneous routes. Mucosal immunisation has recently been explored as it represents an attractive manner of delivering vaccines. It is fast, simple, non-invasive and can be carried out by unskilled individuals. The use of mucosal vaccination seems logical in that most of respiratory viral infections initially start at the mucosal sites and therefore inducing local immunity.

So far, there has been inconclusive evidence to support the use of vitamin C and extracts of the plant Echinacea in common cold prevention. Daily supplementation with large doses of vitamin C does not seem to prevent common colds, however there seems to be a modest (8 to 9%) reduction in the number of symptom days in individuals with established cold symptoms, with larger doses having greater effect (Douglas, Chalker et al. 2000). In vitro studies have shown that Echinacea can activate macrophages, increase phagocytosis, enhance cytokine production (Sharma, Arnason et al. 2006), and natural killer cell activity, and improve lymphocyte and monocyte cell counts (Goel, Lovlin et al. 2005). Current data is available in the adult population and has reported positive findings both in the treatment and prevention of upper respiratory tract infection. However, variations in the design of the clinical trial and in Echinacea preparations have to be taken into account (Giles, Palat et al. 2000).

Zinc has been shown to possess anti-viral properties in vitro and different preparations of zinc have been proposed for the treatment of common cold. Postulated mechanisms in the common cold include interfering with rhinovirus protein cleavage or capsid binding to ICAM-1 in nasal epithelium (Novick, Godfrey et al. 1996). Zinc lozenges appeared to have positive effects on adults but negative effects on children in terms of duration and severity of common cold symptoms (Macknin, Piedmonte et al. 1998; Marshall 2000). Higher doses were found to have a greater impact in reduction of symptom duration and reduced symptom severity (Godfrey, Conant Sloane et al. 1992; Mossad, Macknin et al. 1996). Zinc nasal spray appears to reduce the total symptom score but has no effect on the duration of common cold (Belongia, Berg et al. 2001). Irritation by nasal sprays limits their use; they also seem to have lower concentrations in the nasopharynx (Godfrey 1988).

Amantadine has been the conventional anti-viral against *influenza*. However it is strain specific as it is only effective against *influenza A* and has common side-effects such as insomnia, poor concentration and irritability. It is now largely being replaced by neuraminidase inhibitors such as Zanamivir and Oseltamivir which are licensed for the treatment of *influenza A and B*, including *avian flu H5N1* and *swine flu H1N1*. However, Amantadine still has a role in dealing with Oseltamivir resistant H1N1 virus. In children and adults, early initiation of neuraminidase inhibitors within 48 hours of the onset of symptoms can reduce the duration of flu-like symptoms by 0.5 to 2.5 days (Shun-Shin, Thompson et al. 2009). Early use of these medications can also reduce development of complications such as pneumonia (Yu, Liao et al. 2010). The 2009 pandemic *H1N1* virus remains susceptible to neuraminidase inhibitors, and Oseltamivir has been used extensively for treatment related to this viral infection. Resistance to Oseltamivir has been reported with *H1N1* viral infection but this is mainly restricted to immunocompromised individuals (Bautista, Chotpitayasunondh et al. 2010). Zanamivir has a poor oral bioavailability, and intranasal application has been shown to be effective in treating experimental *influenza* infection with the reduction in symptoms caused, virus shedding and development of otitis media (Hayden, Treanor et al. 1996). Intravenous use of Peramivir or Zanamivir could be lifesaving in critically ill patients with *influenza* infection (Birnkrant and Cox 2009; Harter, Zimmermann et al. 2010).

Ribavarin, a synthetic guanosine nucleoside that has a broad spectrum of antiviral activity, has been used for treatment of infections related to *RSV, metapneumovirus, and parainfluenza and influenza viruses* (Yin, Brust et al. 2009). Potential benefits of ribavarin therapy include the inhibition of RSV-specific IgE production in nasal secretions, which has been associated with the development of hypoxaemia and wheezing (Rosner, Welliver et al. 1987) and it has improved pulmonary functions (Hiatt 1990). Controlled studies also show that the use of ribavarin is effective in reducing the clinical severity score, duration of mechanical ventilation, supplemental oxygen use and days of hospitalisation (Smith, Frankel et al. 1991). Aerosolised ribavarin has been used for the treatment of *RSV* related bronchiolitis and pneumonia. Intravenous formulation could be used for treatment of severe pneumonia, caused by infection *RSV, metapneumovirus, or parainfluenza virus*, on the basis of experience in immunocompromised patients (Hopkins, McNeil et al. 2008). Bonney et al has shown that *metapneumovirus* can be successfully treated with a combination of intravenous ribavarin and immunoglobulin (Bonney, Razali et al. 2009).

Although *rhinovirus* is the major cause of colds, its vast amount of serotypes has made development of anti-virals against it problematic. 90% of *rhinovirus* serotypes gain entry into epithelial cells using ICAM-1 cellular receptors and blockade of these receptors in experimental studies have shown reduced infection severity (Turner, Wecker et al. 1999), but further study is required before this treatment option becomes widely available. Macrolide antibiotics, Bafilomycin A1 and Erythromycin have been shown to inhibit ICAM-1 epithelial expression and hypothesis about their potential as anti-inflammatory agents have yet to be definitive, as clinical proof is either negative or inconclusive (Suzuki, Yamaya et al. 2002).

Recently, an anti-rhinoviral agent known as Plecoranil, which acts by inhibiting the uncoating of Picornaviruses (Ledford, Patel et al. 2004), the RV 3C protease inhibitor, Ruprintrivir(Hayden, Turner et al. 2003) and soluble ICAM-1, Tremacamra(Turner, Wecker et al. 1999) have shown promising results in early-stage clinical trials, but each of these medications was derailed by a combination of cost, pharmacokinetics, toxicity, drug interactions, and limited efficacy (Turner 2005).

6. Conclusion

With the available knowledge regarding the impact of respiratory viruses in the exacerbation of CF, screening for respiratory viruses during pulmonary exacerbations should be implemented as part of routine clinical assessment. This assessment should include obtaining specimens from the respiratory tract and using molecular viral detection methods to reach a rapid diagnosis. The identification of respiratory viruses may allow appropriate anti-virals to be used.

With gene therapy still undergoing further research with regards to its validity and specificity, gaining further understanding in the pathogenesis of virus induced respiratory exacerbations in CF may allow the development of new therapeutic techniques. If viral infection does predispose to bacterial infection, then influencing the interaction between viruses and bacteria could be a next pathway to diminish respiratory morbidity in patients with CF. The development of novel therapies will be exciting and this may further prolong the lifespan of patients with CF and more importantly improve their quality of life.

In light of the above, future research in respiratory viruses in CF is urgently required to address a number of important questions: 1) What is the optimal way for viral sampling? 2) What is the most efficient and rapid method to detect a range of respiratory viruses? 3) How do respiratory viruses influence bacterial behaviour in chronically infected airways? 4) What is the efficacy of *influenza* vaccination in CF? 5) What are the roles of anti-virals in CF?

Further understanding in the pathogenesis of viral infection in CF would be beneficial as this may provide insight to the above unresolved mysteries. At the moment it appears that *influenza* vaccination remains the mainstay of management of viral infections in CF.

7. References

Aaron, S. D., K. Ramotar, et al. (2004). "Adult cystic fibrosis exacerbations and new strains of Pseudomonas aeruginosa." *Am J Respir Crit Care Med* 169(7): 811-5.

Abman, S. H., J. W. Ogle, et al. (1991). "Early bacteriologic, immunologic, and clinical courses of young infants with cystic fibrosis identified by neonatal screening." *J Pediatr* 119(2): 211-7.

Armstrong, D., K. Grimwood, et al. (1998). "Severe viral respiratory infections in infants with cystic fibrosis." *Pediatr Pulmonol* 26(6): 371-9.

Avadhanula, V., C. A. Rodriguez, et al. (2006). "Respiratory viruses augment the adhesion of bacterial pathogens to respiratory epithelium in a viral species- and cell type-dependent manner." *J Virol* 80(4): 1629-36.

Avadhanula, V., Y. Wang, et al. (2007). "Nontypeable Haemophilus influenzae and Streptococcus pneumoniae bind respiratory syncytial virus glycoprotein." *J Med Microbiol* 56(Pt 9): 1133-7.

Barasch, J. and Q. al-Awqati (1993). "Defective acidification of the biosynthetic pathway in cystic fibrosis." *J Cell Sci Suppl* 17: 229-33.

Bautista, E., T. Chotpitayasunondh, et al. (2010). "Clinical aspects of pandemic 2009 influenza A (H1N1) virus infection." *N Engl J Med* 362(18): 1708-19.

Belongia, E. A., R. Berg, et al. (2001). "A randomized trial of zinc nasal spray for the treatment of upper respiratory illness in adults." *Am J Med* 111(2): 103-8.

Birnkrant, D. and E. Cox (2009). "The Emergency Use Authorization of peramivir for treatment of 2009 H1N1 influenza." *N Engl J Med* 361(23): 2204-7.

Bonney, D., H. Razali, et al. (2009). "Successful treatment of human metapneumovirus pneumonia using combination therapy with intravenous ribavirin and immune globulin." *Br J Haematol* 145(5): 667-9.

Brasfield, D., G. Hicks, et al. (1979). "The chest roentgenogram in cystic fibrosis: a new scoring system." *Pediatrics* 63(1): 24-9.

Chattoraj, S. S., S. Ganesan, et al. (2011) "Rhinovirus infection liberates planktonic bacteria from biofilm and increases chemokine responses in cystic fibrosis airway epithelial cells." *Thorax* 66(4): 333-9.

Chiu, C. Y., S. Rouskin, et al. (2006). "Microarray detection of human parainfluenzavirus 4 infection associated with respiratory failure in an immunocompetent adult." *Clin Infect Dis* 43(8): e71-6.

Chrispin, A. R. and A. P. Norman (1974). "The systematic evaluation of the chest radiograph in cystic fibrosis." *Pediatr Radiol* 2(2): 101-5.

Collinson, J., K. G. Nicholson, et al. (1996). "Effects of upper respiratory tract infections in patients with cystic fibrosis." *Thorax* 51(11): 1115-22.

Colombo, C., P. M. Battezzati, et al. (2011). "Influenza A/H1N1 in patients with cystic fibrosis in Italy: a multicentre cohort study." *Thorax* 66(3): 260-1.

Conway, S. P., E. J. Simmonds, et al. (1992). "Acute severe deterioration in cystic fibrosis associated with influenza A virus infection." *Thorax* 47(2): 112-4.

Covalciuc, K. A., K. H. Webb, et al. (1999). "Comparison of four clinical specimen types for detection of influenza A and B viruses by optical immunoassay (FLU OIA test) and cell culture methods." *J Clin Microbiol* 37(12): 3971-4.

de Almeida, M. B., R. M. Zerbinati, et al. (2010). "Rhinovirus C and respiratory exacerbations in children with cystic fibrosis." *Emerg Infect Dis* 16(6): 996-9.

de Vrankrijker, A. M., T. F. Wolfs, et al. (2009). "Respiratory syncytial virus infection facilitates acute colonization of Pseudomonas aeruginosa in mice." *J Med Virol* 81(12): 2096-103.

Dharmaraj, P. and R. L. Smyth (2009). "Vaccines for preventing influenza in people with cystic fibrosis." *Cochrane Database Syst Rev*(4): CD001753.

Dodge, J. A., S. Morison, et al. (1993). "Cystic fibrosis in the United Kingdom, 1968-1988: incidence, population and survival." *Paediatr Perinat Epidemiol* 7(2): 157-66.

Douglas, R. M., E. B. Chalker, et al. (2000). "Vitamin C for preventing and treating the common cold." *Cochrane Database Syst Rev*(2): CD000980.

Elborn, J. S., D. J. Shale, et al. (1991). "Cystic fibrosis: current survival and population estimates to the year 2000." *Thorax* 46(12): 881-5.

Fleming, D. M. (1996). "The impact of three influenza epidemics on primary care in England and Wales." *Pharmacoeconomics* 9 Suppl 3: 38-45; discussion 50-3.

Garcia, D. F., P. W. Hiatt, et al. (2007). "Human metapneumovirus and respiratory syncytial virus infections in older children with cystic fibrosis." *Pediatr Pulmonol* 42(1): 66-74.

Giebels, K., J. E. Marcotte, et al. (2008). "Prophylaxis against respiratory syncytial virus in young children with cystic fibrosis." *Pediatr Pulmonol* 43(2): 169-74.

Giles, J. T., C. T. Palat, 3rd, et al. (2000). "Evaluation of echinacea for treatment of the common cold." *Pharmacotherapy* 20(6): 690-7.

Godfrey, J. C. (1988). "Zinc for the common cold." *Antimicrob Agents Chemother* 32(4): 605-6.

Godfrey, J. C., B. Conant Sloane, et al. (1992). "Zinc gluconate and the common cold: a controlled clinical study." *J Int Med Res* 20(3): 234-46.

Goel, V., R. Lovlin, et al. (2005). "A proprietary extract from the echinacea plant (Echinacea purpurea) enhances systemic immune response during a common cold." *Phytother Res* 19(8): 689-94.

Goss, C. H. and J. L. Burns (2007). "Exacerbations in cystic fibrosis. 1: Epidemiology and pathogenesis." *Thorax* 62(4): 360-7.

Hall, C. B. and R. G. Douglas, Jr. (1975). "Clinically useful method for the isolation of respiratory syncytial virus." *J Infect Dis* 131(1): 1-5.

Hament, J. M., J. L. Kimpen, et al. (1999). "Respiratory viral infection predisposing for bacterial disease: a concise review." *FEMS Immunol Med Microbiol* 26(3-4): 189-95.

Harper, S. A., J. S. Bradley, et al. (2009). "Seasonal influenza in adults and children--diagnosis, treatment, chemoprophylaxis, and institutional outbreak management: clinical practice guidelines of the Infectious Diseases Society of America." *Clin Infect Dis* 48(8): 1003-32.

Harter, G., O. Zimmermann, et al. (2010). "Intravenous zanamivir for patients with pneumonitis due to pandemic (H1N1) 2009 influenza virus." *Clin Infect Dis* 50(9): 1249-51.

Hayden, F. G., J. J. Treanor, et al. (1996). "Safety and efficacy of the neuraminidase inhibitor GG167 in experimental human influenza." *Jama* 275(4): 295-9.

Hayden, F. G., R. B. Turner, et al. (2003). "Phase II, randomized, double-blind, placebo-controlled studies of ruprintrivir nasal spray 2-percent suspension for prevention and treatment of experimentally induced rhinovirus colds in healthy volunteers." *Antimicrob Agents Chemother* 47(12): 3907-16.

Haynes, L. M., D. D. Moore, et al. (2001). "Involvement of toll-like receptor 4 in innate immunity to respiratory syncytial virus." *J Virol* 75(22): 10730-7.

Heikkinen, T., J. Marttila, et al. (2002). "Nasal swab versus nasopharyngeal aspirate for isolation of respiratory viruses." *J Clin Microbiol* 40(11): 4337-9.

Heinonen, S., H. Silvennoinen, et al. (2010). "Effectiveness of inactivated influenza vaccine in children aged 9 months to 3 years: an observational cohort study." *Lancet Infect Dis* 11(1): 23-9.

Hiatt, P. T., D Laber, L (1990). "Pulmonary function (PF) following treatment with ribavarin in infants hospitalised with RSV bronchiolitis." *Am Rev Respir Dis* 141: A624.

Hiatt, P. W., S. C. Grace, et al. (1999). "Effects of viral lower respiratory tract infection on lung function in infants with cystic fibrosis." *Pediatrics* 103(3): 619-26.

Hopkins, P., K. McNeil, et al. (2008). "Human metapneumovirus in lung transplant recipients and comparison to respiratory syncytial virus." *Am J Respir Crit Care Med* 178(8): 876-81.

Hordvik, N. L., P. Konig, et al. (1989). "Effects of acute viral respiratory tract infections in patients with cystic fibrosis." *Pediatr Pulmonol* 7(4): 217-22.

http://genet.sickkids.on.ca/cgi-bin/WebObjects/MUTATION.

Igarashi, Y., D. P. Skoner, et al. (1993). "Analysis of nasal secretions during experimental rhinovirus upper respiratory infections." *J Allergy Clin Immunol* 92(5): 722-31.

Jiang, Z., N. Nagata, et al. (1999). "Fimbria-mediated enhanced attachment of nontypeable Haemophilus influenzae to respiratory syncytial virus-infected respiratory epithelial cells." *Infect Immun* 67(1): 187-92.

Johansen, H. K. and N. Hoiby (1992). "Seasonal onset of initial colonisation and chronic infection with Pseudomonas aeruginosa in patients with cystic fibrosis in Denmark." *Thorax* 47(2): 109-11.

Johnston, S. L., P. K. Pattemore, et al. (1995). "Community study of role of viral infections in exacerbations of asthma in 9-11 year old children." *Bmj* 310(6989): 1225-9.

Katpally, U., T. M. Fu, et al. (2009). "Antibodies to the buried N terminus of rhinovirus VP4 exhibit cross-serotypic neutralization." *J Virol* 83(14): 7040-8.

Kim, E. Y., J. T. Battaile, et al. (2008). "Persistent activation of an innate immune response translates respiratory viral infection into chronic lung disease." *Nat Med* 14(6): 633-40.

Kim, H. W., J. G. Canchola, et al. (1969). "Respiratory syncytial virus disease in infants despite prior administration of antigenic inactivated vaccine." *Am J Epidemiol* 89(4): 422-34.

Kurt-Jones, E. A., L. Popova, et al. (2000). "Pattern recognition receptors TLR4 and CD14 mediate response to respiratory syncytial virus." *Nat Immunol* 1(5): 398-401.

Ledford, R. M., N. R. Patel, et al. (2004). "VP1 sequencing of all human rhinovirus serotypes: insights into genus phylogeny and susceptibility to antiviral capsid-binding compounds." *J Virol* 78(7): 3663-74.

Macknin, M. L., M. Piedmonte, et al. (1998). "Zinc gluconate lozenges for treating the common cold in children: a randomized controlled trial." *Jama* 279(24): 1962-7.

Marshall, I. (2000). "Zinc for the common cold." *Cochrane Database Syst Rev*(2): CD001364.

Mearns, M. (1993). Cystic fibrosis: the first 50 years: a review of the clinical problems anf theit management. *Cystic Fibrosis Current Topics*. J. A. Dodge, D. J. H. Brock and J. H. Widdicombe, John Wiley and Sons Ltd. 1.

Mossad, S. B., M. L. Macknin, et al. (1996). "Zinc gluconate lozenges for treating the common cold. A randomized, double-blind, placebo-controlled study." *Ann Intern Med* 125(2): 81-8.

Murphy, T. F. and S. Sethi (1992). "Bacterial infection in chronic obstructive pulmonary disease." *Am Rev Respir Dis* 146(4): 1067-83.

Nash, E. F., R. Whitmill, et al. (2011). "Clinical outcomes of pandemic (H1N1) 2009 influenza (swine flu) in adults with cystic fibrosis." *Thorax* 66(3): 259.

Nixon, G. M., D. S. Armstrong, et al. (2001). "Clinical outcome after early Pseudomonas aeruginosa infection in cystic fibrosis." *J Pediatr* 138(5): 699-704.

Novick, S. G., J. C. Godfrey, et al. (1996). "How does zinc modify the common cold? Clinical observations and implications regarding mechanisms of action." *Med Hypotheses* 46(3): 295-302.

Nutting, P. A., D. S. Main, et al. (1996). "Toward optimal laboratory use. Problems in laboratory testing in primary care." *Jama* 275(8): 635-9.

Ohrui, T., M. Yamaya, et al. (1998). "Effects of rhinovirus infection on hydrogen peroxide-induced alterations of barrier function in the cultured human tracheal epithelium." *Am J Respir Crit Care Med* 158(1): 241-8.

Olesen, H. V., L. P. Nielsen, et al. (2006). "Viral and atypical bacterial infections in the outpatient pediatric cystic fibrosis clinic." *Pediatr Pulmonol* 41(12): 1197-204.

Oliver, B. G., S. Lim, et al. (2008). "Rhinovirus exposure impairs immune responses to bacterial products in human alveolar macrophages." *Thorax* 63(6): 519-25.

Oppenheimer, E. H. and J. R. Esterly (1975). "Pathology of cystic fibrosis review of the literature and comparison with 146 autopsied cases." *Perspect Pediatr Pathol* 2: 241-78.

Ortiz, J. R., K. M. Neuzil, et al. (2010). "Influenza-associated cystic fibrosis pulmonary exacerbations." *Chest* 137(4): 852-60.

Petersen, N. T., N. Hoiby, et al. (1981). "Respiratory infections in cystic fibrosis patients caused by virus, chlamydia and mycoplasma--possible synergism with Pseudomonas aeruginosa." *Acta Paediatr Scand* 70(5): 623-8.

Pittet, L. A., L. Hall-Stoodley, et al. "Influenza virus infection decreases tracheal mucociliary velocity and clearance of Streptococcus pneumoniae." *Am J Respir Cell Mol Biol* 42(4): 450-60.

Pribble, C. G., P. G. Black, et al. (1990). "Clinical manifestations of exacerbations of cystic fibrosis associated with nonbacterial infections." *J Pediatr* 117(2 Pt 1): 200-4.

Przyklenk, B., A. Bauernfeind, et al. (1988). "Viral infections in the respiratory tract in patients with cystic fibrosis." *Serodign Immunother Infect Dis*(2): 217-25.

Punch, G., M. W. Syrmis, et al. (2004). "Method for detection of respiratory viruses in the sputa of patients with cystic fibrosis." *Eur J Clin Microbiol Infect Dis.*

Qureshi, S. T. and R. Medzhitov (2003). "Toll-like receptors and their role in experimental models of microbial infection." *Genes Immun* 4(2): 87-94.

Rajan, S. and L. Saiman (2002). "Pulmonary infections in patients with cystic fibrosis." *Semin Respir Infect* 17(1): 47-56.

Ramsey, B. W., E. J. Gore, et al. (1989). "The effect of respiratory viral infections on patients with cystic fibrosis." *Am J Dis Child* 143(6): 662-8.

Raza, M. W., S. D. Essery, et al. (1999). "Infection with respiratory syncytial virus and water-soluble components of cigarette smoke alter production of tumour necrosis factor alpha and nitric oxide by human blood monocytes." *FEMS Immunol Med Microbiol* 24(4): 387-94.

Riordan, J. R., J. M. Rommens, et al. (1989). "Identification of the cystic fibrosis gene: cloning and characterization of complementary DNA." *Science* 245(4922): 1066-73.

Rosner, I. K., R. C. Welliver, et al. (1987). "Effect of ribavirin therapy on respiratory syncytial virus-specific IgE and IgA responses after infection." *J Infect Dis* 155(5): 1043-7.

Saiman, L. and J. Siegel (2004). "Infection control in cystic fibrosis." *Clin Microbiol Rev* 17(1): 57-71.

Sanford, B. A., A. Shelokov, et al. (1978). "Bacterial adherence to virus-infected cells: a cell culture model of bacterial superinfection." *J Infect Dis* 137(2): 176-81.

Sawicki, G. S., L. Rasouliyan, et al. (2008). "The impact of incident methicillin resistant Staphylococcus aureus detection on pulmonary function in cystic fibrosis." *Pediatr Pulmonol* 43(11): 1117-23.

Schmid, M. L., G. Kudesia, et al. (1998). "Prospective comparative study of culture specimens and methods in diagnosing influenza in adults." *Bmj* 316(7127): 275.

Schmidt, A. C., J. M. McAuliffe, et al. (2001). "Recombinant bovine/human parainfluenza virus type 3 (B/HPIV3) expressing the respiratory syncytial virus (RSV) G and F proteins can be used to achieve simultaneous mucosal immunization against RSV and HPIV3." *J Virol* 75(10): 4594-603.

Seki, M., Y. Higashiyama, et al. (2004). "Acute infection with influenza virus enhances suspectibility to fatal pneumonia following Streptococcus pneumoniae infection in mice with chronic pulmonary colonisation with Psudomonas aeruginosa." *Clin Exp Immunol* 137(1): 35-40.

Sharma, M., J. T. Arnason, et al. (2006). "Echinacea extracts modulate the pattern of chemokine and cytokine secretion in rhinovirus-infected and uninfected epithelial cells." *Phytother Res* 20(2): 147-52.

Shun-Shin, M., M. Thompson, et al. (2009). "Neuraminidase inhibitors for treatment and prophylaxis of influenza in children: systematic review and meta-analysis of randomised controlled trials." *BMJ* 339: b3172.

Shwachman, H. and L. L. Kulczycki (1958). "Long-term study of one hundred five patients with cystic fibrosis; studies made over a five- to fourteen-year period." *AMA J Dis Child* 96(1): 6-15.

Smith, D. W., L. R. Frankel, et al. (1991). "A controlled trial of aerosolized ribavirin in infants receiving mechanical ventilation for severe respiratory syncytial virus infection." *N Engl J Med* 325(1): 24-9.

Smyth, A. R., R. L. Smyth, et al. (1995). "Effect of respiratory virus infections including rhinovirus on clinical status in cystic fibrosis." *Arch Dis Child* 73(2): 117-20.

Stark, J. M., M. A. Stark, et al. (2006). "Decreased bacterial clearance from the lungs of mice following primary respiratory syncytial virus infection." *J Med Virol* 78(6): 829-38.

Suzuki, T., M. Yamaya, et al. (2002). "Erythromycin inhibits rhinovirus infection in cultured human tracheal epithelial cells." *Am J Respir Crit Care Med* 165(8): 1113-8.

Swierkosz, E. M., D. D. Erdman, et al. (1995). "Isolation and characterization of a naturally occurring parainfluenza 3 virus variant." *J Clin Microbiol* 33(7): 1839-41.

Taylor, L., M. Corey, et al. (2006). "Comparison of throat swabs and nasopharyngeal suction specimens in non-sputum-producing patients with cystic fibrosis." *Pediatr Pulmonol* 41(9): 839-43.

Thomassen, M. J., C. A. Demko, et al. (1985). "Pseudomonas cepacia colonization among patients with cystic fibrosis. A new opportunist." *Am Rev Respir Dis* 131(5): 791-6.

Thompson, C. I., W. S. Barclay, et al. (2006). "Infection of human airway epithelium by human and avian strains of influenza a virus." *J Virol* 80(16): 8060-8.

Thompson, W. W., D. K. Shay, et al. (2004). "Influenza-associated hospitalizations in the United States." *JAMA* 292(11): 1333-40.

Turner, R. B. (2005). "New considerations in the treatment and prevention of rhinovirus infections." *Pediatr Ann* 34(1): 53-7.

Turner, R. B., M. T. Wecker, et al. (1999). "Efficacy of tremacamra, a soluble intercellular adhesion molecule 1, for experimental rhinovirus infection: a randomized clinical trial." *Jama* 281(19): 1797-804.

van den Hoogen, B. G., J. C. de Jong, et al. (2001). "A newly discovered human pneumovirus isolated from young children with respiratory tract disease." *Nat Med* 7(6): 719-24.

Vawter, G. F. and H. Shwachman (1979). "Cystic fibrosis in adults: an autopsy study." *Pathol Annu* 14 Pt 2: 357-82.

Walsh, J. J., L. F. Dietlein, et al. (1961). "Bronchotracheal response in human influenza. Type A, Asian strain, as studied by light and electron microscopic examination of bronchoscopic biopsies." *Arch Intern Med* 108: 376-88.

Wang, E. E., C. G. Prober, et al. (1984). "Association of respiratory viral infections with pulmonary deterioration in patients with cystic fibrosis." *N Engl J Med* 311(26): 1653-8.

Wat, D., C. Gelder, et al. (2008). "Is there a role for influenza vaccination in cystic fibrosis?" *J Cyst Fibros* 7(1): 85-8.

Wat, D., C. Gelder, et al. (2008). "The role of respiratory viruses in cystic fibrosis." *J Cyst Fibros* 7(4): 320-8.

White, A. J., S. Gompertz, et al. (2003). "Chronic obstructive pulmonary disease . 6: The aetiology of exacerbations of chronic obstructive pulmonary disease." *Thorax* 58(1): 73-80.

Wilson, R. and P. J. Cole (1988). "The effect of bacterial products on ciliary function." *Am Rev Respir Dis* 138(6 Pt 2): S49-53.

Winther, B., J. Gwaltney, et al. (1990). "Respiratory virus infection of monolayer cultures of human nasal epithelial cells." *Am Rev Respir Dis.* 141(4 Pt 1): 839-45.

Yin, M., J. Brust, et al. (2009). Antiherpes, anti-hepatitis virus, and anti-respiratory virus agents. *Clinical virology, 3rd edition.* D. Richman, R. Whiyley and F. Hayden. Washington, ASM Press: 217-64.

Yu, H., Q. Liao, et al. (2010). "Effectiveness of oseltamivir on disease progression and viral RNA shedding in patients with mild pandemic 2009 influenza A H1N1: opportunistic retrospective study of medical charts in China." *BMJ* 341: c4779.

Zheng, S., B. De, et al. (2003). "Impaired innate host defense causes suspectibility to respiratory virus infections in cystic fibrosis." *Immunity* 18(5): 619-30.

Zheng, S., W. Xu, et al. (2004). "Impaired nitirc oxide synthase-2 signaling pathway in cystic fibrosis airway epithelium." *Am J Physiol Lung Cell Mol Physiol* 287(2): L374-81.

Permissions

The contributors of this book come from diverse backgrounds, making this book a truly international effort. This book will bring forth new frontiers with its revolutionizing research information and detailed analysis of the nascent developments around the world.

We would like to thank Dinesh D. Sriramulu, for lending his expertise to make the book truly unique. He has played a crucial role in the development of this book. Without his invaluable contribution this book wouldn't have been possible. He has made vital efforts to compile up to date information on the varied aspects of this subject to make this book a valuable addition to the collection of many professionals and students.

This book was conceptualized with the vision of imparting up-to-date information and advanced data in this field. To ensure the same, a matchless editorial board was set up. Every individual on the board went through rigorous rounds of assessment to prove their worth. After which they invested a large part of their time researching and compiling the most relevant data for our readers. Conferences and sessions were held from time to time between the editorial board and the contributing authors to present the data in the most comprehensible form. The editorial team has worked tirelessly to provide valuable and valid information to help people across the globe.

Every chapter published in this book has been scrutinized by our experts. Their significance has been extensively debated. The topics covered herein carry significant findings which will fuel the growth of the discipline. They may even be implemented as practical applications or may be referred to as a beginning point for another development. Chapters in this book were first published by InTech; hereby published with permission under the Creative Commons Attribution License or equivalent.

The editorial board has been involved in producing this book since its inception. They have spent rigorous hours researching and exploring the diverse topics which have resulted in the successful publishing of this book. They have passed on their knowledge of decades through this book. To expedite this challenging task, the publisher supported the team at every step. A small team of assistant editors was also appointed to further simplify the editing procedure and attain best results for the readers.

Our editorial team has been hand-picked from every corner of the world. Their multi-ethnicity adds dynamic inputs to the discussions which result in innovative outcomes. These outcomes are then further discussed with the researchers and contributors who give their valuable feedback and opinion regarding the same. The feedback is then collaborated with the researches and they are edited in a comprehensive manner to aid the understanding of the subject.

Apart from the editorial board, the designing team has also invested a significant amount of their time in understanding the subject and creating the most relevant covers. They scrutinized every image to scout for the most suitable representation of the subject and create an appropriate cover for the book.

The publishing team has been involved in this book since its early stages. They were actively engaged in every process, be it collecting the data, connecting with the contributors or procuring relevant information. The team has been an ardent support to the editorial, designing and production team. Their endless efforts to recruit the best for this project, has resulted in the accomplishment of this book. They are a veteran in the field of academics and their pool of knowledge is as vast as their experience in printing. Their expertise and guidance has proved useful at every step. Their uncompromising quality standards have made this book an exceptional effort. Their encouragement from time to time has been an inspiration for everyone.

The publisher and the editorial board hope that this book will prove to be a valuable piece of knowledge for researchers, students, practitioners and scholars across the globe.

List of Contributors

Patrick Lebecque
Cliniques St-Luc, Université de Louvain, Brussels, Belgium

Maria do Carmo Pimentel Batitucci, Angela Maria Spagnol Perrone and Giselle Villa Flor Brunoro
Federal University of Espírito Santo, Brazil

Iara Maria Sequeiros and Nabil A. Jarad
University Hospitals Bristol NHS Foundation Trust, United Kingdom

Sanjay H. Chotirmall, Catherine M. Greene and Noel G. McElvaney
Respiratory Research Division, Department of Medicine, Ireland

Brian J. Harvey
Department of Molecular Medicine, Royal College of Surgeons in Ireland, Ireland

Marco Lucarelli, Silvia Pierandrei, Sabina Maria Bruno and Roberto Strom
Dept. of Cellular Biotechnologies and Haematology - Sapienza University of Rome, Italy

Donovan McGrowder
Department of Pathology, Faculty of Medical Sciences, University of the West Indies, Mona Campus, Kingston, Jamaica

Gregory G. Anderson
Indiana University Purdue University Indianapolis, USA

Gabriel Mitchell and François Malouin
Université de Sherbrooke, Canada

Marchandin Hélène, Michon Anne-Laure and Jumas-Bilak Estelle
University Montpellier 1, Equipe Pathogènes et Environnements, UMR 5119 ECOSYM, France

Marchandin Hélène and Michon Anne-Laure
University Hospital of Montpellier, Bacteriology Laboratory, France

Jumas-Bilak Estelle
University Hospital of Montpellier, Hygiene Laboratory, France

Yaqin Xu and Stefan Worgall
Weill Cornell Medical College, Department of Pediatrics, New York, NY, USA

Dennis Wat
Adult Cystic Fibrosis Unit, Papworth Hospital, Cambridge, United Kingdom

www.ingramcontent.com/pod-product-compliance
Lightning Source LLC
Chambersburg PA
CBHW070738190326
41458CB00004B/1215